ANALYTICAL METHODS IN HUMAN TOXICOLOGY

ANALYTICAL METHODS IN HUMAN TOXICOLOGY

Part 1

Edited by

A. S. CURRY

MACMILLAN

First published 1984 by
Scientific and Medical Division
THE MACMILLAN PRESS LTD
London and Basingstoke
Companies and representatives throughout the world

Printed in Hong Kong

British Library Cataloguing in Publication Data
Analytical methods in human toxicology.
Part 1.
1. Toxicology—Technique
I. Curry, A. S.
615.9′0028 RA1211
ISBN 0-333-34866-4

Contents

The contributors

E. Bailey
MRC Toxicology Unit
Carshalton
Surrey SM5 4EF

R. J. Flanagan
Consultant Biochemist
Poisons Unit
Guy's Hospital
St Thomas's Street
London SE1 9RT

D. J. Harvey
University Department of Pharmacology
South Parks Road
Oxford OX1 3QT

L. V. Jones
Forensic Science Laboratory
Washington Hall
Euxton
Chorley
Lancs PR7 6HJ

A. V. Kovatsis
Department of Toxicology
University of Thessalonika
Thessalonika
Greece

M. S. Lennard
Wellcome Lecturer in Pharmacology and Therapeutics
University Department of Therapeutics
Royal Hallamshire Hospital
Sheffield S10 2JF

R. F. Metcalfe
Biology Division
CDE, Porton Down
Salisbury
Wiltshire SP4 0JQ

M. Morley
Department of Forensic Medicine
Clinical Sciences Building
St James's Hospital
Beckett Street
Leeds LS9 7TF

J. S. Oliver
Lecturer in Forensic Medicine (Toxicology)
Department of Forensic Medicine and Science
University of Glasgow
Glasgow G12 8QQ

B. S. Thomas
Department of Clinical Endocrinology
Imperial Cancer Research Fund Laboratories
P.O. Box 123
Lincoln's Inn Fields
London WC2A 3PX

G. T. Tucker
Reader in Clinical Pharmacology and Therapeutics
University Department of Therapeutics
Royal Hallamshire Hospital
Sheffield S10 2JF

R. Whelpton
Department of Pharmacology and Therapeutics
The London Hospital Medical College
Turner Street
London E1 2AD

B. Widdop
Consultant Biochemist
Poisons Unit
Guy's Hospital
St Thomas's Street
London SE1 9RT

Introduction

Analytical toxicology encompasses a vast range of techniques. There will therefore be two types of readers who use these volumes: those who wish to find out the methods that are being used to solve a problem that has occurred in a particular area and those who need to see which technique is most pertinent to their area of research. The volumes reflect both approaches.

One theme is common, and this is the astonishingly small quantities of foreign materials that can be localised, identified and measured in the human body. One picogram is to one gram what one gram is to two hundred thousand five-ton elephants, and this analogy emphasises that the purity of all handling preparations in analytical toxicology must be ensured at all stages. So often a researcher may spend months, even years, tracking down a material that turns out to be a plasticiser, a wax or even a contaminant from the operator, possibly diurnal or sex-related. There is no easy way to overcome such problems except to read in depth the work of experts who have the greatest experience and it is the intention of these volumes to present such work.

Analytical toxicology does not stop when a particular compound has been traced and its metabolism followed in the body. The way in which it affects the normal action of the body can lead to dramatic consequences in medicine and some of the most modern advances concern toxicology at the cellular level. Indeed the entry of drugs into genetic pathways is being tracked by the analytical techniques that are described in these volumes.

Both the generalist and the specialist are concerned with the living and the dead, as are those who wish to produce better drugs to treat disease. Every lifesaving or post-mortem analysis is a step towards understanding the very nature of life itself. The techniques now available cover the whole spectrum from the disintegration of molecules in mass spectroscopy to the immunological properties of the body and the effect of light and radiation to reveal compounds within a cell.

The subject is fascinating in that there are so many ways to tackle a new problem. This, coupled with the high cost of 'black box' instruments, means that all of us need periodically to review the latest state of the art to help us decide which way to go.

It is the hope of the editor that the reader will find much of interest and of help in these volumes.

Reading, 1984 A. S. C.

1

The detection of drugs by histochemical procedures

M. MORLEY

1.1 INTRODUCTION

Many methods of analysis are available to the toxicologist for determining the type and amount of drug within human tissues, but few have the potential of histochemistry for enabling the precise site of action of a drug to be defined. Histochemistry is essentially the examination of the chemical as opposed to the morphological structure of tissue preparations. Nondiffusible coloured or fluorescent reaction products which can be visualised under the microscope indicate the cellular localisation of the endogenous or exogenous substances under investigation.

Autoradiography has provided a useful histochemical tool in investigations with laboratory animals, but such procedures are obviously of limited use to the morbid anatomist. Few people obligingly imbibe radiolabelled drugs before their death! The application of other histochemical procedures to the problem of drug localisation within tissues would provide invaluable information about the toxic actions of a drug in man and would ultimately enable more precise determination of the cause of death. At present such conclusions have to be drawn from relatively gross toxicological data, as few poisons produce notable lesions within the body.

All of the published literature has concentrated on the development of fluorescence methods of detection but other types of histochemical reactions may prove equally suitable. In addition the use of microspectrofluorimeters and microdensitometers may allow some quantification of the data. The field is wide and needs to be exploited. I hope that the ensuing paragraphs will give some insight into the problems that will be encountered in developing such techniques and will excite the imagination of those interested in becoming active participants in this area of research.

1.2 PROCESSING TECHNIQUES

Before any tissue sample can be subjected to a histochemical staining procedure it must first be processed in such a manner that minimal disruption occurs in the morphological and chemical characteristics of the specimen. Procedures which preserve tissue morphology are not necessarily compatible with those which preserve tissue histochemistry and a compromise has to be reached between the two. Drugs may be soluble in the chemicals used for fixation, embedding and dehydration. Further problems arise if immunological methods are employed, for these chemicals may destroy the immunoreactive groups.

Although the precise method of tissue preparation is ultimately dependent upon the physico-chemical properties of the particular substance under investigation it should be noted that the characteristics of a pure drug may be different from those pertaining in the histochemical environment. For example, Δ-tetrahydrocannabinol (Δ-THC) could be considered as being suitable for processing by the aqueous technique of immunofluorescence because of its extreme degree of lipophilicity, but leaching from tissue section still occurs because it forms a water-soluble complex with its antibody (Morley and Gee, 1982). There are no precisely defined rules for the development of such procedures. Success is largely a matter of trial and error.

1.2.1 Fixation

The ultimate purpose of fixation in drug histochemistry is to prevent diffusion of the substances under investigation away from their sites of localisation at the time of tissue death. The type of fixative required will be determined both by the nature of the drug being investigated and the proposed histochemical staining procedure. For example, the presence of mercury salts in fixatives may be unsuitable for use with fluorescence techniques as they act as quenching agents. Similarly, fixatives which alter the reactive groups of a drug will be of little value when combined with methods involving chemical staining reactions.

No formal studies have been carried out on the suitability of different types of fixatives for use with drugs. The fixatives that have been used are those which are usually encountered in histochemical procedures for demonstrating biological molecules. Pertschuk and his colleagues have used ethanol as a fixative in the immunofluorescent detection of both phenobarbital (Pertschuk *et al.*, 1976) and methadone (Pertschuk and Sher, 1975; Pertschuk *et al.*, 1977). The high degree of water solubility of sodium phenobarbital was considered to be incompatible with drug retention during the aqueous processing procedures of immunofluorescence but this factor is much less critical with methadone. Methadone has been localised in both alcohol-fixed and unfixed human brain tissue. Very little is known about the chemistry of fixation by alcohol. It acts as a protein precipitant. The denaturation resulting from this action may alter the solubility characteristics of the drug-receptor complex, so reducing the amount of leaching of the water-soluble drug from the tissue during processing.

Lipid-soluble compounds may not require fixation in tissues if aqueous processing techniques are to be employed. For example, Balkon and his colleagues (1980) have successfully localised morphine in rat brain by immunofluorescence. However, lipophilicity cannot always be taken as suitable property for using unfixed material with aqueous staining methods. As has been mentioned previously, Δ-THC cannot be detected by a simple indirect immunofluorescence technique because the drug forms a water-soluble complex with its antibody. 19% of the drug is leached from tissue sections after incubation with the primary antiserum and a further 7% is lost following incubation with the secondary antiserum (Figure 1.1). Intermediary fixation steps after each antiserum incubation may help to alleviate this problem but care should then be taken that a fixative is chosen which does not destroy the immunoreactive groups of the drug-antibody complexes. Much has been written about the effect of fixatives on protein immunoreactivity. Reviews published by Nairn (1976a), Pearse (1968a)

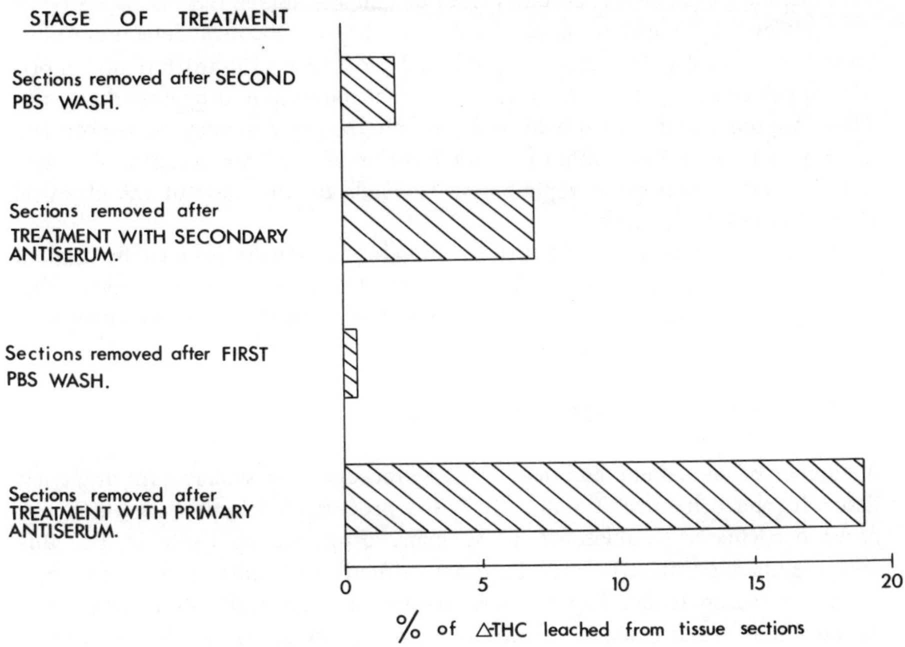

Figure 1.1 Estimation of the amount of Δ-THC leached from sections of spiked human liver during processing by the indirect immunofluorescence technique. Tissue sections spiked with 1 μg of radioactive Δ-THC were processed by the indirect immunofluorescence technique. Five sections were removed for scintillation counting at each stage of the procedure. The figure shows the amount of Δ-THC leached from the tissue sections at each stage of the procedure. (© ASTM, 1916 Race Street, Philadelphia, PA 19103, USA. Reprinted with permission.)

and Feteanu (1978a) are recommended for consultation. Other aspects of the effects of fixatives on immunofluorescent staining will be dealt with in the ensuing section on this technique.

Stora (1980a, b) has used both Carnoy's and Bouin's fixatives for the examination of the histological localisation of the chemical carcinogens aflatoxin B1, *N*-2-fluorenylacetamide and benzo(α)pyrene. Bouin's fixative is a mixture of picric acid, formaldehyde, glacial acetic acid and acetone, while Carnoy's fixative contains chloroform, glacial acetic acid and absolute ethanol. The intracellular pattern of distribution of the carcinogens was not affected by the choice of fixative. The efficiency of fixation proved to be limited, however, for subsequent deparaffinisation procedures removed all weakly bound molecules from the cells.

Some drugs may be totally unsuitable for use with liquid fixatives of any sort, as they may be leached from the tissue as soon as they come into contact with any aqueous or nonaqueous solvents. In these instances vapour fixation may provide a suitable alternative. Formaldehyde and osmium tetroxide vapours are most commonly encountered in histochemistry but others that have been used include glutaldehyde, chromyl chloride and alcohol.

A review of the use of vapour fixation in the histochemical detection of biological macromolecules has been published by Pearse (1968b) but no reports have appeared in the literature of the use of such methods in drug histochemistry. Those vapours, such as formaldehyde, which fix proteins may be appropriate as they may alter the solubility characteristics of the drug–receptor complex. Other suitable choices of vapour may be made on the basis of the chemical characteristics of the drug.

Advice on the choice of fixative for drug histochemistry is inevitably limited by the lack of research that has been carried out in this area. Conventional fixatives may prove suitable for this purpose but completely new ones may have to be developed for use with specific drugs.

1.2.2 Embedding and dehydration

A number of embedding and dehydration procedures are available for preparing tissue for histochemical staining. It is the process of dehydration which can prove particularly troublesome, as so many drugs are lipid-soluble. For this reason embedded material may be more difficult to handle than simple solid blocks of frozen tissue. The nonpolar nature of many embedding compounds dictates that water must be removed from the tissue before the embedding compound can penetrate into the tissue block. Similarly the embedding compound must be removed to allow penetration of the staining reagents. The use of organic solvents as dehydrating agents leaches many lipid-soluble drugs from the tissues.

The technique of freeze drying is a neat way of sidestepping this problem. Water is removed under vacuum from tissues which have been frozen rapidly at temperatures as low as −190°C. This material can then be embedded directly without recourse to dehydration by organic solvents. The technique has been used successfully in the detection of antibiotics such as terramycin (Helander and Böttiger, 1953), tetracycline (Böttiger, 1955a), chlortetracycline (Böttiger, 1955b) and doxycycline (Liss and Norman, 1975). Water-soluble waxes are available which may be used in conjunction with freeze-dried material should the drug under investigation be soluble in either nonpolar embedding agents or the organic solvents required for removal of these materials from the tissue before histological staining can begin. They are also useful for embedding materials which may be affected by the relatively high temperatures required for embedding in paraffin wax (56 to 60 °C), as the procedure can be carried out at 20 to 30 °C.

Unfortunately, freeze drying is a time-consuming process which requires the use of expensive apparatus that may not be available in all laboratories. Although simple unembedded frozen sections may provide a suitable alternative, some dehydration is still necessary in order to observe cytological detail. Sufficient dehydration may occur when such sections are thaw-mounted onto microscope slides. Egorin *et al.* (1974) describe the localisation of adriamycin and daunorubicin by virtue of their autofluorescent characteristics in thaw-mounted frozen sections of hamster kidney, heart and lung mounted in a phosphate-buffered saline–glycerol solution and similar dehydration procedures have been used in the immunofluorescent detection of phenobarbital (Pertschuk *et al.*, 1976), methadone (Pertschuk *et al.*, 1977) and morphine (Balkon *et al.*, 1980). This method of dehydration has not, however, proved satisfactory in our laboratory. The autofluorescence of both tetracycline and chlorpromazine was found to be masked by an opaque film overlying sections of simple thaw-mounted tissue. Pearse (1968c) notes that some kind of protein film forms on thaw-mounted preparations which interferes with the penetration of some staining reagents. This may be responsible for the quenching of fluorescence in our preparations.

The technique of section freeze-substitution (Chang and Hori, 1961) may provide a suitable alternative to either freeze drying or simple freeze–thaw procedures. Although in this process the ice crystals present in frozen sections of biological material are dissolved by floating the tissue sections in cold liquid dehydrating agents, the dehydration process is completed much more rapidly than it is with embedded material, thus reducing the amount of exposure of the drug to organic solvents. Obviously, a dehydrating agent has to be chosen in which the drug under investigation has little or no solubility. Both tetracycline and chlorpromazine have been localised satisfactorily by this method using acetone cooled to −20 °C as the dehydrating agent (Gelder and Gee, 1979). Even though chlorpromazine has a solubility of about 1 in 100 in acetone, sufficient quantities of this drug are retained in the sections to allow visualisation of its luminescence in the cortical region of the brain (Figure 1.2).

Section freeze-substitution would seem to be particularly suitable for use with water-soluble drugs. After dehydration the floating sections are sufficiently stretched for direct mounting on cover slips or microscope slides. Flotation and expansion of embedded materials in heated water baths can remove water-

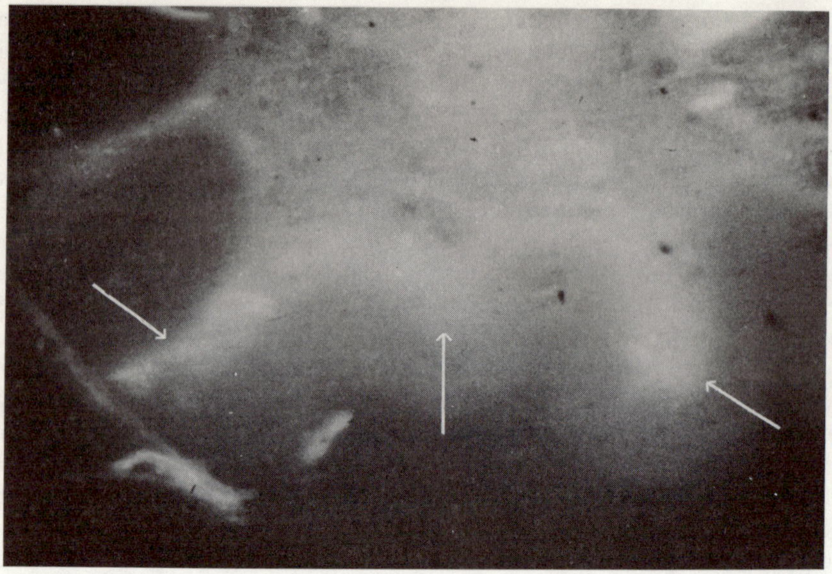

Figure 1.2 Distribution of chlorpromazine in the subcortical layer of mouse brain. Sections of mouse brain were prepared by the freeze-substitution technique. The specimen was maintained at $-195\,^{\circ}C$ and excited with u.v. light. The areas of luminescence characteristic of the drug are arrowed (Gelder and Gee, 1979). (© *Journal of the Forensic Science Society*.)

soluble material. For example, Gelder and Gee (unpublished observations) have observed that such procedures leach tetracycline from soft paraffin-embedded tissues such as the liver and the kidney, although the drug is retained at sites of strong binding such as the areas of mineralisation in bone.

Ultimately the choice of embedding and dehydration procedures will be limited by the solubility characteristics of the drug in question and the amount of time available before the results are required. Although freeze-drying procedures would seem to offer an easy solution to the problem of dehydration, they can take up to a week to complete, whereas sections prepared by freeze substitution are ready for staining within a few minutes.

1.2.3 Mounting procedures

On completion of histochemical staining the tissue sections must be mounted in some material for subsequent observation on the microscope. It is important that a mountant should be chosen in which the drug is not soluble. Liquid paraffin has proved to be a suitable mountant for many of the antibiotics and for chlorpromazine. It has the added advantage that when it is used in conjunction with paraffin-embedded material it dissolves the paraffin wax surrounding the biological tissues. This obviates the need for exposure of the sections to organic deparaffinisation agents which may leach drugs from the tissue. All but strongly bound molecules of the chemical carcinogens aflatoxin B1, *N*-2-fluorenylacelamide and benzo(α)pyrene, for example, are removed at this stage of the processing procedure (Stora, 1980a). Other properties of the mountant may also affect its suitability for use with a particular histochemical procedure. Fluorescent mountants will obviously be incompatible for use with fluorescent staining techniques. Many different mountants are available commercially and each should be considered carefully before the final choice is made.

1.3 FLUORESCENCE METHODS OF EXAMINATION

Spectrofluorimetric techniques for analysing drugs are well established in toxicology. Similarly, fluorescence microscopy is widely used for examining tissue structures. It seems logical that a combination of these two procedures should provide a means of localising drugs within tissue sections and successful histofluorescence techniques for a number of drugs have been described in the literature. Their position has been detected both by virtue of their autofluorescence characteristics (e.g. Gelder and Gee, 1979; Stora, 1980a, b) and by indirect procedures such as immunofluorescence (e.g. Pertschuk *et al.*, 1977; Balkon *et al.*, 1980). Other indirect procedures such as induced fluorescence may also prove to be of value, but these are entirely speculative at present.

Detailed theoretical descriptions of fluorescence will not be dealt with here. A comprehensive review of the subject has been published by Udenfriend (1962). It is simplest terms fluorescence can be defined as the radiation emitted by certain substances when they are irradiated or 'excited' with ultraviolet or short-wavelength visible light. A spectrum can be recorded of both excitation and emission radiations. The wavelengths at the peaks of these spectra are referred to as the excitation and emission maxima (Ex_{Δ} and Em_{Δ}). Use of the excitation maximum for irradation results in maximum fluorescence emission. The excitation and emission maxima are characteristic of each substance and consequently the conditions of examination can be controlled in such a way that only the substance in question is detected. The degree of control that can be exerted in fluorescence microscopy is more limited than it is in spectrofluorimetry because many naturally occurring cellular constituents autofluoresce. For this reason some drugs and flurochromes lend themselves more readily to this type of investigation than others. These problems are dealt with in the forthcoming section together with a brief discussion of the various types of equipment available to the microscopist.

1.3.1 Fluorescence microscopy

The ultimate aim of a histoflorescence technique is to produce an intense and specific image in the microscope of the fluorescent molecules under study. The attainment of this goal will be aided if the contributions made by the components of the microscope are understood.

1.3.1.1 Factors affecting image intensity

1. Type of illumination Two types of illumination systems are available with fluorescence microscopes. They involve the use of either transmitted or incident light (Figure 1.3). For transmitted illumination the light source is positioned below the microscope stage and the section is excited by transmitting u.v. light through the tissue. For incident (epi-) illumination the light source is positioned above the microscope stage and the exciting radiations are directed onto the upper surface of the section.

Maximal fluorescence intensity is never observed with either of these systems because the biological tissues absorb light from both the excitation and the emission beams. With transmitted illumination the intensity of fluorescence from molecules in the upper cellular layers is reduced as a result of absorption of some of the excitation light during passage through the tissue. Similarly, fluorescence from molecules in the lower layers of cells is reduced as a result of tissue absorption of some of the emitted light. In epi-illuminated systems the intensity of fluorescence from these low-lying molecules may be reduced even further because wavelengths from both the excitation and the emission beams are absorbed by the tissues, but little attenuation of either of these radiations occurs in the upper cell layers. This results in a much brighter image than can be obtained with transmitted illumination, particularly when dealing with thick specimens.

Optimal visualisation of the fluorescence image is easier to achieve in epi-illuminated instruments because a single lens acts as both condenser (focusing the excitation light onto the section) and objective (collecting the light emitted by the section). Focusing of this lens onto the specimen results in the proper alignment of this part of the microscope. With transmitted illumination two separate lenses, each with an independent optical axis, are required for these purposes. These axes must be perfectly aligned before optimal visualisation can be attained and such alignment will not always be easy to maintain in routine use.

Other features of epi-illuminated instruments aid the ease with which a bright image can be obtained. For example, oil-immersion objectives are easier to use because a drop of oil on the specimen is sufficient for observation of fluorescence; in transmitted systems oil is also required on the surface of the condenser. In addition, since substage illumination is fully available in epi-illuminated instruments, fluorescence microscopy can be combined with transmitted brightfield microscopy. This can be extremely useful as it permits selection of the area of examination before irradiation of the specimen, and so reduces image fading.

The design features of epi-fluorescence microscopes thus allow a bright fluorescence image to be easily obtained. It is perhaps for this reason that the use of these instruments has become extremely popular in recent years.

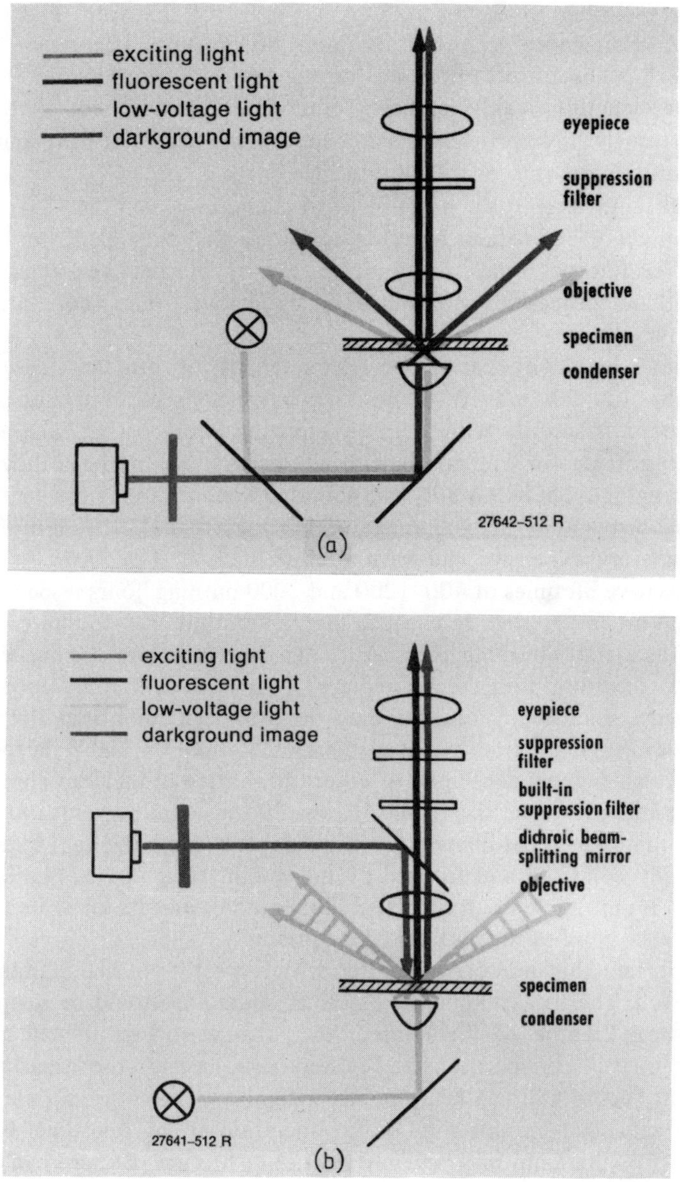

Figure 1.3 A comparison of transmitted and epi-illumination. In transmitted illumination (a) the specimen is excited by passing u.v. light through the tissue. The excitation beam is focused onto the section by means of a substage condenser. Emitted light is collected by the objective lens and observed through the eyepiece. In epi-illumination (b) the excitation beam is directed onto the upper surface of the section. The objective acts as both a condenser and a collecting lens. (*Courtesy E. Leitz (Instruments) Ltd.*)

2. Light sources The function of a light source is to provide light at a wavelength corresponding to the excitation maximum of the drug. The resulting intensity of fluorescence depends both upon the emission intensity of the light source and the absorption efficiency of the drug (or fluorochrome) for the emitted wavelength. Weakly emitting fluorochromes need more excitation light than strongly fluorescent ones. An inappropriate choice of light source may severely limit the intensity of the fluorescence image.

Some light sources emit a continuum of wavelengths while others have distinct peaks of emission. The former have the advantage that they can be used with a wide range of fluorochromes. The emission spectra and relative intensities of a number of light sources commonly used in fluorescence microscopy are shown in Figure 1.4.

Continuous emission spectra are characteristic of tungsten–halogen and xenon lamps. 12-, 50- and 100-W tungsten–halogen lamps are inexpensive and may be used satisfactorily with intensely emitting fluorochomes such as FITC. They are unsuitable for irradiation with u.v. light, however, since they do not emit wavelengths of between 300 and 400 nm. Xenon burners can be used for illumination throughout the full range of the spectrum (i.e. from u.v. to red) but they are very expensive and have a short lifetime. The 75-W, 110-W and 450-W bulbs have lifetimes of 400, 1200 and 2000 burning hours respectively.

Mercury burners are slightly cheaper than xenon but they too have a limited lifetime of about 200 burning hours. Although their characteristic line spectrum may restrict their use with certain materials, they are commonly encountered in fluorescence microscopy because they do emit high intensities over a wide range of wavelengths. They are available as 50-, 100- or 200-W burners, the choice of which is dependent upon whether transmitted or incident illumination is to be used. The large arc size of the 50- and 200-W lamps prevents optimal use of the light intensity in epi-illuminated instruments because the light bundle cannot be totally collected and focused by the intermediate optics. Similarly, the 100-W lamp is unsuitable for transmitted illumination since its small arc does not fill the entrance pupil of the darkfield condenser.

It is important that burners are treated with respect if optimal illumination is to be achieved. The total number of hours of operation should be restricted to the theoretical lifetime of the burner. Many lamps still ignite well past this period, but their continued use is to be discouraged because the intensity of the emitted light becomes dramatically reduced. Similarly, attention should be paid to the recommended minimum hours for operation at any one time. Frequent switching off of the lamp may severely restrict its lifetime. Burners can explode under these conditions and this is not only extremely noisy but it can cause extensive damage to the lamphouse!

3. Magnification and numerical aperture The intensity of the fluorescence image is affected by both the magnification and the numerical aperture of the lenses of the microscope. Maximal brightness is obtained by using minimal

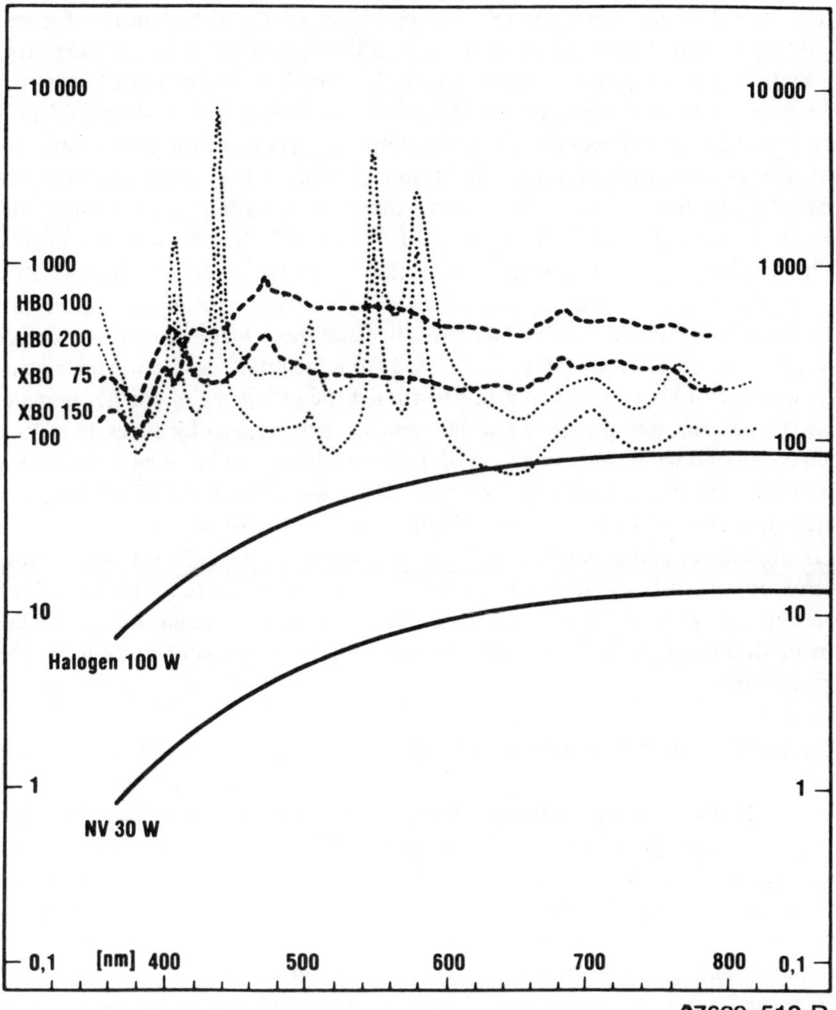

Figure 1.4 Emission spectra for lamps commonly used in fluorescence microscopy. The x-axis corresponds to the wavelength in nm. The y-axis shows the light intensity on a logarithmic scale. *Courtesy of E. Leitz (Instruments) Ltd.*)

magnification together with high numerical aperture. The choice of objectives and eyepieces which will fulfil these conditions is determined by the type of illumination being used.

With transmitted-light microscopes this choice is dependent ultimately upon the characteristics of the substage condenser. Darkfield condensers are more usually employed in fluorescence microscopy because they give much better image contrast than brightfield systems. This is because the cone of excitation light does not enter the microscope objective directly when it is focused on the specimen. Light can enter the objectives only when it is refracted from the section. However, this is strictly true only when low- to moderate-power dry objectives are used. Oil-immersion objectives with a numerical aperture of more than 0.95 can still collect light from the illuminating cone of the condenser. This is visible as unwanted excitation light and it reduces the image contrast. The numerical aperture of the system can be increased by using oil-immersion condensers. Such condensers with numerical apertures of 1.20 and 1.40 are available.

In epi-illuminated systems the illumination of the specimen and the collection of the emitted fluorescence is performed by the objective alone. Immersion objectives are preferable to dry objectives because more incident light is reflected from glass-to-air interfaces than is reflected from the interfaces between glass and oil, glycerine or water. Originally this restricted the efficiency of epi-fluorescence microscopes for low-power work but special immersion objectives have now been developed which have low to moderate magnifications but greater numerical apertures than dry lenses, e.g. 10 x NA = 0.45, oil immersion; 25 x NA = 0.60, water immersion; 40 x NA = 1.30, oil immersion (Leitz, Wetzlar).

It should be remembered that not all objectives are suitable for fluorescence microscopy as they are sometimes equipped with many extra lenses for correction of imaging errors. These extra lenses reduce transmission and thus the brightness of fluorescence. Achromat and fluorite objectives are very suitable for this type of work.

1.3.1.2 Factors affecting image specificity

The specificity of the fluorescence image observed in the microscope is largely dependent upon the filters used in the system. Ideally the drug or fluorochrome under study should be excited at its excitation maximum so that the fluorescence of the surrounding biological tissue is kept to a minimum. In conventional spectrofluorimetry this is readily achieved by using monochromators in the excitation and emission beams. Selective wavelength excitation in fluorescence microscopy can never be so precise because of the limitations imposed by filter technology. However, vast improvements have been made in this area in recent years and these have aided the attainment of image specificity as well as increasing image contrast.

Selective wavelength excitation is achieved by placing (1) an excitation filter between the light source and the specimen which filters out unwanted excitation light and (2) a barrier or suppression filter between the specimen and the observer which transmits only the wavelengths of fluorescence characteristic of the drug or fluorochrome (Figure 1.5). An understanding of filter characteristics is obviously required if appropriate excitation and barrier filters are to be chosen.

Two main types of filter are currently in use in fluorescence microscopy. These are coloured glass and interference filters. They differ in the way in which they are constructed and in their transmission characteristics. *Coloured glass*

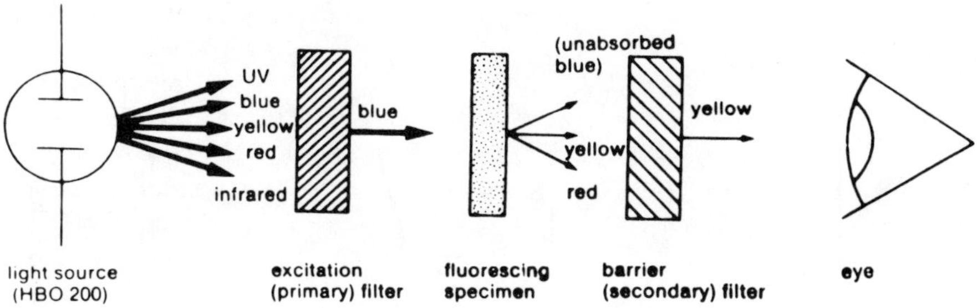

Figure 1.5 Selective wavelength excitation in fluorescence microscopy. Selective wavelength excitation is achieved by placing, first, an excitation filter between the light source and the specimen which filters out unwanted excitation light from the light source and, second, a barrier or suppression filter between the specimen and the observer which transmits only the fluorescence wavelength of the drug under study. The diagram shows the elements in a fluorescence microscope required for blue excitation. (*Courtesy Carl Zeiss Instruments*.)

filters have been used for many years. They transmit light of their own colour and absorb light of complementary colours but their transmission characteristics are not very selective. *Interference filters* are composed of glass substrates onto which thin layers of a salt compound are deposited. Multilayered filters are produced by repeating this deposition process several times. They are much more selective than simple glass filters because their transmission characteristics depend upon the interference of light rays by individual layers. The thickness and the refractive index of the coatings can be chosen for selective enhancement or suppression of transmission and reflection of specific wavelengths.

The transmission characteristics of an individual filter determines whether it is to be described as a short-pass, long-pass or a band-pass filter. Some transmission curves of commonly used filters are given in Figure 1.6.

1. Short-pass filters These are almost always interference filters. They transmit lower wavelengths but block higher wavelengths of light. They are identified by the abbreviations SP (short pass) or KP (Kurz pass), together with the maximum wavelength of light that the filter will transmit; e.g. KP440 is a short-pass filter which will transmit only wavelengths below 440 nm.

2. Long-pass filters These have a high transmission for the longer wavelengths but block the lower wavelengths of light. Until recently they were all made of coloured glass but now interference long-pass filters are also available. They are identified by abbreviations LP (long pass) or K (Kanten filter) together with the minimum wavelength of light which the filter will transmit. Older types of glass filter are often used in their construction, e.g. GG (green glass), OG (orange glass), RG (red glass), BG (blue glass).

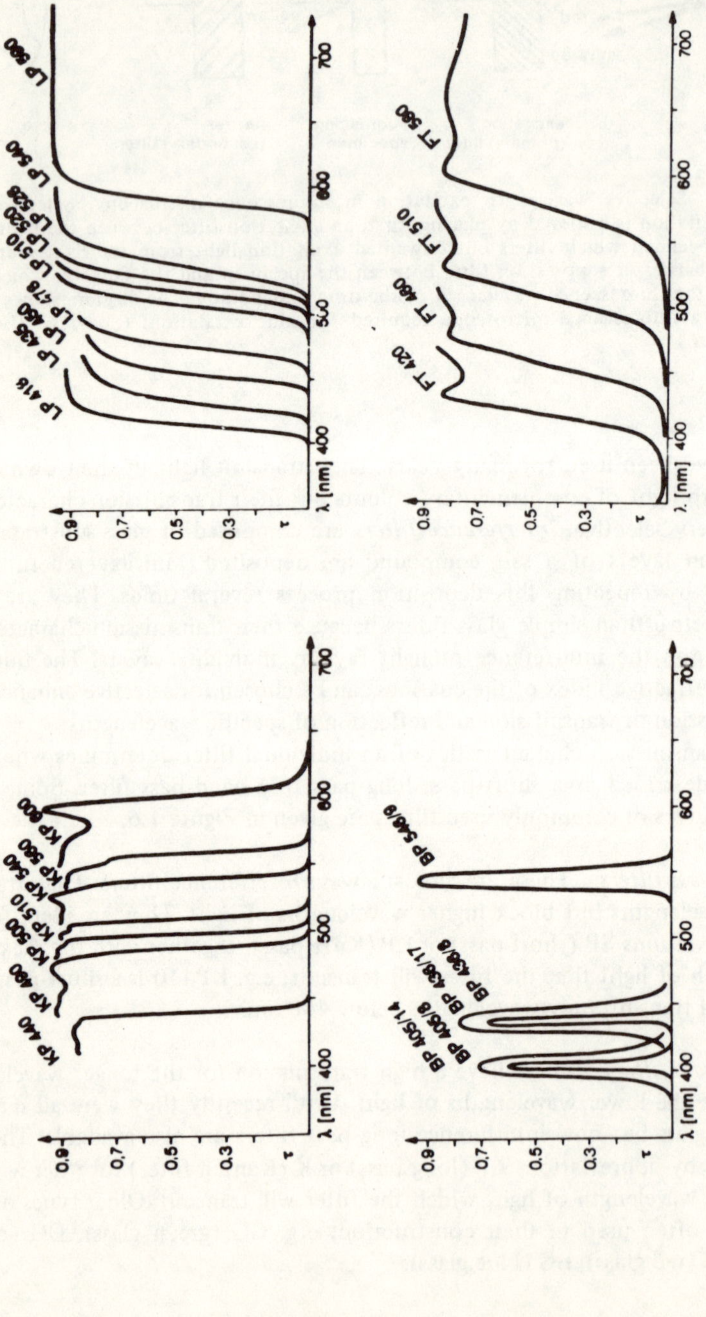

Figure 1.6 Transmission characteristics of some short-pass (KP), long-pass (LP), band-pass (BP) and chromatic beam splitters (FT). (*Courtesy Carl Zeiss Instruments.*)

3. Band-pass filters These transmit one particular area or band of the spectrum. Both glass and interference band-pass filters are available but the former have rather broad transmission characteristics and thus excite more background autofluorescence than the interference types. In the past a disadvantage of the interference band-pass filters was that they had low (50 to 60%) transmission values, but much higher transmissions (90%) are now available from this type of filter. Band-pass filters are identified by the abbreviations BP, SAL, AL, TAL or PIL.

The half-width of a band-pass filter is the width of the main transmission curve at 50% of the peak transmission. Filters are considered to have a broad transmission curve if half the half-width is greater than 50 nm. Such filters are termed wide-band filters. Narrow-band filters have a half-width of less than 20 nm.

4. Chromatic beam splitters (dichroic mirrors) Chromatic beam splitters or dichroic mirrors are used in epi-fluorescence microscopes where they are positioned at an angle of 45° between the excitation and the suppression filters (Figure 1.3). They reflect the excitation light down onto the specimen and transmit the wavelengths of fluorescence collected by the objective. They should not be confused with normal 50–50% beam splitters which only separate the incident beam into two perpendicular beams of 50% light intensity each and do not effect the wavelength composition of the light. Chromatic beam splitters are identified by the terms CBS (chromatic beam splitters), DM (dichroic mirror), TK (Teiler Kante) or FT (Farb Teiler). Their characteristics are always given for incident light falling under 45°. Standard chromatic beam splitters are available at 400 or 420 nm for u.v.-excitation, at 455 or 460 nm for violet excitation, at 500 or 510 nm for blue excitation and at 580 nm for green excitation.

5. Combinations of filters suitable for excitation The specificity of a fluorescence image depends partly upon the combination of filters used to produce excitation. The main requirement is for a specific narrow-band filter which will select the wavelength of the excitation peak of the fluorochrome or drug but in epi-illuminated instruments an appropriate dichroic mirror will also have to be chosen. In addition, heat filters are required to protect both the specimen and the other filters from the heat produced by the lamp.

Narrow-band excitation is much more readily achieved by using combinations of short-pass and long-pass filters than by using coloured glass filters. Short-pass filters determine the lower wavelengths of transmission while long-pass filters determine the higher wavelengths of transmission.

6. Combinations of filters suitable for wavelength suppression The function of a barrier filter is to transmit only the wavelength of light specific to the fluorochrome or drug under study. It thus has to absorb any background fluorescence and any stray excitation light. In epi-illuminated microscopes this function is fulfilled partly by the chromatic beam splitter, but in both transmission and epi-illumination systems specific barrier filters are also required. LP filters are used predominantly for this purpose as they transmit light of longer wavelengths and select or absorb light of shorter wavelengths.

7. Adaptability of microscope systems In choosing a fluorescence microscope the types of filter combinations likely to be required should be kept in mind. Although all illumination systems can be modified to suit particular requirements, there is some variation in the cost and ease with which this can be done.

1.3.2 Autofluorescence procedures

Although a number of drugs have autofluorescent properties, not all are suitable for visualisation by fluorescence microscopy. Only those which emit fluorescence in the visible region of the spectrum can be discerned by the human eye. Microspectrofluorimetry could be used to record u.v. emission spectra but transmission of the short wavelengths (i.e. < 300 nm) requires the use of quartz optics, which may prove prohibitively expensive. The moving stages and automatic measuring devices which would also be necessary for detecting these short wavelengths would add further to the cost. Obviously, similar limitations are imposed upon the excitation characteristics of the drug.

These limitations severely restrict the use of this technique in forensic toxicology. Of the drugs known to be involved in fatal poisoning cases in England and Wales in 1979, for example, only three have emission maxima in the visible region of the spectrum (Tables 1.1 and 1.2). The method has provided useful information in other toxicological and pharmacological fields, however, as the fluorescence characteristics of a number of carcinogens, antibiotics and therapeutic agents for cancer are suitable for direct visualisation (Table 1.3).

It is evident from these studies that the success of the technique depends upon a high intensity of fluorescence emission by the drug together with a good colour contrast against the surrounding tissues. As discussed below the former property is perhaps the most important of the two.

1.3.2.1 Colour Contrast

Many biological molecules fluorescence when excited with u.v. light. Animal tissues generally have a blue or grey-blue autofluorescence under such conditions and this can prove troublesome if the drug under investigation has a similar fluorescence emission. Antibiotics such as tetracycline and terramycin which fluoresce in the yellow and yellow-green areas of the spectrum are easily detected by fluorescence microscopy (Helander and Böttiger, 1953; Böttiger, 1955a) but the technique becomes more difficult with drugs such as sodium salicylate (Helander, 1949) and chlorpromazine (Gelder and Gee, 1979) which emit blue light.

Table 1.1 Abstract of the drugs involved in fatal poisoning in England and Wales in 1979 (as reported by the Office of Population Censuses and Surveys)

Drug	Number of fatal poisonings
barbiturates	880
paracetamol	551
dextropropoxyphene	331
amitriptyline	181
acetylsalicylic acid*	148
diazepam	120
chlormethiazole	97
nitrazepam	93
dothiepin	76
flurazepam	73
trimipramine	51
imipramine*	44
orphenadrine	41
chlorpromazine*	40
propranolol	33
carbromal	32

*The three drugs asterisked are the only ones with emission maxima in the visible region of the spectrum

Table 1.2 The excitation and emission wavelength maxima of acetylsalicylic acid, imipramine and chlorpromazine in 0.2 M phosphate buffer, pH 7.0

Drug	Concentration	Excitation maximum, Ex_{Δ} (nm)	Emission maximum, Em_{Δ} (nm)
acetylsalicylic acid	1.25	320	400
imipramine	0.25	315	400
chlorpromazine	0.25	345	456

Ex_{Δ} = excitation maximum.
Em_{Δ} = emission maximum.

Modification of the conditions of examination may sometimes alleviate these problems. This has been demonstrated most dramatically with chlorpromazine (Gelder and Gee, 1979). In this study whole-body sections of chlorpromazine-injected mice were prepared by bisecting animals frozen at −20 °C. The cut surfaces of these frozen preparations showed no evidence of the drug's auto-fluorescence when illuminated with u.v. light. The distribution of the drug

Table 1.3 The use of fluorescence microscopy for detecting autofluorescent drugs*

Drug	Colour of emission	Reference
Antibiotics		
tetracycline	yellow	Böttiger, 1955a; Gelder and Gee, 1979
chlortetracycline	yellow	Böttiger, 1955b
terramycin	yellow–green	Helander and Böttiger, 1953
doxycycline	yellow–green	Liss and Norman, 1975
Carcinogens		
aflatoxin B1	blue	Stora, 1980a
benzo(α)pyrene	blue	Stora, 1980a
N-2-fluoroenylacetamide	yellow–green	Stora, 1980a
Anti-cancer		
adriamycin	orange–red	Egorin *et al.*, 1974
daunorubicin	orange–red	Egorin *et al.*, 1974
Others		
sodium salicylate	blue–violet	Helander, 1949
chlorpromazine	yellow	Gelder and Gee, 1979

*The table lists the autofluorescent drugs which have been detected by fluorescence microscopy together with descriptions of the colour of emission when the drugs are excited with u.v. or blue light.

became readily visible, however, when the temperature was reduced to −195 °C by immersing the mice in liquid nitrogen. A bright-yellow luminescence was evident in the walls of the ascending vena cava, the heart and blood vessels in the thoracic region, the dorsal thoracic muscles, the tongue, the spinal cord and the cortical regions of the brain. Autoradiographs using ^{35}S chlorpromazine confirmed these sites of localisation.

Observation of histological preparations at such low temperatures requires the development of cold stages for the microscope. Gelder (1978) describes a simple stage which consists of a polystyrene trough into which liquid nitrogen is poured. The microscope slide is supported above the surface by two brass blocks. A 10× objective can be used quite safely with this system. Obviously, mountants cannot be used with such histological preparations as they freeze, but the distribution of drugs can still be visualised and measured microspectrofluorimetrically (Figure 1.2).

It is likely that chlorpromazine is phosphorescing at the low temperatures used in this study, as the emission continues on removal of the excitation light. If this is so then the use of such low-temperature techniques may have interesting implications for future studies on drug localisation since many drugs, such as diazepam, phosphoresce but do not fluoresce in the visible region of the spectrum.

1.3.2.2 Intensity of fluorescence emission

Although a good colour contrast between drug and tissue autofluorescence aids the detection of the former in histological preparations it is not of paramount importance. This is exemplified by the studies by Stora (1980a–c) on the intracellular localisation of the chemical carcinogens aflatoxin B1 and benzo(α) pyrene, both of which have a blue autofluorescence. The preparative techniques used with these compounds leached all but strongly bound molecules of the carcinogens from the tissue. Stora suggests that the bound fluorescent molecules may have been rendered insoluble by the formation of complexes between the carcinogen and cellular macromolecules. With some drugs such as tetracycline the formation of such complexes can result in a dramatically increased intensity of fluorescence emission (Kohn, 1961; Morley *et al.*, 1982) and this may explain why these blue autofluorescing carcinogens can be visualised so readily.

Kohn (1961) was the first person to report this effect with tetracylcine using solutions of the drug and macromolecules such as DNA and albumin buffered to physiological pH. These results were confirmed both in solutions and histological preparations by Morley *et al.* (1982). Divalent metal ions are necessary for this binding, possibly because they serve as a connecting bridge between the macromolecules and the drug. The effect may also be due partly to a photochemical reaction, as the degree of enhancement of drug fluorescence by the macromolecules is dependent upon the wavelength of the excitation light. Preliminary examinations of the fluorescence characteristics of drug-macromolecule mixtures may thus yield valuable information about the optimal conditions required for detection of a drug in a histological preparation.

In this context it is interesting to note that at room temperature protein molecules have no effect on the fluorescence emission from either imipramine or chlorpromazine in buffered solutions (Morley *et al.*, 1982) and that under the same conditions of temperature neither of these drugs can be detected by fluorescence microscopy (Gelder and Gee, 1979; Gee *et al.*, 1981). Similarly, the fluorescence intensity of sodium salicylate is enhanced only in the presence of specific macromolecules such as albumin and this drug is not easily visualised in histological preparations (Gee *et al.*, 1981; Morley *et al.*, 1982).

Although the intensity of emission can be enhanced by modifying the temperature and the pH of a tissue section, the property of complex formation with macromolecules appears to be of overriding importance for successful detection of autofluorescent drugs with low colour-contrast against the surrounding tissues. Thus although reduction of the ambient temperature to $-195\,^{\circ}$C can enhance the fluorescence intensities of imipramine and salicylate crystals by a factor of four (Morley, unpublished observations) this is insufficient to enable detection of these drugs in histological sections. It should be noted that the fluorescence intensity of chlorpromazine is increased by as much as 33 times by such a reduction in temperature. This increase, together with the shift from blue to yellow emission wavelengths, is sufficient to allow visualisation of the drug.

It may be possible to produce an effective increase in emission intensity by decreasing the intensity of tissue autofluorescence. A simple way of doing this is to use fixed instead of frozen sections, for in general fixed tissues have a lower autofluorescence than do frozen tissues. Both formol–saline and absolute ethanol reduce the intensity of tissue autofluorescence without affecting the wavelength of emission (Gelder and Gee, unpublished observations). Similar observations have been made by Stora (1980a) using Carnoy's fixative.

Such procedures may be inappropriate for use with some drugs because of their solubility characteristics. In these instances, careful selection of the wavelength of light used for excitation may prove to be an appropriate step. Mixtures of u.v. and violet light, for example, result in an extremely low intensity of autofluorescence from freeze-substituted sections of liver tissue (Gelder and Gee, 1979). The intensity is so low that it lies below the visible threshold (Figure 1.7). Any detectable fluorescence in sections excited in this manner must thus be due entirely to drug-laden material. The possible sacrifice of reduced emission intensity from the drug by not using the Ex_{Δ} for excitation may be far outweighed by the abolition of tissue autofluorescence.

1.3.2.3 Recommended scheme of study

It may be helpful if the information on autofluorescence procedures is summarised and presented in the form of a scheme of study for the development of such a technique.

Step 1: Spectrofluorimetric examination of the fluorescence characteristics of the drug Preliminary examination of the fluorescence characteristics of the drug is required in order that appropriate excitation and suppression filters can be chosen for the microscope. This should be done using buffered solutions of the drug in both the presence and the absence of biological macromolecules such as proteins and DNA. Some drugs form complexes with these macromolecules and the fluorescence characteristics of these complexes may differ from those of the free drug. Only those drugs which fluoresce in the visible region of the spectrum are suitable for direct visualisation by fluorescence microscopy. Unless quartz optics are available at least some of the excitation spectrum should also lie in the visible range.

Step 2: Preparation of whole-body fluorograms from laboratory animals The preparation of whole-body fluorograms may be helpful, as they enable the choice of tissue for subsequent histological processing to be made without having to

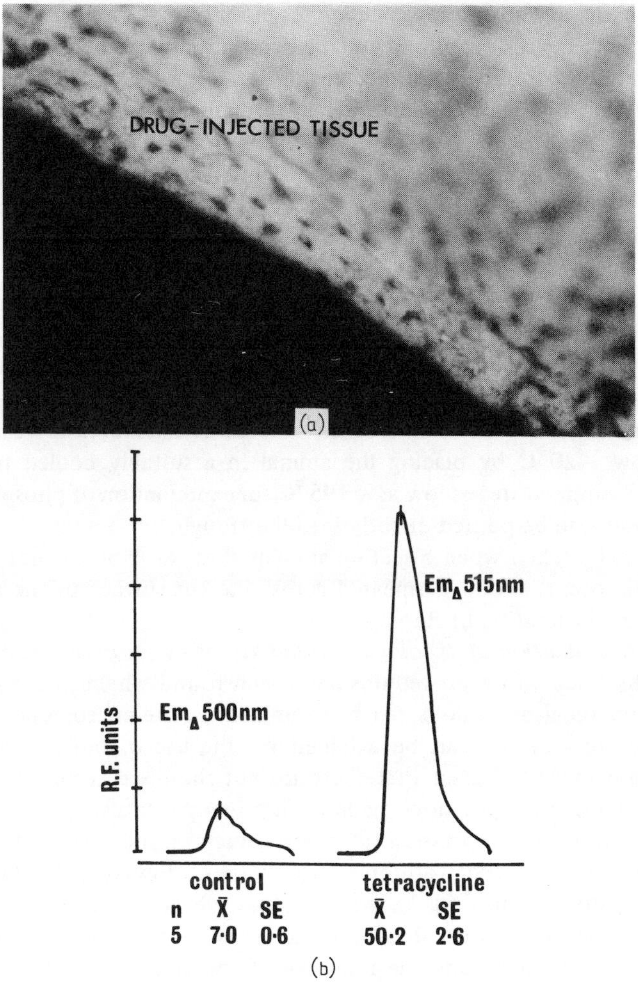

Figure 1.7 It is possible to produce an effective increase in the emission intensity from a drug in a tissue section by decreasing the intensity of tissue autofluorescence. The use of violet light for exciting liver tissue from tetracycline-injected mice and normal mice, for example, only allows visualisation of the drug-injected tissue (a). The autofluorescence of the control tissue–recorded by microspectrofluorimetry (b)–is not visible to the naked eye. (*Courtesy Journal of the Forensic Science Society*.)

resort to expensive and time-consuming procedures such as whole-body autoradiograph or chemical extraction. They have the added advantage that the effect of extremely low temperatures on the luminscence characteristics of a drug can easily be examined. The intensity of fluorescence emission is often greatly enhanced at low temperatures and this may aid detection of the drug. Reduction of temperature may also result in the production of phosphorescent emissions.

The wavelengths of phosphorescence are often longer than those of fluorescence. Consequently either the emission from the drug may be shifted from the u.v. into the visible region of the spectrum (e.g. diazepam) or the colour contrast against the surrounding biological molecules may be enhanced (e.g. chlorpromazine).

Whole-body fluorograms are easily prepared from laboratory animals such as mice. The drug is administered to an animal and after a period of time appropriate for uptake but not excretion the animal is killed by cervical dislocation. The carcase is then rapidly frozen, for example in liquid nitrogen or acetone cooled with solid carbon dioxide, allowed to warm to $-20\,^{\circ}$C and bisected sagitally using a sharp knife. The cut surface of the animal can then be examined under u.v. excitation in a dark room. Illumination is achieved by using two lamps positioned on either side of the animal in such a way that the excitation light hits the cut surface at an angle of approximately 45°. This positioning also allows photographic records to be made of the results. The temperature can be maintained below $-20\,^{\circ}$C by placing the animal in a suitably cooled trough. For reduction to temperatures as low as $-195\,^{\circ}$C for examination of phosphorescence liquid nitrogen can be poured directly into the trough.

Care must be taken when bisecting animals that the blood is not allowed to thaw. If this occurs blood is smeared across the cut surface of the animal and this results in obliteration of fluorescence.

Step 3: Examination of histological preparations by fluorescence microscopy. Once suitable preparative procedures have been found which retain the drug in the tissue, histological sections can be examined on the microscope. The appropriate conditions of pH can be attained by the use of buffered mountants, although care must be taken that these do not fluoresce. Temperature can be controlled by using temperature-regulated microscope stages.

The excitation and suppression filters are chosen on the basis of data obtained from the preliminary spectrofluorescence studies. However, should the fluorescence intensity of the drug be weak, it may be advantageous to choose an excitation wavelength which does not excite tissue autofluorescence. This has the same effect as increasing the intensity of emission from the drug. The use of fixed as opposed to frozen tissue is also useful in this respect.

1.3.2.4 Future developments of the technique in toxicology

Although autofluorescence procedures have provided useful information in clinical toxicology they are of more limited use in forensic fields. This is primarily because few drugs of interest to the forensic sciences have fluorescence characteristics in the visible region of the spectrum. Additional problems arise when the technique is applied to human material. In such studies, unlike those involving the use of laboratory animals, difficulties are encountered in obtaining suitable control material because the autofluorescence of human tissue is quite variable from one individual to another. Further complications arise in forensic toxicology because tissue autofluorescence may be affected by decomposition. No formal studies have as yet been carried out on this aspect of the procedure. They would yield valuable information which would enable extension of the technique into the field of forensic toxicology.

1.3.3 Immunofluorescence procedures

The techniques of immunofluorescence have greater potential than autofluorescence methods for detecting the sites of drug localisation in tissue preparations. The fluorescence characteristics of the drug itself are unimportant as its position is located indirectly by means of a specific antibody conjugated to a fluorochrome. In addition, provided that nonspecific staining of the tissues by the conjugate is kept to a minimum it is much easier to discriminate between drug-free and drug-laden material.

The available methods have been extensively discussed by Nairn (1976) and Feteanu (1978b). Two basic procedures have been developed and both are applicable to the histological localisation of drugs. They are referred to as the direct and the indirect techniques and they differ only in the stage at which fluorochrome-labelled antiserum is applied to the tissue (Figure 1.8). In the direct technique the position of the drug is located by staining the material with a drug-specific antiserum which has been conjugated to a fluorochome. In the indirect technique this antiserum (the primary antiserum) is left unlabelled and the site of its binding are detected by means of a second incubation step in which the tissue is stained with a fluorochrome-labelled secondary antiserum raised against the immunoglobulins of the species used to produce the primary antiserum.

The direct technique is preferred by some workers because staining is completed more rapidly. However, each time a different drug is studied the antiserum to that drug must be conjugated to a fluorochrome. This problem is not so acute with the indirect procedure because a single fluorochrome-labelled secondary antiserum can be used to detect a wide range of drug antibodies, provided that these antibodies have been raised in the same species of animal. A number of suitable fluorescent secondary antisera are available commercially and the use of these may considerably reduce the amount of time involved in setting up an indirect technique.

The indirect method is particularly useful when stocks of primary antiserum are limited. In addition it may enhance the brightness of the fluorescent image because more fluorochrome molecules can bind to a single molecule of antigen than in the direct procedure (Figure 1.9). It must be remembered, however, that the observed intensity of the fluorescence image is partly dependent upon the level of nonspecific binding of the antisera to other tissue components. Such binding must be kept to a minimum if the full potential of the indirect technique to enhance image brightness is to be exploited.

All the work that has been carried out on the immunofluorescent detection

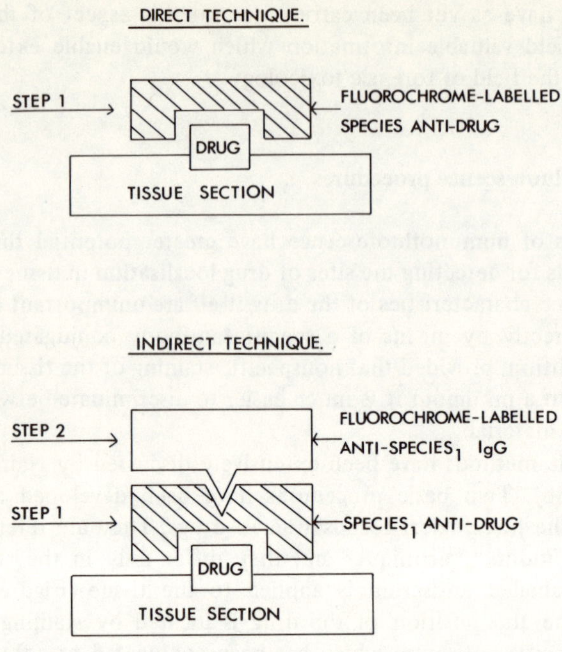

Figure 1.8 The direct and indirect immunofluorescence technique.

Direct technique

(a) Step 1: apply diluted fluorochrome-labelled species anti-drug to the section.
(b) Wash in phosphate-buffered saline (PBS), pH 7.2.
(c) Mount in buffered glycerol.

Indirect technique

(a) Step 1: apply diluted species anti-drug to the section (the primary antiserum).
(b) Wash in PBS, pH 7.2.
(c) Step 2: stain with diluted fluorochrome-labelled anti-species immunoglobulin (the secondary antiserum).
(d) Wash in PBS, pH 7.2.
(e) Mount in buffered glycerol.

of drugs has involved the use of the indirect procedure and on the whole it has proved successful. It has enabled the histological localisations of methadone (Pertschuk and Sher, 1975; Pertschuk *et al.*, 1977), phenobarbital (Pertschuk *et al.*, 1976) and morphine (Balkon *et al.*, 1980) to be described. In theory these aqueous processing procedures should be ideally suited to detecting lipophilic drugs, but experience with tetrahydrocannabinol has shown that this is not always true (Morley and Gee, 1982). The conclusions drawn from this study will be discussed in greater detail later in the section. First, an outline will be given for an approach to setting up an immunofluorescence technique.

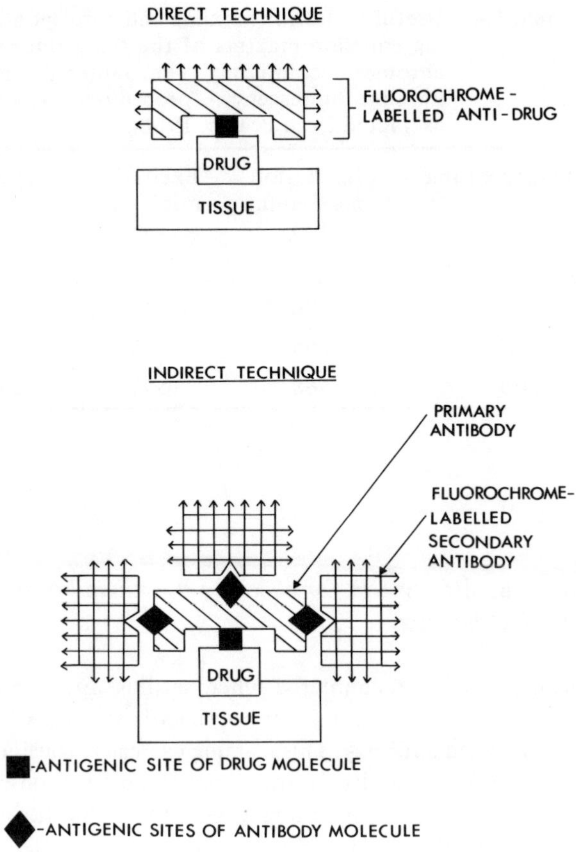

Figure 1.9 Amplification of image brightness in the indirect immunofluorescence technique. In theory the use of the indirect procedure can increase the brightness of the fluorescence image. This is illustrated for the detection of a drug with a single binding site for its specific antibody. The large protein molecules of the antibody to the drug will have many more antigenic sites than the drug itself. Consequently, a greater number of fluorochrome-labelled molecules are involved in localising the drug in the indirect procedure. This amplifies the brightness of the image.

1.3.3.1 Choice of fluorochrome

Although a number of fluorochomes are suitable for linkage to proteins, only three are commonly encountered in the immunofluorescence procedure. These are fluorescein isothiocyanate (FITC), tetramethylrhodamine isothiocyanate (TRITC) and lissamine-rhodamine B (RB200). Commercially prepared conjugates and specific filter systems are available for all these materials. Their excitation and emission maxima are given in Table 1.4.

Table 1.4 Useful excitation maxima and corresponding emission maxima of the three fluorochromes commonly encountered in immunofluorescence procedures (data extracted from Pearse, 1968d)

Fluorochrome	Excitation maximum, Ex_{Δ} (nm)	Excitation minimum, Em_{Δ} (nm)	pH
FITC	490	517	7.6
TRITC	555	580	8.0
RB200	568	597	8.0

1.3.3.2 Use of an in vitro *system for checking the suitability of immunofluorescence for detecting the drug*

One of the main problems encountered when settling upon an immunofluorescence technique lies in eliminating any nonspecific staining of the tissues by the fluorochrome-labelled antibody. This staining can cause considerable difficulties in the interpretation of results. In the direct technique, nonspecific binding is largely the result of electrostatic interaction between the tissue proteins and conjugated globulins in the antisera. In the indirect technique both the primary and secondary antisera can bind nonspecifically to the tissue. It is useful to run preliminary trials with an *in vitro* system from which tissue protein is absent in order to get a rapid assessment of the suitability of the immunofluorescence procedure for detecting the drug.

One such system has been developed for the immunofluorescent detection of protein antigens such as botulinum toxin (Allen, 1963). It involves the entrapment of antigen from solution by gelling agar. Once gelled the agar is treated as a tissue sample for the purposes of processing. The effects of fixatives on the immunoreactivity of the antigens and the optimal length of time required for the detection of specific staining can then be determined. Such information provides valuable guidelines for the application of the technique to biological tissues.

The method has not yet proved useful for the detection of small drug molecules such as Δ-THC (Morley, unpublished observations). However, this may be due to the unsuitability of the immunofluorescence procedure for detecting this drug rather than to problems inherent to the system, such as diffusion of the antigen out of the agar strands.

1.3.3.3 Detection of nonspecific staining in biological tissue

Two basic controls can be introduced into preliminary experiments which allow the detection of nonspecific staining. Steps may then be taken to reduce the intensity of this nonspecific fluorescence after which further experiments can be conducted using more stringent controls. Each of these stages will be discussed in detail.

1. Substrate and antiserum controls The use of these two types of control in preliminary experiments enables rapid detection of nonspecific staining of the tissues by the antisera. They are outlined in Figure 1.10, where they are described for the indirect technique. Similar principles are involved when controlling the direct technique.

In substrate-controlled experiments the same primary antiserum (species anti-drug) is used to stain either drug-laden or drug-free tissue. No specific binding will occur in the latter. In antiserum-controlled experiments variations are made in the specifications of the primary antiserum. Drug-laden tissue is stained with either species anti-drug or nonimmune serum from the same species of animal used to produce the antiserum to the drug. Nonimmune serum will not bind to the drug. Any fluorescence in either of these control tissues is indicative of nonspecific staining.

2. Reduction of nonspecific staining Nonspecific staining is caused mainly by electrostatic interaction between basic proteins within the tissue section and conjugated proteins within the antisera. The intensity of this staining varies between different tissues and different batches of antisera. It is also partly dependent upon the processing procedures used to prepare the tissue section. Fresh-frozen cryostat sections exhibit the greatest degree of nonspecific staining, even after post-fixation in fixatives such as alcohol and acetone. Freeze-drying reduces the intensity of nonspecific staining, as does fixation in formalin. Formalin can also reduce the intensity of specific staining, but this problem can sometimes be overcome by pretreating sections from such material with 1% ammonium hydroxide or 25% sodium bisulphite (Maestrone, 1963). Such procedures have proved effective with protein toxins such as ricin (Morley, unpublished observations). The way in which these reagents neutralise the effect of formalin on antigens is not clear.

The intensity of nonspecific staining is also partly dependent upon the dilution of the antisera used to stain the tissues. A range of antiserum dilutions should always be used when setting up any technique in order to determine the effective working solution at which the ratio between the respective intensities of specific and nonspecific staining is optimal. In indirect procedures the dilutions of both the primary and secondary antisera must be considered and it has become conventional to use chessboard systems of staining in the making of these assessments for the indirect technique (Figure 1.11).

Figure 1.10 Controlling immunofluorescence procedures. The controls which should be included in immunofluorescence experiments are explained for use with the indirect technique. The same principles are involved when controlling the direct technique. Any fluorescence in the control tissue is indicative of nonspecific staining.

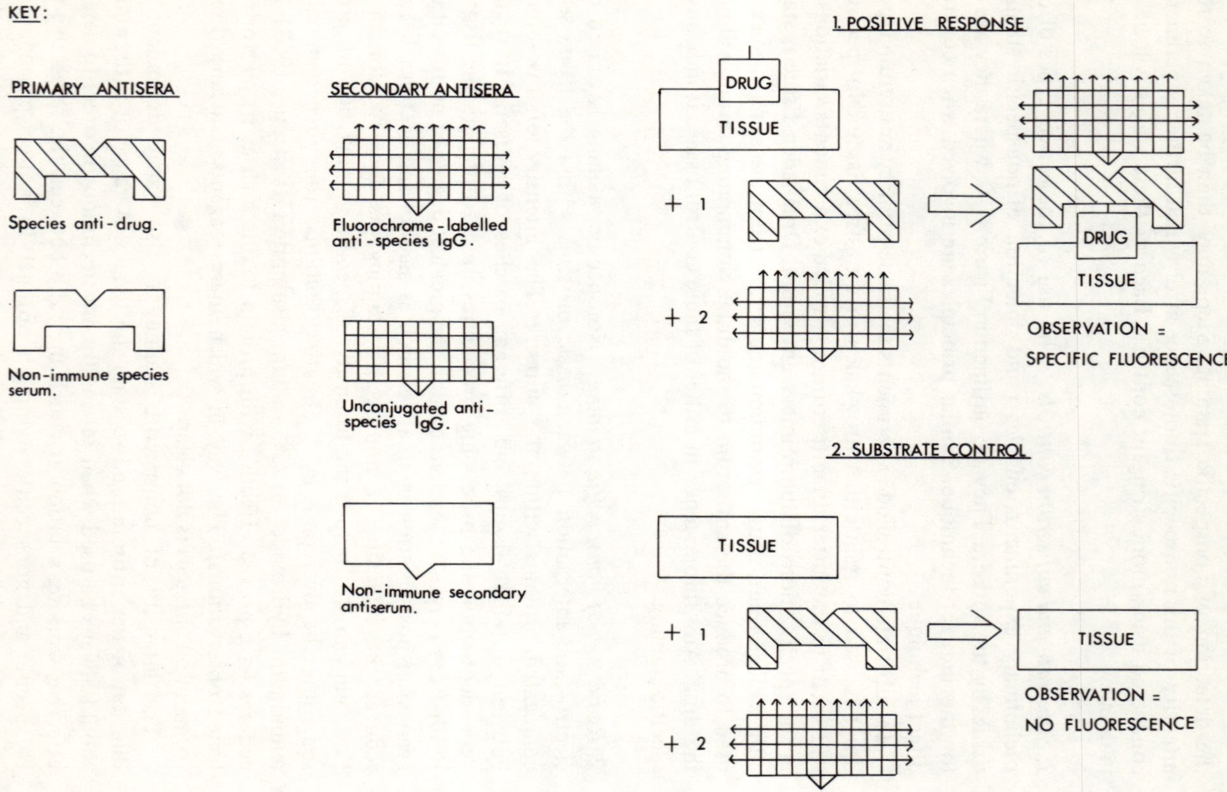

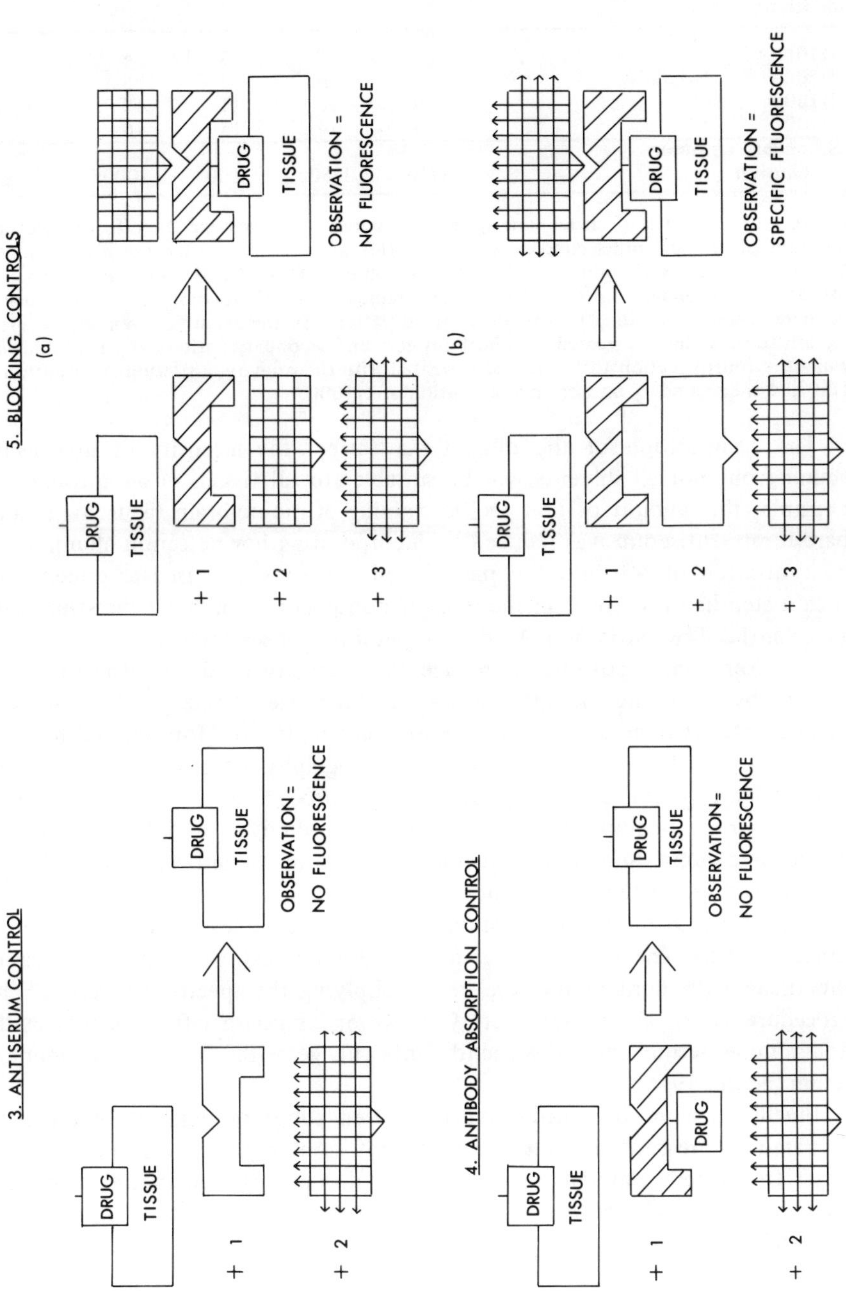
3. ANTISERUM CONTROL
DRUG
TISSUE
+ 1
+ 2
OBSERVATION = NO FLUORESCENCE
4. ANTIBODY ABSORPTION CONTROL
DRUG
TISSUE
+ 1
+ 2
OBSERVATION = NO FLUORESCENCE
5. BLOCKING CONTROLS
(a)
DRUG
TISSUE
+ 1
+ 2
+ 3
OBSERVATION = NO FLUORESCENCE
(b)
DRUG
TISSUE
+ 1
+ 2
+ 3
OBSERVATION = SPECIFIC FLUORESCENCE

Primary antiserum dilution	Section number			
1/10	1	2	3	4
1/50	5	6	7	8
1/1000	9	10	11	12
1/100	13	14	15	16
Secondary antiserum dilution	1/10	1/50	1/100	1/1000

Figure 1.11 The use of chessboard systems of staining for assessing the effective working dilutions of primary and secondary antisera in the indirect immunofluorescence technique. Chessboard systems of staining enable easy assessment of the effective working dilutions of primary and secondary antisera. Sections are stained with various combinations of dilutions of these antisera according to a predetermined pattern. In the example given here the first section to be stained is treated with both primary and secondary antisera at a 1/10 dilution, while the fourth section to be stained is treated with the primary antiserum at a dilution of 1/10 and the secondary antiserum at a dilution of 1/1000.

The composition of the diluent may affect the intensity of nonspecific staining but not all diluents will be suitable for all tissues or all antisera. For example, the amount of nonspecific staining of mouse-brain tissue by an anti-barbiturate antiserum was reduced by incorporating bovine serum albumin to a concentration of 4% into the phosphate-buffered saline used as diluent, but such a step had no effect on the level of nonspecific staining of the same tissue by an anti-Δ-THC antiserum (Morley, unpublished observations).

It is sometimes possible to reduce the intensity of the nonspecific fluorescence by absorbing the antisera with acetone-dried tissue powders or tissue homogenates (Coons and Kaplan, 1950; Kaplan, 1958). More refined purifications may be achieved with column chromatography. Affinity chromatography is particularly useful for this purpose. In this procedure the antigen is coupled to a supporting medium. It binds to its specific antibody as the antiserum is passed down the column. Subsequent chemical splitting of the antigen–antibody complex allows use of the specific antibody in the immunofluorescence technique.

Reductions in nonspecific staining may also be achieved by modifying the tissue proteins. The receptor sites for such binding can be blocked by treating the tissue with nonimmune sera before applying the specific antiserum. This procedure is not always satisfactory, however, as nonspecific elements in the nonimmune serum can subsequently interchange with those in the immune serum (Nairn, 1976b).

Finally, a word of warning must be given about the use of commercially prepared fluorescent antisera. The amount of nonspecific staining that can result from these materials varies widely, and it is suggested that as many products as possible should be examined when developing an immunofluorescence technique.

3. The use of more stringent controls Once nonspecific staining has been reduced to a minimum, more stringent controls can be introduced into the experiments. These ensure that the remaining fluorescence is specifically localising the antigen under study.

(a) Antibody absorption controls. The specificity of the antiserum for the drug can be tested by using antibody absorption controls. These can be used with both the direct and indirect techniques. In such controls the intensity of staining should be either reduced or abolished when the primary antiserum has previously been incubated with the antigen (Figure 1.10). This can be either the free drug alone or the drug in combination with the ligand to which it was linked during the initial process of raising the antisera. It should be noted that when the antigen forms a soluble complex with its antibody the fluorescence of the control tissue may only be reduced and not abolished. This is because exchanges of antibody may take place between the drug molecules in the soluble complex and the drug molecules bound to the tissue. Obviously no such problem arises when the antigen–antibody complex precipitates out of the incubation mixture.

(b) Blocking controls. These can be used in both direct and indirect immunofluorescence experiments. In such controls the fluorescence resulting from binding of the conjugated antiserum should be inhibited by pretreating the tissue with unconjugated antiserum but not by pretreatment with nonimmune serum. The procedures are outlined in Figure 1.10. They provide a check that the binding is specific either to fluorochrome-labelled anti-drug immunoglobulins (in the direct technique) or to fluorochrome-labelled antispecies immunoglobulins (in the indirect technique) and that it is not caused by the binding of any fluorochrome-labelled nonspecific proteins to the tissue.

(c) Assessments of method specificity. This type of assessment may be introduced into experiments using the indirect technique. It provides a check that the areas of fluorescence are specific to some substance in the primary antiserum and do not result from any nonspecific binding of the secondary antiserum. Consequently it is a useful preliminary to antibody absorption controls, as it may prevent the wastage of valuable material in the absorption procedure.

Sections of drug-laden material are stained with progressive dilutions of primary antiserum (e.g. 1/10, 1/50, 1/100, 1/1000, 1/10 000), while the dilution of the secondary antiserum is kept constant. Any variations which occur in the intensity of staining will thus be attributable to the primary antiserum alone. Nonspecific binding of the secondary antiserum to the tissue will be evident if the intensity of the fluorescence is not progressively reduced.

1.3.3.4 Problems specific to the immunofluorescence detection of drugs

The aqueous processing procedures of the immunofluorescence technique would seem to be ideally suited for use with lipophilic compounds such as drugs. Indeed, the indirect technique has been used successfully for localising methadone (Pertschuk and Sher, 1975; Pertschuk *et al.*, 1977), phenobarbital (Pertschuk *et al.*, 1976) and morphine (Balkon *et al.*, 1980). Less success has been achieved with Δ-THC, the active constituent of cannabis (Morley and Gee, 1982), and a number of points have been raised in this study which may be of relevance to work with other drugs.

1. The solubility characteristics of the drug–antibody complex The solubility characteristics of the drug–antibody complex may be more important than those of the drug itself from the point of view of retaining the drug in the tissue during processing. For example, Δ-THC is an extremely lipophilic substance and, indeed, radiotracer experiments have shown that at least 70 per cent of this drug remains bound to sections of liver tissue after staining by the indirect technique. However, large losses of Δ-THC from the tissue occur immediately after incubation with the primary antiserum, indicating that the drug forms a water-soluble complex with its antibody (Figure 1.1). The formation of similar water-soluble complexes between the primary and secondary antibodies may account for the further losses of Δ-THC encountered after incubation with the secondary antiserum. It is therefore important that consideration is given to the solubility characteristics of such complexes when designing an experimental protocol for the immunofluorescent detection of drugs.

2. The site attachment of the drug to its receptor site in the tissue Many drugs are composed of small molecules and thus it is likely that they have only one antigenic site. It is possible that the position of attachment of the drug to its receptor may mask part of this antigenic site. Should this occur then the drug would be inaccessible for binding with its antibody. It is thus advisable to use a number of antisera raised against a variety of antigens which differ in the position of the hapten–ligand linkage.

3. Cross-reactivity of the primary antiserum with drug metabolites Some of the drug in a tissue section may be present in the form of metabolites rather than in that of the parent compound. These metabolites will be detected only if they cross-react with the primary antiserum. The importance of such cross-reactivity will depend upon the particular drug being studied and the purpose of the study. Obviously it will be detrimental to investigations of the sites of drug action where the parent compound is the pharmacologically active molecule. It will be less of a problem in studies of general distribution.

1.4 FIELDS REQUIRING FURTHER EXAMINATION

All of the published literature on the detection of drugs by histochemical procedures has concentrated on fluorescence methods of detection, but other histochemical techniques may prove equally suitable. The production of coloured rather than fluorescent reaction products would obviate the need for expensive fluorescent microscopes.

It is possible that conventional colorimetric methods of detection may be modified for the purposes of histochemical staining. Ferric chloride, for example, has been used for many years as a means of rapidly detecting salicylate in body fluids. A characteristic purple reaction product is produced. A similar response is observed when frozen sections of kidney from salicylate-injected mice are stained with ferric chloride but as yet no method has been devised of preventing diffusion of the reaction product away from the sites of drug distribution (Morley, unpublished observations). This response does not occur with kidney tissue from control animals.

The use of substrate film techniques may overcome the problem of reaction-product diffusion. These procedures are discussed by Pearse (1972). They have been used mainly to localise enzymes within tissue sections but it may be possible to devise suitable modifications for the purposes of localising drugs. The techniques have been developed for use with enzymes whose substrates are insoluble in water but whose chromogenic products are capable of removal by aqueous washing. In the simpler methods the substrate is incorporated into an inert medium such as agar gel or gelatin, a thin film of which is then placed in contact with the tissue section. The areas of enzyme distribution can be observed as translucent regions after subsequent washing of the reaction product from the supporting medium.

If immunological methods prove suitable for localising a drug then immuno-enzyme procedures may be used in the place of immunofluorescent techniques. The same principles operate in both but in the former the conjugated antibody is linked to an enzyme, such as horseradish peroxidase, instead of to fluorochrome. The position of the conjugated enzyme is subsequently located by means of a coloured reaction product resulting from the reaction between the enzyme and a suitable substrate. These procedures have an additional advantage in that they can be used in conjunction with electron microscopy.

Another aspect of drug histochemistry which has not been examined is that of quantification. Microspectrofluorimeters and microdensitometers are now widely available and provide the possibility of at least semi-quantifying the data. In the systems currently in use in other histochemical fields the intensity of the fluorescence or the optical density of a coloured reaction product is compared with the fluorescence or the optical density of a set of standards which have been treated in as close a manner as possible to the biological tissue being examined. The area is too wide to be discussed here and the reader is referred to the reviews cited in the list of further reading for further information on the subject.

The use of histochemical procedures for localising drugs has great potential for broadening our understanding of toxicological reactions in man. Much work remains to be done and I hope that at least some readers will be encouraged to pursue investigations into this area of research.

REFERENCES

Allen, J. (1963). Immunofluorescence applied to protein solutions. *J. Lab. Clin. Med.* **62**, 517–24.

Balkon, J., Bidanset, J. H., and Lynch, V. D. (1980). Immunofluorescence detection of drugs in postmortem assessment of drug influence in cause of death. *J. Forens. Sci.* **25**, 88–94.

Böttiger, L. E. (1955a). On the distribution of tetracycline in the body. *Antibiotics Chemother.* **5**, 332–9.

Böttiger, L. E. (1955b). On the distribution of chlortetracycline in the body. *Acta. Med. Scand.* **151**, 343–8

Chang, J. P., and Hori, S. H. (1961). The section freeze-substitution technique. 1: Method. *J. Histochem. Cytochem.* **9**, 292–300.

Coons, A. H., and Kaplan, M. H. (1950). Localisation of antigen in tissue cells. 2: Improvements in a method for the detection of antigen by means of fluorescent antibody. *J. Exper. Med.* **91**, 1–13.

Egorin, M. J., Hildebrand, R. C., Cimino, E. F., and Bachur, N. R. (1974). Cytofluorescence localization of adriamycin and daunorubicin. *Cancer Res.* **34**, 2243–5.

Feteanu, A. (1978a). Special technology and applications. In *Labelled Antibodies in Biology and Medicine*, 2nd edn. Abacus, Tunbridge Wells, p. 94.

Feteanu, A. (1978b). *Ibid*., pp. 95–114.

Gee, D. J., Gelder, S. R., Morley, M., and Sivaloganathan, S. (1981). Applications of microspectrofluorimetry to forensic medicine. *UV Spectrometry Group Bulletin* **9**, 53–63.

Gelder, S. R. (1978). A cold stage for observing an autoluminescent drug in tissue sections at 77 K using a DIALUX microscope. *Leitz. M. H. Wiss v Techn.* **8**, No. 7.

Gelder, S. R., and Gee, D. J. (1979). The visualisation of two autofluorescent drugs in tissue sections by fluorescent microscopy. *J. Forens. Sci. Soc.* **19**, 107–116.

Helander, S. (1949). On the distribution of some salicylic acid derivatives in the tissues. *Acta. Pharmacol.* **6**, 97–106.

Helander, S., and Böttiger, L. E. (1953). On the distribution of terramycin in different tissues. *Acta. Med. Scand.* **47**, 71–5.

Kaplan, M. H. (1958). Immunologic studies of heart tissue. 1: production in rabbits of antibodies reactive with an autologous myocardial antigen following immunisation with heterologous heart tissue. *J. Immun.* **80**, 254–67.

Kohn, K. W. (1961). Mediation of divalent metal ions in the binding of tetracycline to macromolecules. *Nature*, Lond. **191**, 1156–8.

Liss, R. H., and Norman, J. C. (1975). Visualisation of doxycycline in lung tissue and sinus secretions by fluorescent techniques. *Chemotherapy* **21** (suppl. 1), 27–35.

Maestrone, G. (1963). Demonstration of leptospiral and viral antigens in formalin-fixed tissues. *Nature*, Lond. **197**, 409–10.

Morley, M., and Gee, D. J. (1982). An assessment of the immunofluorescence technique as a method of demonstrating the histological localisation of tetrahydrocannabinol in post-mortem tissues. *J. Forens. Sci.* **27**, 837–43.

Morley, M., Gee, D. J., Moffat, A., and Gaunt, P. J. (1982). The effect of proteins on drug autofluorescence: forensic applications. In preparation.

Nairn, R. C. (1976a). Immunological tracing: general considerations. In *Fluorescent Protein Tracing*, 4th edn. Churchill Livingstone, Edinburgh and New York, pp. 132–4; 142–5.

Nairn, R. C. (1976b). *Ibid*., p. 158.

Pearse, A. G. E. (1968a). Fluorescent methods (immunofluorescence). In *Histochemistry: Theoretical and Applied*, 3rd edn. Williams and Wilkins, Baltimore, vol. 1, p. 203.

Pearse, A. G. E. (1968b). The chemistry of fixation. *Ibid*., vol. 1, pp. 86–8.

Pearse, A. G. E. (1968c). Cold knife and microtome methods. *Ibid*., vol. 1, p. 25.

Pearse, A. G. E. (1968d). Fluorescent antibody methods (immunofluorescence). *Ibid*., vol. 1, pp. 188–95.

Pearse, A. G. E. (1972). Substrate film techniques. *Ibid*., vol. 2, pp. 1009–15.

Pertschuk, L. P., and Sher, J. H. (1975). Demonstration of methadone in the human brain by immunofluorescence. *Res. Commun. Chem. Pathol. Pharmacol.* **11**, 319–22.

Pertschuk, L. P., Ford, D. H., Rainfold, E. A., and Brigati, D. J. (1976). Localization of phenobarbital in mouse central nervous system by immunofluorescence. *Acta Neurol. Scand.* **53**, 325–34.

Pertschuk, L. P., Ford, D. H., and Rainford, E. A. (1977). Localization of methadone in fetal rat eye by the immunofluorescence technic. *Expl. Eye Res.* **24**, 547–52.

Stora, C. (1980a). Histofluorescence technique for the intracellular localization of chemical carcinogens. *Histochem. J.* **12**, 631–40.

Stora, C. (1980b). Cellular localization of chemical carcinogens studied by fluorescence microscopy. *Oncology* **37**, 20–2.

Stora, C. (1980c). Comparative study of the cellular localization of three polycylic hydrocarbons differing in their carcinogenicity. *Ibid.* **37**, 23–6.

Udenfriend, S. (1962). *Fluorescence Assay in Biology and Medicine*. Academic, New York, vol.1.

FURTHER READING

Affinity chromatography

Affinity Chromatography, Principles and Methods (undated). Pharmacia Fine Chemicals, Uppsala.

Fluorescence

(a) General principles

Udenfriend, S. (1962). *Fluorescence Assay in Biology and Medicine*, Academic, New York, San Francisco, London, vol 1.

(b) Microscopy

Nairn, R. C. (1976). Fluorescence microscopy and photomicography. In *Fluorescent Protein Tracing*, 4th edn. Churchill Livingstone, Edinburgh, pp. 68–108.

Pearse, A. G. E. (1972). Fluorescence microscopy. In *Histochemistry, Theoretical and Applied*, 3rd edn. Churchill Livingstone, Edinburgh, vol. 2, pp. 1171–206.

Ploem, J. S. (1977). Quantitative fluorescence microscopy. In Meek, G. A., and Elder, H. Y. (eds), *Analytical and Quantitative Methods in Microscopy*, 1st edn. Cambridge University Press, Cambridge, pp. 55–90.

Histochemistry

Pearse, A. G. E. (1968). *Histochemistry, Theoretical and Applied*, 3rd edn. Williams and Wilkins, Baltimore, vol. 1.

Pearse, A. G. E. (1972). *Ibid*., vol. 2.

Immunoenzyme techniques

Feteanu, A. (1978). *Labelled Antibodies in Biology and Medicine*. Abacus, Tunbridge Wells.

Heyderman, E. (1979). Immunoperoxidase technique in histopathology: applications, methods and controls. *J. Clin. Pathol.* **32**, 971–8.

Immunofluorescence

Feteanu, A. (1978). *Labelled Antibodies in Biology and Medicine*. Abacus, Tunbridge Wells.

Nairn, R. C. (1976). *Fluorescent Protein Tracing*. Churchill Livingstone, Edinburgh.

Pearse, A. G. E. (1968). Fluorescent antibody methods (immunofluorescence). In *Histochemistry, Theoretical and Applied*, 3rd edn. Williams and Wilkins, Baltimore, vol. 1, pp. 180–213.

Quantitative histochemistry

Meek, G. A., and Elder, H. Y. (eds) (1977). *Analytical and Quantitative Methods in Microscopy*. Cambridge University Press, Cambridge.

Pearse, A. G. E. (1972). Quantitative histochemistry. In *Histochemistry, Theoretical and Applied*, 3rd edn. Churchill Livingstone, Edinburgh, vol. 2, pp. 1225–59.

2
Clinical toxicology

R. J. FLANAGAN and B. WIDDOP

2.1 INTRODUCTION

Clinical toxicology is concerned with the diagnosis, treatment and also the prevention of poisoning in man. Self-poisoning with drugs remains the problem encountered most frequently by the physician. It has been estimated that within the U.K. some three hundred thousand patients per year ingest poisons either by accident or with suicidal intent and of these some forty to fifty per cent are admitted to hospital. A total of 120 640 admissions from this cause were recorded in England and Wales in 1978, which represents a sixfold increase over the corresponding figure for 1958 (Vale and Meredith, 1981). Over this same period a wide range of drugs, notably those with psychotropic activity, became available and these agents have now emerged as the poisons ingested by most patients. Barbiturates and other sedative-hypnotic agents such as the benzodiazepines, tricyclic antidepressants, analgesics such as paracetamol and salicylate and also narcotics such as codeine and dextropropoxyphene are the predominant compounds involved, although the incidence of barbiturate poisoning has decreased in the UK following the success of CURB (Campaign for the Use and Restriction of Barbiturates) (Proudfoot and Park, 1978).

2.2 TREATMENT OF POISONING–ROLE OF THE LABORATORY

2.2.1 Introduction

Most poisoned patients admitted to hospital are mildly intoxicated and make a complete physical recovery with supportive treatment. Even in more severe cases, supportive therapy alone is often successful in bringing about a satisfactory outcome. In such instances toxicological analyses are not required. However, with certain severely poisoned patients, the detection, identification and in some instances measurement of the poison(s) ingested can make a valuable contribution to diagnosis, management or prognosis.

2.2.2 Diagnosis of acute poisoning

Few centrally depressant drugs produce characteristic diagnostic features when taken in overdose, and even where clinical signs have become associated with a particular poison, there are often many alternative explanations for the patient's condition. In one study of 208 patients presenting with coma of unknown aetiology in whom toxicological investigations were performed, poisoning was found to be the cause of coma in 108 patients (52%) and alternative diagnoses, mainly neurological, were eventually established in 90 (Helliwell *et al.*, 1979).

In addition to the differential diagnosis of coma, there are a number of other instances where toxicological analyses can aid diagnosis. The detection of salicylate or ethylene glycol, for example, may help to provide the diagnosis in the case of a patient with a severe acidosis, while the detection of agents such as chlorpropamide may be important in establishing the reason for hypoglycaemia. It may also be important to establish whether a clinical diagnosis of self-poisoning was correct in the face of denial of this possibility either from relatives or indeed from the patient.

2.2.3 Management of the poisoned patient

Some severely poisoned patients may require active treatment in the form of either antidotes or procedures designed to increase the rate of elimination of the poison. Antidotes are available for a number of poisons and these are normally given when the clinical diagnosis has been made (Meredith and Vale, 1981). On the other hand, laboratory tests may help to establish the diagnosis and thus prompt the administration of the antidote in such instances as acute methanol or ethylene glycol poisoning (Vale *et al.*, 1982) or in paracetamol poisoning where there is no circumstantial indication that this has occurred (Canalese *et al.*, 1981). Once antidotal therapy has begun, analytical information may be valuable in guiding treatment. For example, the clinical management of organophosphate poisoning may be simplified by measurement of serum and erythrocyte cholinesterase activity when giving massive infusions of atropine. Plasma ethanol concentrations are useful in the management of poisoning with methanol or ethylene glycol (ethanediol) to ensure that effective doses of the antidote are given (Vale *et al.*, 1982). Toxicological analyses can sometimes assist in limiting unnecessary treatment, as in patients undergoing intravenous therapy with *N*-acetylcysteine who are found not to be at risk following the ingestion of paracetamol.

When the active removal of a drug by techniques such as forced diuresis, haemodialysis or charcoal haemoperfusion is contemplated, toxicological investigations are necessary to identify the poison(s) and to assess the amount available for removal. Only a limited number of drugs and poisons can be removed by these procedures (Table 2.1), which are themselves not without risk and should only be used if warranted by the clinical condition of the patient. Serial plasma-concentration measurements can help to assess whether active therapy is needed, especially where delayed absorption of the drug is likely as in the case of poisoning with sustained-release theophylline (Helliwell and Berry, 1979). They serve also to monitor the efficacy of the technique adopted (Raper *et al.*, 1982).

Table 2.1 Poisons removed in significant amounts by active-elimination treatment

Procedure	Poison	Minimum plasma concentration for effective removal ($mg\ l^{-1}$ unless otherwise stated)
forced alkaline diuresis	salicylate	500
	phenobarbitone	100
	barbitone	100
forced acid diuresis	quinine	20
peritoneal dialysis	ethylene glycol	$0.5\ g\ l^{-1}$
	lithium	$3\ mmol\ l^{-1}$
haemodialysis	ethanol	$5\ g\ l^{-1}$
	methanol	$0.5\ g\ l^{-1}$
	ethylene glycol	$0.5\ g\ l^{-1}$
	lithium	$3\ mmol\ l^{-1}$
	phenobarbitone	100
	barbitone	100
	salicylate	500
charcoal haemoperfusion	phenobarbitone	100
	barbitone	100
	other barbiturates	40
	glutethimide	40
	methaqualone	40
	meprobamate	100
	ethchlorvynol	150
	trichloroethanol	80
	theophylline	60
	salicylate	500
	paracetamol	100

Toxicology analyses may help to suggest appropriate conservative management. For example, the identification and measurement of cardiotoxic agents such as tricyclic antidepressants can indicate the need to monitor cardiac function in patients poisoned with these agents and thus give warning of treatable but potentially fatal complications.

2.2.4 Diagnosis of brain-stem death

The vital functions of severely brain-damaged patients can now be maintained almost indefinitely by mechanical means. This has generated a medical dilemma in formulating criteria according to which the support systems can be withdrawn. The physician must be confident that the damage is irreversible and recovery therefore not possible. The criteria adopted in the UK (Conference of Medical Royal Colleges, 1976) emphasised the need to exclude the presence of CNS depressant drugs, especially in patients whose primary cause of coma was drug overdose. By the same token, the continued presence of drugs such as benzodiazepines or thiopentone, which are often infused in an attempt to avoid anoxic cerebral damage, should also be excluded.

2.2.5 Diagnosis of chronic poisoning

Continued exposure to poisonous substances, particularly those which accumulate in the body, leads ultimately to pathological damage. Chronic poisoning is most prevalent in the occupational environment and frequently involves toxic metals such as lead, mercury and cadmium. The detection of abnormally high concentrations of these substances in the blood confirms the diagnosis and indicates the need to avoid further exposure. Lead poisoning is so common in young children, especially in those with pica, that many clinical chemistry departments have the facility to measure blood lead concentrations. Excessive accumulation of aluminium by renal dialysis patients can lead to severe deterioration in bone structure and a lethal encephalopathy (Parkinson *et al.*, 1981). The need to monitor levels of this element in serum and dialysis fluid is now regarded as almost mandatory.

Carbon monoxide is perhaps the most insidious of all poisons and accounts for many fatalities each year. Less well known is its ability to induce a multitude of neurological symptoms in patients chronically exposed to sub-lethal concentrations (*Lancet* editorial 1981; Thompson and Henry, 1983). Blood carboxyhaemoglobin measurements form a vital part of the diagnosis.

Concern as to the frequency and severity of adverse reactions to drugs has increased in recent years (Jick, 1977). For some drugs, clinical effects are related to plasma concentrations, and thus regular plasma concentration monitoring can minimise toxicity and at the same time optimise the therapeutic response. This area, known as therapeutic drug monitoring (TDM), has expanded enormously over the last 10 years and regular services are now available in most large hospital laboratories (Marks, 1979).

2.2.6 Diagnosis and treatment of drug, ethanol or solvent abuse

Clinicians specialising in the treatment of drug dependence have come to rely on laboratory tests to monitor drug taking in their patients. The analyses guard against the issuing of drugs to patients who may not, in fact, be dependent upon them and help to assess the progress or otherwise of treatment of genuinely dependent patients (Widdop, 1980). The abuse of psychotomimetic agents such as cannabis, LSD or amphetamines can lead to symptoms or signs indistinguishable from those due to an acute mental disorder. In these circumstances laboratory tests can provide crucial diagnostic evidence. Similarly, the measurement of blood or urinary ethanol concentrations has become almost standard practice in monitoring compliance with abstinence therapy (Hamlyn *et al.*, 1975).

Covert ingestion of anticoagulants to create fictitious disease can occur in patients treated previously with these drugs (O'Reilly and Aggeler, 1976). Most, though not all, have a psychiatric history; some are doctors or nurses with easy access to the drugs. Diagnosis of the problem can be baffling and patients often undergo complex haematological investigations before the real cause is suspected. The detection and measurement of an anticoagulant in the plasma clinches the diagnosis. Similarly, analytical tests to detect laxatives and diuretics in patients taking these surreptitiously can avoid months of fruitless clinical and biochemical investigations (De Wolff *et al.*, 1983).

Maternal drug abuse during the last stages of pregnancy can hold drastic consequences for the neonate. Infants born to mothers using opiate drugs invariably undergo an acute withdrawal syndrome. Benzodiazepines can produce floppy, unresponsive babies, although this occurs most frequently when the mother has received large intravenous doses of diazepam to combat eclamptic fits. Over-indulgence in tea or coffee can produce neonates with substantial blood concentrations of caffeine and corresponding features of jitteriness and lack of appetite. These situations are compromised by the neonate's restricted ability to metabolise drugs and the symptoms can persist for several days (Myers and Myers, 1979). Quantitative analysis of the suspected drug in the child's blood can confirm the cause of the condition and reassure the clinician that no organic disorder is present.

Solvent abuse ('glue sniffing') carries a risk of sudden death and at least 169 such fatalities occurred within the UK in the 10 years from 1971 (Anderson *et al.*, 1982). Acutely poisoned patients admitted to hospital may present with a variety of neurological signs such as drowsiness or convulsions and again the detection of the agent abused in blood specimens can be a valuable diagnostic aid (King *et al.*, 1981).

2.2.7 Forensic aspects of clinical toxicology

The fundamental role of the analyst in clinical toxicology is to assist the physician in the diagnosis and treatment of intoxicated patients. In so doing he may occasionally become involved in cases with medico-legal implications. This can be quite straightforward as, for example, when a self-poisoned patient dies in hospital. Toxicological data from ante-mortem samples are very often used by the pathologist or coroner in establishing the cause of death.

Unlawful administration of drugs or other poisons to adults is rare, but by no means unknown. A high proportion of patients who attribute their symptoms to this cause have a psychiatric disorder. Nevertheless, the physician often feels obligated to satisfy himself that the patient's claims are unfounded by seeking the help of the laboratory. With children the situation is much more complex and several reports have suggested that unauthorised drug administration by parents or guardians may often go unrecognised (Rogers *et al.*, 1976; Lorber *et al.*, 1980; Flanagan *et al.*, 1981). Some paediatricians have gone as far as to advocate laboratory testing for drugs in all children who present with bizarre symptoms for which no obvious pathological cause can be detected.

Evidence for unlawful poisoning belongs, in the first instance, to the physician and the hospital analyst is beholden to maintain strict medical confidentiality in dealings with the police and other interested parties. If legal proceedings ensue, the analyst may be called upon to present written or verbal evidence in a court of law. All records relating to the receipt, subsequent handling and analysis of the samples must be carefully preserved. Any residual sample material should be carefully stored, preferably frozen, pending repeat analyses by police laboratories or other agencies. Indeed, it is sensible to refrigerate and retain all samples submitted for emergency analysis for an appropriate period (say three to four weeks) in case further clinical or forensic investigations are required.

2.2.8 Research in clinical toxicology

Information relating to the acute toxicity in man of newly introduced drugs and also some of the less frequently encountered drugs and other poisons is often inadequate. Toxicological investigations in patients thought to have ingested an overdose of these agents can provide useful data to assist in the management of future cases and also in the evaluation of the safety of the agent in normal use. Chemical analyses are vital in this context in order to establish that the agent suspected had in fact been ingested, since there are often major discrepancies between the drug or drugs thought to have been ingested on clinical or circumstantial grounds and the results of toxicological tests (Widdop, 1974). Analyses also ensure that significant amounts of the agent were present in the blood or urine, since estimation of the dose ingested by other means such as tablet counting is notoriously inaccurate. Toxicological investigations can also help to establish the contribution of metabolites to the overall toxicity, as exemplified by the finding that 4-hydroxyglutethimide is largely responsible for the persistence of coma in acute glutethimide poisoning (Ambre and Fischer, 1974).

Some poisons have a delayed effect and only produce serious toxic symptoms several hours after ingestion. For some of these, plasma concentrations can be useful prognostic aids, as in the examples of paracetamol (Prescott, 1978) and paraquat (Proudfoot *et al*., 1979). However, these guidelines can be established only by collecting analytical data from large numbers of asymptomatic, moderately affected and severely poisoned patients.

The development of good analytical methods for new compounds and improved techniques to deal with the older drugs and poisons is a major feature of research in this area. Not only should the analytical method(s) used have adequate speed, sensitivity and selectivity, but due attention must be paid to possible sources of error or confusion. The use of methods which measure pharmacologically inactive metabolites in addition to the parent drug has given a totally erroneous impression of the efficacy of active-removal techniques such as forced diuresis or haemodialysis when applied to certain drugs such as barbiturates, and can be equally misleading where paracetamol overdosage is suspected (Stewart *et al*., 1979). Continued improvement in the scope, selectivity and reliability of the analytical methods used is also desirable in view of the forensic implications of many of the analyses undertaken.

2.3 SPECIMEN COLLECTION

2.3.1 Introduction

Due to the wide range of analytes which may be encountered and the variety of circumstances in which toxicological analyses may be needed it is not possible to give universally applicable specimen requirements. Nevertheless, in the case of an adult patient in whom general toxicological investigations are required, heparinised blood (10 ml), urine (30 to 50 ml) and gastric contents (30 to 50 ml) (if available) should often prove adequate. Whenever possible, the specimens should be obtained before drug administration takes place in hospital in order to avoid any interference in the analyses. Drugs may be administered during investigative procedures, e.g. sedatives prior to CAT scans, or inadvertently during therapeutic manoeuvres; for example lignocaine lubricants are frequently used during urinary catheterisation or gastric lavage. Some treatments can invalidate subsequent toxicological examinations, for example the use of hyperbaric oxygen will rapidly dissociate carboxyhaemoglobin. In the following paragraphs, some recommendations on the collection and storage of specimens are made.

2.3.2 Blood

Collection into heparinised tubes is advisable in most instances where drugs are involved, although these are not recommended for aminoglycoside antibiotic assays (gentamicin, kanamycin) and EDTA is a suitable alternative anticoagulant. EDTA is also preferred for carboxyhaemoglobin, lead and cadmium measurements. Preservatives are unnecessary if the analyses are to be performed on the day of collection. If samples are to be stored for longer periods, blood containing ethanol should be preserved with sodium fluoride (1 ml of blood added to approximately 10 mg of sodium fluoride). Physicians should be dissuaded from using venepuncture swabs containing alcohols such as isopropanol which might contaminate the specimen. Mucous heparin preparations containing cresol BP or chlorbutol are also best avoided. Contamination from the environment or the specimen container should be guarded against, especially when aluminium, lead, cadmium, mercury or iron are to be measured. Careless discharge of blood through a syringe needle can cause sufficient haemolysis to invalidate a serum iron assay and may affect immunoassays which rely on scintillation counting.

Some years ago it was found that certain commercial blood tubes with soft rubber stoppers released plasticisers which could displace basic drugs from plasma α_1-acid glycoprotein and cause a redistribution into the erythrocytes, although manufacturers now take steps to prevent this. Samples for paraquat assay should always be dispensed into plastic tubes since this compound is adsorbed on to glass. Conversely, organic solvents may be absorbed into plastic and therefore blood from suspected cases of 'glue sniffing' should be collected into glass tubes.

Finally, the stability of drugs in plasma should always be considered if samples are to be stored for retrospective analyses. Several drugs are known to decompose in plasma at room temperature, especially in daylight (e.g. paracetamol, nitrazepam, phenothiazines) and specimens should be stored deep-frozen.

2.3.3 Gastric contents

This includes vomit and gastric aspirate or stomach washings. It is important to obtain the first sample of washings rather than a later sample which may be considerably diluted. This is the most useful sample for qualitative analyses since the poison(s) may be present in high concentrations and the sample is usually devoid of metabolites which can complicate certain assays. At least 30 to 50 ml of sample should be obtained in order to carry out a wide range of tests, and no preservative should be added.

2.3.4 Urine

This sample is also valuable for qualitative screening since it is usually available in large volumes and often contains higher concentrations of drugs and some other poisons than the blood. The presence of drug metabolites can be helpful if chromatographic techniques which characterise the parent drug and its metabolites are applied. A 30 to 50 ml specimen is sufficient for a comprehensive series of tests and no preservative should be added. It should be noted that it is possible to obtain a urine specimen too soon after an overdose, i.e. before appreciable amounts of the ingested poison(s) have been excreted, particularly if the patient is in shock.

2.3.5 Other specimens

Any materials (tablets, powders, liquids, solvent containers, tablet bottles, syringes etc.) found with the patient should be retained for possible toxicological examination. However, it may be the case that such ancillary material has played no part in the episode and the biological specimens should be analysed preferentially. Other specimens such as breast milk or saliva may sometimes be available, and the use of these fluids in toxicological analyses has been discussed by Wilson *et al*. (1980) and by Idowu and Caddy (1982).

2.4 ANALYTICAL TECHNIQUES USED IN CLINICAL TOXICOLOGY

2.4.1 Introduction

The use of physico-chemical techniques in the detection, identification and measurement of drugs and other poisons in body fluids or tissues has its origins in forensic toxicology. Major advances in analytical methodology followed the application of physico-chemical techniques such as spectrophotometry and chromatography in the late 1940s. In particular, ultraviolet (u.v.) and infrared (i.r.) spectrophotometry, together with visible spectrophotometry (colorimetry), and paper and ion-exchange column chromatography were widely used. Paper chromatography has been largely superceded by thin-layer chromatography (TLC) since this latter technique offers advantages of speed of analysis and lower detection limits. Improved instrumentation for u.v. spectrophotometry (including facilities for derivative spectroscopy), spectrophotofluorimetry, atomic absorption spectrophotometry, anode stripping voltammetry and electrochemistry has led to these techniques being widely applied to particular problems.

Gas–liquid chromatography (GLC) has made a notable contribution to both the qualitative and quantitative analysis of drugs and other organic poisons, especially since the introduction of sensitive detectors such as the flame-ionisation detector (FID) and the electron-capture detector (ECD). These two detection systems are complementary, since the ECD shows in normal use an enhanced but selective response to certain compounds, in practice those containing either a halogen or some other 'electron-capturing' species such as a nitro moiety. The FID responds to most organic compounds. More recently, the scope of GLC has been further extended by the introduction of practical nitrogen-phosphorus detectors which have an enhanced and selective response to organic nitrogen or phosphorus compounds. The use of gas chromatography in combination with mass spectrometry (GC–MS) provides high sensitivity together with unparalleled selectivity, and can identify unequivocally many compounds using only nanograms of material.

Immunoassays, ranging from the classical radioimmunoassay (RIA) to the latest developments involving immunofluorescence techniques, have found wide application. They have the advantage of high sensitivity, are reasonably selective, and can often be applied directly to plasma or urine samples without prior purification.

High-performance liquid chromatography (HPLC) has emerged in recent years as the most versatile technique available to the toxicological analyst. In contrast to GLC, which is restricted to analysing compounds or derivatives which are both stable and volatile at temperatures up to about 350 °C, HPLC can tackle almost any organic analyte. As a qualitative screening device, however, HPLC is rather limited by the lack of a universal detector analogous to the FID in GLC, although a range of sensitive and reliable detectors (u.v. absorption, fluorimetric and electrochemical) is now available. A great advantage of the technique is the ease with which column effluent fractions corresponding to chromatographic peaks can be collected and further scrutinised by, for example, immunoassay or probe-injection mass-spectrometry.

2.4.2 Qualitative tests

The circumstantial evidence surrounding acute poisoning cases is often dubious and much analytical time can be saved by screening specimens before embarking on quantitative exercises. Simple presumptive colour tests are always useful (Table 2.2) and details of these and additional procedures are given by Meade

Table 2.2 Qualititative tests for drugs and other poisons (see also Meade *et al.*, 1972)

Analyte	Sample	Analytical principle	Approximate limit of sensitivity ($mg\ l^{-1}$)
ethchlorvynol	urine/gastric aspirate	Forms red colour with diphenylamine sulphate.	5
imipramine	urine/gastric aspirate	Forms yellow–green–blue colour with Forrest reagent.	50
paracetamol	urine/gastric aspirate	Hydrolysis to *p*-aminophenol and forms blue indophenol dye with *o*-cresol–ammonia.	5
paraquat	urine/gastric aspirate	Forms blue complex with alkaline dithionite (NB: diquat–yellow–green colour).	1
phenothiazines	urine/gastric aspirate	Form coloured complexes with FPN reagent.	50
salicylates	plasma/serum or urine	Form purple colour with ferric salts.	50
trichloro-compounds (e.g. chloral hydrate)	urine/gastric aspirate	Fujiwara reaction (see Maehly, 1967).	1

et al. (1972) and Widdop (1985). U.V. spectrophotometric scanning of sample extracts is still widely used, although the increased incidence of multiple drug overdose in recent years has reduced its appeal in favour of chromatographic and immunoassay procedures. Comprehensive analytical schemes largely based upon TLC of solvent or solid-phase extracts of urine have been described both for emergency toxicology (Berry and Grove, 1973) and addiction screening (Widdop, 1980). Recent papers have discussed the use of standardised TLC systems in toxicological analysis (Franke *et al.*, 1982; Stead *et al.*, 1982). A unique TLC kit (Toxi-Lab), specifically designed as a broad-spectrum drug-detection system for use in the emergency toxicology laboratory, has been described by Michand and Jones (1980).

Specialised toxicological laboratories rely heavily on analytical schemes involving a combination of TLC and GLC procedures (Widdop, 1985). Ardrey and Moffat (1981) have presented GLC retention-index data on 1318 compounds of toxicological interest on SE-30/OV-1 columns. The application of polysiloxane-deactivated capillary columns as a means of identifying compounds on the basis of retention indices has been discussed by Schepers *et al.* (1982). The recent development of cheaper 'mass-selective' detectors (Hewlett-Packard, Finnegan) will increase the use of GC–MS systems in clinical toxicology laboratories.

Qualitative immunoassay tests for drugs tend to be group-selective, e.g. towards opiates, barbiturates, benzodiazepines or cannabinoids (Table 2.3). Syva have led the field here with the conventional EMIT system, and more recently the EMIT-St designed for use by nonlaboratory personnel (Sutheimer *et al.*, 1982). Agglutination inhibition assays are becoming more reliable and find particular application in the monitoring of patients attending drug-dependence treatment clinics (Vanzeiti *et al.*, 1983). Qualitative screening procedures for heavy metals (Blacklock and Sadler, 1981), pesticides (Fysh and Jones, 1980) and organic solvents (Ramsey and Flanagan, 1982) have also been described.

2.4.3 Quantitative methods

These are conveniently considered in terms of 'chromatographic' and 'nonchromatographic' techniques. A summary of some useful nonchromatographic methods is given in Table 2.3. The list is not exhaustive since additional immunoassay procedures aimed at the therapeutic drug monitoring market produced by the Syva, Abbott, Ames, Beckman and Seward laboratories have appeared over the last two to three years and the reader is advised to consult these organisations for up-to-date information. There are drawbacks with these immunoassays, however, not least the high cost per assay, although some kits can be 'stretched' if suitable apparatus is available (Conard *et al.*, 1981). Moreover, the antibodies used in these assays may recognise a basic chemical structure which is common not only to the parent drug and its metabolites, but also to other drugs in the same chemical group. Interference from metabolites or

Table 2.3 Nonchromatographic methods used in analytical toxicology

Analyte (s)	Sample	Analytical technique	Limit of sensitivity	Reference or kit manufacturer
amphetamine	urine	EMIT*	2 mg l^{-1}	Syva
antiarrhythmics	plasma/ serum	EMIT	1 mg l^{-1}	Syva
anticonvulsants	plasma/ serum	EMIT	2 mg l^{-1}	Syva
barbiturates	plasma/ urine	EMIT	2 mg l^{-1}	Syva
benzodiazepines	plasma/ urine	EMIT	0.5 mg l^{-1}	Syva
cannabinoids	urine	EMIT*	15 μg l^{-1}	Syva
carboxyhaemoglobin	blood	spectrophotometry	5% CoHb	Blackmore (1970)
cholinesterase activity	serum	enzyme assay (colorimetric)	–	Sigma Chemical Company
cocaine	urine	EMIT*	1.6 mg l^{-1}	Syva
diazepam	blood/ urine	^{3}H RIA	0.3 μg l^{-1}	Rutterford and Smith (1980)
digoxin	plasma/ serum	^{125}I RIA	0.2 μg l^{-1}	Wellcome Reagents
ethanol	plasma/ serum	enzyme assay (spectrophotometric)	10 ml l^{-1}	Sigma Chemical Company
ethanol	blood/ urine	electrochemical	0.5 mg l^{-1}	Knepil and Fergie (1980)
gentamicin	plasma/ serum	EMIT	2 mg l^{-1}	Syva
iron	plasma/ serum	colorimetry	0.1 mg l^{-1}	Hyland Laboratories
lithium	plasma/ serum	atomic absorption or flame emission spectrophotometry	0.1 mmol l^{-1}	Fry (1981)
lysergic acid diethylamide	serum/ urine	^{3}H RIA	0.03 μg l^{-1}	Ratcliffe *et al.* (1977)
methotrexate	plasma/ serum	EMIT	1 μg l^{-1}	Syva
morphine	plasma/ urine	^{3}H RIA	25 μg l^{-1}	Roche Diagnostics
opiates	urine	EMIT*	0.5 mg l^{-1}	Syva
opiates	urine	haemagglutination* inhibition		Boehringer Corporation
paracetamol	plasma/ serum	enzyme assay (calorimetric)	10 mg l^{-1}	Cambridge Life Sciences
paraquat	plasma/ serum	^{3}H RIA	2 μg l^{-1}	Levitt (1979)

Table 2.3 (continued)

paraquat	plasma/serum	calorimetry	50 μg l^{-1}	Jarvie and Stewart (1979)
phencyclidine	urine	EMIT*	150 μg l^{-1}	Syva
salicylates	plasma/serum	calorimetry	20 mg l^{-1}	Trinder (1954)
tetrahydrocannabinol	plasma/urine	^{3}H RIA	6 μg l^{-1}	Teale *et al.* (1974)
theophylline	plasma/serum	EMIT	2 mg l^{-1}	Syva

*Qualitative only.

other drugs (or even from haemolysed or uraemic specimens) can sometimes be minimised by, for example, solvent extraction or column chromatography prior to the assay, but separate measurements of pharmacologically active metabolites or other drugs are still required.

High-performance thin-layer chromatography (HPTLC) has been advocated for quantitative work by some authors, but the high cost of the fluorescence scanners and of the plates themselves, together with dispersion and/or reflection problems has discouraged its use in clinical laboratories. On the other hand, elution chromatography (primarily GLC and HPLC) has been used extensively. The development of simple microextraction procedures using small (50 to 100 μl) specimens of plasma/serum or urine followed by GLC–FID (or ECD detection for benzodiazepines) and their applications in clinical toxicology have been described by Flanagan (1983). These procedures, when applied to plasma or serum for compounds such as barbiturates, glutethimide, chlormethiazole and benzodiazepines, yield both qualitative and quantitative information simultaneously, and their incorporation into an analytical scheme together with spot-tests and TLC has been described by Widdop (1985). The use of nitrogen-phosphorus detection has enhanced the selectivity and sensitivity of some GLC analyses, but a number of practical considerations in the use of this type of detector have become apparent. First, many nitrogen- or phosphorus-containing compounds such as plasticisers show a good response and may be mistaken for drugs or interfere with quantitation (Ramsey *et al.*, 1980). Second, small changes in the position or temperature of the bead or in the carrier-gas or hydrogen/air flow-rates or changes in the column-oven temperature may all influence either the selectivity or sensitivity of the system, even using modern electrically-heated bead systems.

HPLC has been applied widely in the quantitative analysis of particular drugs. Stationary-phase materials such as octadecylsilyl (ODS) or trimethylsilyl (TMS), chemically bonded to a 5- or 10-μm particle-size silica matrix, together with an aqueous buffer–methanol or acetonitrile eluent, are satisfactory for the analysis of many acidic and neutral compounds. However, these systems are less useful for basic analytes and the separations obtained differ little from those achieved on silica columns (Wheals, 1980). In both instances the major influence on retention is probably the presence of underivatised silanol groups on the silica surface which act as cation-exchange sites. A better approach to the HPLC of basic drugs uses underivatised silica together with a nonaqueous eluent such as methanol modified by the addition of compounds which are highly ionised in organic media (Flanagan *et al.*, 1982). The major factors influencing both the selectivity of such systems and the retention volumes of individual analytes are the pH and the ionic strength of the eluent. Changes in the organic component of the eluent can also alter the selectivity towards certain analytes, as can the use of chemically bonded stationary phases.

The following paragraphs give examples of recent chromatographic approaches to measuring a few of the more important drugs and poisons.

Paracetamol has been measured by GLC–FID as the acetylated derivative using a simple extractive derivatisation procedure which uses *N*-butyryl-*p*-aminophenol as a reactive internal standard (Huggett *et al.*, 1981). This is useful since confirmation of peak identity may be obtained either by performing the extraction without addition of the derivatisation reagent or by using a different acetylating agent such as butyric anhydride (Flanagan, 1983). This method for plasma paracetamol measurement has advantages of small sample requirement and enhanced selectivity and sensitivity when compared with the popular spectrophotometric method of Glynn and Kendal (1975). This is especially important in cases presenting many hours after ingestion of the drug where the diagnosis may depend upon accurate measurement of the residual plasma paracetamol concentration. The simultaneous HPLC assay of paracetamol and salicylate in plasma has been described by Widdop (1985).

Porter and Auansakul (1982) have described an improved method for the measurement of ethylene glycol (ethanediol) in plasma or serum. This is based on the reaction of phenylboronic acid with ethylene glycol to form a cyclic phenylboronate ester. This derivative is then analysed by GLC–FID using a 2-m column packed with 3 per cent OV-101 on Chromosorb W HP. Propane-1, 3-diol (trimethylene glycol) is used as a reactive internal standard. The phenylboronate derivative of propane-1, 2-diol (propylene glycol) is resolved from the derivatives of both ethylene glycol and the internal standard on this system. This is important, since propylene glycol may be a vehicle in certain intravenous preparations (Robinson *et al.*, 1983). However, studies in our laboratory have shown that the final reaction mixture used by Porter and Auansakul is a two-phase system and that markedly different peak heights and/or peak areas can be obtained upon replicate injection, depending on the phase composition of the portion obtained for GC analysis. This problem can be obviated and the whole method simplified by adding both the internal standard solution in acetonitrile (2 vols) and the phenylboronate reagent also in acetonitrile (2 vols) to the specimen (1 vol.). After vortex mixing (30 s) and centrifugation (9950*g*, 2 min), a portion (1 to 2 μl) of the supernatant may be taken for direct GLC analysis. It is very important to be aware of 'ghost' ethylene glycol peaks when using either method, however.

Although RIA for plasma paraquat (Table 2.3) provides good selectivity and sensitivity, a simple HPLC method has been developed which gives equivalent selectivity and sensitivity and can also measure diquat in the presence of paraquat (I. Jane, personal communication). The method is based on the oxidation of paraquat to a dipyridone using potassium ferricyanide. This is then extracted using chloroform–isopropanol (9 : 1, v/v) and analysed using a 15-cm ODS-modified 5-μm silica column with 0.8 $g\,l^{-1}$ ammonium nitrate in methanol-water (1 : 2 v/v) (pH 9) as eluent, together with fluorescence detection (excitation 335 nm, emission 435 nm). Ethyl paraquat is used as a reactive internal standard, and the retention volumes of the oxidation products of diquat, paraquat and ethylparaquat are approximately 5.5, 7 and 13 ml, respectively.

2.5 QUALITY ASSURANCE

In any analytical procedure it is important that all reasonable steps are taken to ensure the reliability of the results obtained. This is of special importance in clinical toxicology where the analyses may have a profound effect on patient care. Even apparently trivial omissions, such as failure to quote clearly the units used in the analysis, can have serious consequences, for example if the clinician wrongly assumes the result to be expressed in terms of mass rather than molar units, or vice versa.

The primary consideration in ensuring that the results of an analysis will serve their intended purpose is to use only those methods which have adequate scope, selectivity and sensitivity, and reliability. Moreover, the limitations of these methods should be fully understood and considered together with the clinical situation when interpreting the result obtained. In accord with this view, most drug detection and identification procedures developed in our laboratory have involved chromatographic methods and have been applied to plasma whenever possible, to obtain both qualitative and quantitative information simultaneously. In order to minimise analytical errors, simple extraction procedures are employed, with direct analysis of the resulting extract, and all qualitative measurements are performed relative to an internal standard. Solutions containing a number of known drugs are chromatographed either daily or with each specimen on each analytical system to ensure consistent performance, and quantitative standards are chromatographed in conjunction with all plasma concentration measurements. Quality-assurance sera for toxicological assays are available from several commercial sources. Unfortunately, the manufacturers tend to incorporate too many drugs into one sample such that resolution by routine chromatographic methods is difficult, if not impossible.

External quality-assurance schemes play an important role in monitoring the routine performance of established methods. In the UK only one scheme for toxicological assays other than those for certain metals is currently in regular operation, namely that for paracetamol, salicylate and barbiturates organised at the Regional Toxicology Laboratory at Dudley Road Hospital in Birmingham (Epton, 1979). In the near future these assays may also be incorporated into the National External Quality Assurance Scheme for clinical chemistry.

Qualitative proficiency testing programs for drugs of abuse have been established in the USA since 1964 (Guerrant and Hall, 1977) and participation is mandatory for all laboratories receiving government money for servicing the Drug Addict Rehabilitation Programs. State and interstate programs for quantitative toxicology have been described by Buhl *et al.* (1978) and Sohn (1977). In Europe a drugs-of-abuse quality-control scheme has been established by Professor Ferrara of the Institute of Legal Medicine, University of Padova, Italy. The most comprehensive and relevant scheme for clinical toxicology laboratories, however, is that devised in the Netherlands by Dijkhuis (1979). Samples are despatched together with a concise case-history. Participants are asked to carry out a search for (often unknown) substances, to quantitate these, to interpret the clinical significance of the results and to provide advice for patient treatment. Notwithstanding these efforts, it is fair to say that the general standard of performance in toxicology assays is low in many laboratories. This fact has been highlighted particularly in surveys where quality-assurance material has been inserted surreptitiously into several laboratories in the guise of authentic clinical samples. These surveys revealed alarming discrepancies in the drugs detected and in the results of quantitative assays (Pippenger *et al.*, 1976; Ingelfinger *et al.*, 1981). It is to be hoped that this situation will improve with the growing recognition that analytical toxicology can make an important contribution to medical care.

2.6 INTERPRETATION OF RESULTS

Factors such as individual tolerance, age, coingestion of other poisons and the presence of organic disease must always be considered when relating toxicological data to the patient's clinical condition. Nevertheless, for those drugs and poisons where the blood concentration bears a relationship to the clinical effect, useful interpretative guidelines can be formulated (Table 2.4). Other publications, notably those of Taylor *et al.* (1981), Baselt (1982), Osselton (1984) and Moffat (1984) contain additional information for many compounds.

CONCLUSION

Analytical toxicology is a complex discipline, and many of the exercises described in the foregoing pages are feasible only in specialised laboratories which are adequately equipped with modern instruments and trained personnel. These units can offer emergency coverage to numerous hospitals in a densely populated urban area where the rapid transport of samples presents no problems. Such laboratories are few and far between, however (at least in the UK), and the onus for providing local emergency toxicological services still rests largely on the clinical chemist. Fortunately, the list of drugs and poisons for which laboratory diagnosis has a direct bearing on the management of an acutely intoxicated patient is short (Table 2.5) and can be handled by a relatively small number of qualitative and quantitative tests.

Commercial kits based on colorimetric, enzymatic or immunochemical principles are now available for some of these poisons, but they vary in selectivity and reliability and the clinical chemist must be aware of their limitations in these respects. For example, a kit for serum paracetamol measurement based on the method of Glynn and Kendal (1975) produces spurious results in the presence of high concentrations of salicylate (Mace and Walker, 1976) and in samples contaminated with *o*-cresol (Pitts, 1979). This method is also insensitive to paracetamol concentrations below 50 mg l^{-1}. The enzymatic paracetamol assay kit (Cambridge Life Sciences, Cambridge, UK) is highly selective and produces quick and accurate results for plasma paracetamol concentrations down to at least 10 mg l^{-1} (Brown *et al.*, 1983).

The EMIT system for serum barbiturates (Syva, Palo Alto, California, USA) is only semi-quantitative and can only differentiate between short-acting barbiturates and phenobarbitone. Ultraviolet spectrophotometric methods for barbiturate drugs are also unselective although Walberg (1981) has described a procedure which differentiates phenobarbitone from shorter-acting barbiturates after quantitation. Chromatographic techniques (GLC and HPLC) are far superior since they can distinguish and measure these drugs and related hypnotics such as glutethimide simultaneously.

Ethanol can be measured conveniently and accurately in plasma by kits based on oxidation by alcohol dehydrogenase and estimation of reduced NAD production (Lundquist, 1959). Alternatively, a reasonable measure of blood ethanol concentration can be gained by using breath analysers which can be connected to unconscious patients via a nasal tube (Knepil and Fergie, 1980). A pocket-size battery-operated version (Alcolmeter, S-D2, Lion Laboratories Ltd, Cardiff, UK) is particularly suited to this purpose. The instrument detects all primary and secondary alcohols and there is no interference from other volatile substances such as ketones and esters. Ideally, the clinical chemist should perform this test, although it is feasible to devolve the duty to medical and nursing personnel provided they are given adequate training and the laboratory retains overall control of the calibration and maintenance of the equipment.

Clinical chemistry laboratories involved in therapeutic drug monitoring will already have immunoassay systems available for theophylline estimation and it is a simple matter to adapt these for a stat overdose assay. Reliable commercial kits for serum iron estimation have been around for many years. The colorimetric method of Trinder (1954) is still the method of choice for plasma sali-

Table 2.4 Guide to the interpretation of the results of toxicological analyses (analytes measured in plasma unless otherwise stated)

Substance		'Therapeutic' or normal concentrations (less than)	Concentrations associated with serious toxicity
acetaminophen (paracetamol)		20 mg l^{-1} (0.13 mmol l^{-1})	200 mg l^{-1} (1. 32 mmol l^{-1}) (4 h post-ingestion) 70 mg l^{-1} (0.46 mmol l^{-1}) (10 h post-ingestion)
acetylsalicylic acid (as salicylates)		250 mg l^{-1} (1.8 mmol l^{-1})	900 mg l^{-1} (6.5 mmol l^{-1}) (6 h post-ingestion) 450 mg l^{-1} (3.2 mmol l^{-1}) (24 h post-ingestion)
alprenolol		0.2 mg l^{-1}	40 mg l^{-1}
aluminium		15 μg l^{-1}	200 μg l^{-1}
amiodarone		2 mg l^{-1}	not known
amitriptyline (+ nortriptyline)		0.2 mg l^{-1}	1 mg l^{-1}
amylobarbitone		5 mg l^{-1}	40 mg l^{-1}
amoxapine		0.2 mg l^{-1}	5 mg l^{-1}
amphetamine		0.1 mg l^{-1}	0.5 mg l^{-1}
arsenic	blood	30 μg l^{-1}	50 μg l^{-1}
	serum/plasma	20 μg l^{-1}	50 μg l^{-1}
	urine	40 μg l^{-1}	200 μg l^{-1}
	hair and nail	1 μg g^{-1}	2 μg g^{-1}
atenolol		0.5 mg l^{-1}	2.5 mg l^{-1}
azapropazone		50 mg l^{-1}	not known
barbitone		15 mg l^{-1}	100 mg l^{-1}
bromazepam		0.15 mg l^{-1}	not known

butobarbitone		10 mg l^{-1}	80 mg l^{-1}
butriptyline (+ norbutriptyline)		0.2 mg l^{-1}	1 mg l^{-1}
cadmium	blood	5 μg l^{-1}	20 μg l^{-1}
	urine	5 μg l^{-1}	20 μg l^{-1}
caffeine		15 mg l^{-1}	60 mg l^{-1}
camphor		–	1 mg l^{-1}
carbamazepine		10 mg l^{-1}	50 mg l^{-1}
carbon monoxide (carboxyhaemoglobin)		5% (smokers)	30%
chloral hydrate (as trichloroethanol)		10 mg l^{-1}	80 ml l^{-1}
chloramphenicol		20 mg l^{-1}	40 mg l^{-1}
chlordiazepoxide (+ norchlordiazepoxide)		2 mg l^{-1}	10 mg l^{-1}
chlormethiazole		2 mg l^{-1}	20 mg l^{-1}
chlormezanone		8 mg l^{-1}	50 mg l^{-1}
chloroquine		0.4 mg l^{-1}	1 mg l^{-1}
chlorpromazine		0.1 mg l^{-1}	1 mg l^{-1}
clobazam (+ norclobazam)		2 mg l^{-1}	10 mg l^{-1}
clomipramine (+ norclomipramine)		0.5 mg l^{-1}	1 mg l^{-1}
clonazepam		0.05 mg l^{-1}	1 mg l^{-1}
clonidine		1 μg l^{-1}	10 μg l^{-1}
clorazepate dipotassium (as nordiazepam)		2 mg l^{-1}	5 mg l^{-1}

Table 2.4 (continued)

Substance		'Therapeutic' or normal concentrations (less than)	Concentrations associated with serious toxicity
cocaine		0.3 mg l^{-1}	3 mg l^{-1}
codeine		0.1 mg l^{-1}	1 mg l^{-1}
cyanide	blood	0.04 mg l^{-1}	1 mg l^{-1}
cyclobarbitone		5 mg l^{-1}	40 mg l^{-1}
desalkylflurazepam (from flurazepam)		0.2 mg l^{-1}	2 mg l^{-1}
desipramine		0.2 mg l^{-1}	1 mg l^{-1}
dextropropoxyphene		0.3 mg l^{-1}	1 mg l^{-1}
diazepam (+ nordiazepam)		2.5 mg l^{-1}	10 mg l^{-1}
diflunisal		150 mg l^{-1}	500 mg l^{-1}
digoxin		2 μg l^{-1}	4 μg l^{-1}
dihydrocodeine		0.1 mg l^{-1}	1 mg l^{-1}
dinitro-ortho-cresol (DNOC)		–	50 mg l^{-1}
diphenhydramine		0.5 mg l^{-1}	5 mg l^{-1}
diquat		–	0.4 mg l^{-1}
disopyramide		3 mg l^{-1}	8 mg l^{-1}
dothiepin (+ nordothiepin)		0.3 mg l^{-1}	1 mg l^{-1}
doxepin (+ nordoxepin)		0.3 mg l^{-1}	1 mg l^{-1}
ethchlorvynol		20 mg l^{-1}	100 mg l^{-1}
ethosuximide		80 mg l^{-1}	250 mg l^{-1}

ethyl alcohol (ethanol)		0.8 g l^{-1} (legal driving limit in blood in UK)	3.0 g l^{-1}
ethylene glycol		–	0.5 g l^{-1}
fenfluramine		0.2 mg l^{-1}	0.5 mg l^{-1}
flecainide		0.8 mg l^{-1}	not known
flunitrazepam		0.05 mg l^{-1}	1 mg l^{-1}
fluoride		0.1 mg l^{-1}	2.5 mg l^{-1}
flurazepam		0.02 mg l^{-1}	1 mg l^{-1}
gentamicin		12 mg l^{-1}	20 mg l^{-1}
glutethimide		4 mg l^{-1}	30 mg l^{-1}
haloperidol		0.1 mg l^{-1}	0.5 mg l^{-1}
heptabarbitone		5 mg l^{-1}	40 mg l^{-1}
hexobarbitone		5 mg l^{-1}	40 mg l^{-1}
heroin (as morphine, including conjugated)		0.05 mg l^{-1}	0.3 mg l^{-1}
ibuprofen		50 mg l^{-1}	0.5 g l^{-1}
imipramine (+ desipramine)		0.3 mg l^{-1}	1 mg l^{-1}
indomethacin		5 mg l^{-1}	not known
iron children:		1.8 mg l^{-1} (34 μmol l^{-1})	5.0 mg l^{-1} (90 μmol l^{-1})
adults:		1.8 mg l^{-1} (34 μmol l^{-1})	8.0 mg l^{-1} (145 μmol l^{-1})
isoniazid		20 mg l^{-1}	50 mg l^{-1}
isopropyl alcohol (isopropanol)		–	1.5 g l^{-1}
lead children:	blood	250 μg l^{-1} (1.2 μmol l^{-1})	600 μg l^{-1} (2.9 μmol l^{-1})
adults:	blood	300 μg l^{-1} (1.5 μmol l^{-1})	800 μg l^{-1} (3.8 μmol l^{-1})

Table 2.4 (continued)

Substance		'Therapeutic' or normal concentrations (less than)	Concentrations associated with serious toxicity
lignocaine (lidocaine)		5 mg l^{-1}	8 mg l^{-1}
lithium		1.3 mmol l^{-1}	3 mmol l^{-1}
lorazepam		0.2 mg l^{-1}	2 mg l^{-1}
magnesium		2.3 mmol l^{-1}	5 mmol l^{-1}
maprotiline		0.3 mg l^{-1}	0.5 mg l^{-1}
medazepam (+ diazepam and nordiazepam)		2 mg l^{-1}	10 mg l^{-1}
mefenamic acid		10 mg l^{-1}	25 mg l^{-1}
meperidine (pethidine)		0.5 mg l^{-1}	2 mg l^{-1}
meprobamate		10 mg l^{-1}	100 mg l^{-1}
mercury	blood	10 μg l^{-1}	40 μg l^{-1}
	urine	10 μg l^{-1}	100 μg l^{-1}
methadone		1 mg l^{-1} (maintenance therapy)	0.4 mg l^{-1} (single overdose)
methaqualone		4 mg l^{-1}	20 mg l^{-1}
methohexitone		5 mg l^{-1}	20 mg l^{-1}
methyl alcohol (methanol)		–	200 mg l^{-1}
methylamphetamine		0.05 mg l^{-1}	0.3 mg l^{-1}
methylphenidate		0.1 mg l^{-1}	0.5 mg l^{-1}
methyprylone		10 mg l^{-1}	30 mg l^{-1}
metoprolol		0.5 mg l^{-1}	10 mg l^{-1}
mexiletine		1.5 mg l^{-1}	4 mg l^{-1}

mianserin (+ normianserin)	0.1 mg l^{-1}	0.5 mg l^{-1}
morphine (including conjugated)	0.05 mg l^{-1}	0.3 mg l^{-1}
naproxen	100 mg l^{-1}	not known
nitrazepam	0.2 mg l^{-1}	2 mg l^{-1}
nomifensine (total hydrolysed)	4 mg l^{-1}	not known
nordiazepam	2 mg l^{-1}	5 mg l^{-1}
nortriptyline	0.15 mg l^{-1}	1 mg l^{-1}
orphenadrine	0.2 mg l^{-1}	2 mg l^{-1}
oxazepam	1 mg l^{-1}	5 mg l^{-1}
oxprenolol	0.2 mg l^{-1}	2 mg l^{-1}
oxyphenylbutazone	100 mg l^{-1}	200 mg l^{-1}
paracetamol	20 mg l^{-1} (0.13 mmol l^{-1})	200 mg l^{-1} (1.32 mmol l^{-1}) (4 h post-ingestion) 70 mg l^{-1} (0.46 mmol l^{-1}) (10 h post-ingestion)
paraquat	–	0.5 mg l^{-1} (6 h post-ingestion) 0.25 mg l^{-1} (12 h post-ingestion)
pentazocine	0.2 mg l^{-1}	1 mg l^{-1}
pentobarbitone	5 mg l^{-1}	40 mg l^{-1}
pethidine	0.5 mg l^{-1}	2 mg l^{-1}
phencyclidine	–	0.3 mg l^{-1}
phenobarbitone	30 mg l^{-1}	100 mg l^{-1}
phenol	0.1 mg l^{-1} (conjugated)	50 mg l^{-1}

Table 2.4 (continued)

Substance	'Therapeutic' or normal concentrations (less than)	Concentration associated with serious toxicity
phenylbutazone	100 mg l^{-1}	200 mg l^{-1}
phenylpropanolamine	0.1 mg l^{-1}	2 mg l^{-1}
phenytoin	20 mg l^{-1}	40 mg l^{-1}
prazepam (as nordiazepam)	2 mg l^{-1}	5 mg l^{-1}
primidone (phenobarbitone should be measured in addition)	12 mg l^{-1}	50 mg l^{-1}
procainamide	8 mg l^{-1}	16 mg l^{-1}
procyclidine	1 mg l^{-1}	2 mg l^{-1}
propoxyphene (dextropropoxyphene)	0.3 mg l^{-1}	1 mg l^{-1}
propranolol	0.1 mg l^{-1}	2 mg l^{-1}
protriptyline	0.2 mg l^{-1}	1 mg l^{-1}
quinalbarbitone	5 mg l^{-1}	30 mg l^{-1}
quinidine	5 mg l^{-1}	10 mg l^{-1}
quinine	10 mg l^{-1}	15 mg l^{-1}
salicylates	250 mg l^{-1} (1.8 mmol l^{-1})	900 mg l^{-1} (6.5 mmol l^{-1}) (6 h post-ingestion) 450 mg l^{-1} (3.2 mmol l^{-1}) (24 h post-ingestion)

sodium valproate (valproic acid)		80 mg l^{-1}	not known
sulthiame		12 mg l^{-1}	30 mg l^{-1}
temazepam		1 mg l^{-1}	5 mg l^{-1}
thallium	blood urine	10 μg l^{-1} 10 μg l^{-1}	100 μg l^{-1} 500 μg l^{-1}
theophylline		20 mg l^{-1}	40 mg l^{-1}
thioridazine		1 mg l^{-1}	5 mg l^{-1}
tocainide		10 mg l^{-1}	not known
toluene		–	5 mg l^{-1} (acute exposure)
triazolam		0.1 mg l^{-1}	not known
trichloroethanol (from chloral or trichloroethylene)		10 mg l^{-1}	80 mg l^{-1}
trimipramine (+ nortrimipramine)		0.3 mg l^{-1}	1 mg l^{-1}
verapamil		0.25 mg l^{-1}	4 mg l^{-1}
valproic acid		80 mg l^{-1}	not known

Table 2.5 Assays which may be required urgently in cases of severe acute poisoning

Drug or poison	Implications in management
paracetamol	antidotal therapy with oral methionine or i.v. *N*-acetyl cysteine (possibly active elimination therapy in very severe/late cases)
barbiturates	active elimination therapy
glutethimide	active elimination therapy
theophylline	active elimination therapy
ethanol	differential diagnosis (e.g. in presence of head injury); active elimination therapy
iron	antidotal therapy with i.v. desferrioxamine
salicylate	active elimination therapy
paraquat	oral adsorbents; active elimination therapy
methanol	antidotal therapy with i.v. ethanol; active elimination therapy
ethylene glycol	antidotal therapy with i.v. ethanol; active elimination therapy
quinine	minimise ocular damage (e.g. by stellate ganglion block); active elimination therapy
lithium	active elimination therapy

cylate assay (although interference from endogenous ketones should be guarded against) and serum lithium is easily measured by atomic emission flame photometry (Fry, 1981). Plasma paraquat assays are complicated and samples should be referred to a specialised laboratory. However, the detection of paraquat in urine is extremely simple and the test reagents can be packed into gelatine capsules which are viable for at least six months (Widdop, 1976). Poisoning with methanol or ethylene glycol should always be considered in patients who present with a severe increased anion-gap metabolic acidosis. A raised plasma osmolality reading is a further indication, but definitive diagnosis is reached by the detection and measurement of these substances in the blood. Methanol assay by gas chromatography should pose few problems in a modern clinical chemistry laboratory and has the great advantage of detecting ethanol and other primary and secondary alcohols at the same time. A gas-chromatographic method for ethylene glycol has been referred to in section 2.4.3.

A more comprehensive search for drugs and poisons is no longer beyond the capabilities of the clinical chemist, who now has access to standardised TLC systems such as Toxi-Lab and a wide range of immunological assays in addition to the classical 'spot' tests. However, if the frequency of screening requests is low it makes sense, not least from an economic point of view, to refer these directly to the nearest specialised toxicology laboratory. Here a whole battery of techniques, including GLC and HPLC, can be brought to bear immediately and many compounds can be identified and measured in the blood within one or two hours (Widdop, 1982). For hospitals based on outlying rural areas, however, especially in countries with under-developed transport systems, this is impracticable. It is in these isolated laboratories, therefore, that the new simple diagnostic tests, immunological and otherwise, will have most impact.

REFERENCES

Ambre, J. J., and Fischer, J. L. (1974). Identification and activity of the hydroxy metabolite that accumulates in the plasma of humans intoxicated with glutethimide. *Drug Metab. Dispos.* **2**, 151–8.

Anderson, H. R., Dick, B., Palmer, J. C., and Ramsey, J. D. (1982). Deaths associated with the abuse of volatile substances: an investigation of 140 deaths in the United Kingdom 1971–81. *Human Toxicol.* **1**, 207–21.

Ardrey, R. E., and Moffat, A. C. (1981). Gas–liquid chromatographic retention indices of 1318 substances of toxicological interest on SE-30 or OV-1 stationary phase. *J. Chromatogr.* **220**, 195–252.

Baselt, R. C. (1982). *Disposition of Toxic Drugs and Chemicals in Man*, 2nd edn. Biomedical Publications, Davis, California.

Berry, D. J., and Grove, J. (1973). Emergency toxicological screening for drugs commonly taken in overdose. *J. Chromatogr.* **80**, 205–19.

Blacklock, E. C., and Sadler, P. A. (1981). A rapid screening method for heavy metals in biological fluids by emission spectroscopy. *Clin. Chim. Acta* **113**, 89–94.

Blackmore, D. J. (1970). The determination of carbon monoxide in blood and tissue. *Analyst* **95**, 439–58.

Brown, S. S., Campbell, R. S., Price, C. P., Rambohul, E., Widdop, B., Barbour, H. M., Roberts, J. G., Burnett, D., Atkinson, T., Scawen, M. D., and Hammond, P. M. (1983). Collaborative trial of an enzyme-based assay for the determination of paracetamol in plasma. *Ann. Clin. Biochem.* **20**, 353–9.

Buhl, S. N., Kowalski, P., and Vanderlinde, R. E. (1978). Quantitative toxicology. Interlaboratory and Intermethod Evaluation in New York State. *Clin Chem.* **24**, 442–7.

Canalese, J., Gimson, A. E. S., Davis, M., and Williams, R. (1981). Factors contributing to mortality in paracetamol-induced hepatic failure. *Br. Med. J.* **282**, 199–201.

Conard, P. P., Parker, N. C., Cross, R. E., and Wojcieszyn, O. A. (1981). Adaptation of drug enzyme immunoassays to a micro centrifugal analyser. *Clin. Chem.* **27**, 1090.

Conference of Medical Royal Colleges (1976). Diagnosis of brain death. *Br. Med. J.* **2**, 1187–8.

De Wolff, F. A., Edelbroek, P. M., de Haas, E. J. M., and Vermeij, P. (1983). Experience with a screening method for laxative abuse. *Human Toxicol.* **2**, 385–9.

Dijkhuis, I. C. (1979). *Quality Control of Drug Assays in Therapy and Toxicology*. PhD thesis, University of Leiden, The Netherlands.

Epton, J. (1979). Paracetamol: a report of a regional quality control scheme. *Ann. Clin. Biochem.* **16**, 265–70.

Flanagan, R. J. (1983). *Development and Application of Simple Micro-analytical Techniques in Clinical Toxicology*, PhD thesis, University of London.

Flanagan, R. J., Huggett, A., Saynor, D. A., Raper, S. M., and Volans, G. N. (1981). Value of toxicological investigations in the diagnosis of acute drug poisoning in children. *Lancet* **ii**, 682–5.

Flanagan, R. J., Storey, G. C. A., Bhamra, R. K., and Jane, I. (1982). High performance liquid chromatographic analysis of basic drugs on silica columns using non-aqueous ionic eluents. *J. Chromatogr.* **247**, 15–37.

Franke, J. P., Schepers, P., Bosman, J., and de Zeeuw, R. A. (1982). Optimization of thin-layer chromatography for toxicological screening: Applicability of shorter development distances. *J. Analyt. Toxicol.* **6**, 131–4 (see also correction in 7 (1983), 62).

Fry, D. (1981). Lithium–analytical techniques. In Richens, A., and Marks, V. (eds). *Therapeutic Drug Monitoring*. Churchill Livingstone, Edinburgh, pp. 217.

Fysh, R. R., and Jones, L. V. (1980). The screening of pesticides in forensic toxicology. In Oliver, J. S. (ed.), *Forensic Toxicology*. Croom Helm, London. pp. 189–203.

Glynn, J. P., and Kendal, S. E. (1975). Paracetamol measurement. *Lancet* **i**, 1147–8.

Guerrant, G. O., and Hall, C. T. (1977). Drug Abuse Proficiency Testing. *Clin. Toxicol.* **10**, 209–219.

Hamlyn, A. N., Brown, A. J., Sherlock, S., and Baron, D. N. (1975). Casual blood-ethanol estimations in patients with chronic liver disease. *Lancet* **ii**, 345–7.

Helliwell, M., and Berry, D. (1979). Theophylline poisoning in adults. *Br. Med. J.* **2**, 1114.

Helliwell, M., Hampel, G., Sinclair, E., Huggett, A., and Flanagan, R. J. (1979). Value of emergency toxicological investigations in differential diagnosis of coma. *Br. Med. J.* **2**, 819–21.

Huggett, A., Andrews, P., and Flanagan, R. J. (1981). Rapid micro-method for the measurement of paracetamol in blood plasma or serum using gas–liquid chromatography with flame-ionisation detection. *J. Chromatogr.* **209**, 67–76.

Idowu, O. R., and Caddy, B. (1982). A review of the use of saliva in the forensic detection of drugs and other chemicals. *J. Forens. Sci. Soc.* **22**, 123–35.

Ingelfinger, J. A., Isakson, G., Shine, D., Costello, C. E. and Goldman, P. (1981). Reliability of the toxic screen in drug overdose. *Clin. Pharmacol. Ther.* **29**, 570–75.

Jarvie, D. R., and Stewart, M. J. (1979). The rapid extraction of paraquat from plasma using an ion-pairing technique. *Clin. Chim. Acta.* **94**, 241–51.

Jick, H. (1977). The discovery of drug-induced illness. *N. Engl. J. Med.* **296**, 481–5.

King, M. D., Day, R. E., Oliver, J. S., Lush, M., and Watson, J. M. (1981). Solvent encephalopathy. *Br. Med. J.* **283**, 663–5.

Knepil, J., and Fergie, R. (1980). The fuel cell measurement of blood alcohol. In Oliver, J. S. (ed.), *Forensic Toxicology*. Croom Helm, London, pp. 95–103.

Lancet Editorial (1981). Carbon monoxide, an old enemy forgot. *Lancet* **ii**, 75–6.

Levitt, T. (1979). Determination of paraquat in clinical practice using radioimmunoassay. *Proc. Anal. Div. Chem. Soc.* **16**, 72–6.

Lorber, J., Reckless, J. P. D., and Watson, J. B. G. (1980). Non-accidental poisoning: the elusive diagnosis. *Arch. Dis. Childh.* **55**, 643–7.

Lundquist, F. (1959). Ethyl alcohol in blood and tissues. In Glick, D. (ed.), *Methods of Biochemical Analysis*. Interscience, New York, vol. 7, p. 217.

Mace, P. K. K., and Walker, G. (1976). Salicylate interference with plasma-paracetamol method. *Lancet* **ii**, 1362.

Maehly, A. C. (1967). Volatile toxic compounds. In Stolman, A. (ed.), *Progress in Chemical Toxicology*. Academic Press, London, pp. 63–98.

Marks, V. (1979). Clinical monitoring of therapeutic drugs. *Ann. Clin. Biochem* **16**, 370–9.

Meade, B. W., Widdop, B., Blackmore, D. J., Brown, S. S. Curry, A. S., Goulding, R., Higgins, G., Matthew, H. J. S., and Rinsler, M. G. (1972). Simple tests to detect poisons. *Ann. Clin. Biochem.* **9**, 35–46.

Meredith, T. J., and Vale, J. A. (1981). Antidotes. In Vale, J. A., and Meredith, T. J. (eds), *Poisoning: Diagnosis and Treatment*. Update Books, London, pp. 33–45.

Michand, J. D., and Jones, D. W. (1980). Thin-layer chromatography for broad spectrum drug detection. *Amer. Lab.* **12**, 104.

Moffat, A. C. (ed.) (1985). *Clarke's Isolation and Identification of Drugs*, 2nd edn. Pharmaceutical Press, London.

Myers, R. E., and Myers, S. E. (1979). Use of sedative, analgesic and anesthetic drugs during labour and delivery: Bane or boon? *Amer. J. Obstet. Gynecol.* **133**, 83–104.

O'Reilly, R. A., and Aggeler, P. M. (1976). Covert anticoagulant ingestion: study of 25 patients and review of world literature. *Medicine* **55**, 389–99.

Osselton, M. D. (1983). Toxicological tables: A compendium of pharmacological, therapeutic and toxicological data on 136 drugs and chemicals in humans. In Sunshine, I.

(ed.), *Methodology for Analytical Toxicology*, Vol. III. CRC Press, Boca Raton.

Parkinson, I. S., Ward, M. K., and Kerr, D. N. S. (1981). Dialysis encephalopathy, bone disease and anaemia: the aluminium syndrome during regular haemodialysis. *J. Clin. Pathol.*, **34**, 1285–94.

Pippenger, C. E., Penry, J. K., White, B. G., Daly, D. D., and Buddington, R. (1976). Interlaboratory variability in determination of plasma antiepileptic drug concentrations. *Arch. Neurol.* **33**, 351–5.

Pitts, J. (1979). False-positive paracetamol assay. *Lancet* **i**, 213–4.

Porter, W. H., and Auansakul, A. (1982). Gas-chromatographic determination of ethylene glycol in serum. *Clin. Chem.* **28**, 75–8.

Prescott, L. F. (1978). Prevention of hepatic necrosis following paracetamol overdosage. *Hlth Bull.* **36**, 204–12.

Proudfoot, A. T., and Park, J. (1978). Changing pattern of drugs used in self-poisoning. *Br. Med. J.* **1**, 90–93.

Proudfoot, A. T., Stewart, M. J., Levitt, T., and Widdop, B. (1979). Paraquat poisoning: significance of plasma paraquat concentrations. *Lancet* **ii**, 330–32.

Ramsey, J. D., and Flanagan, R. J. (1982). Detection and identification of volatile organic compounds in blood by headspace gas-chromatography as an aid to the diagnosis of solvent abuse. *J. Chromatogr.* **240**, 423–44.

Ramsey, J. D., Lee, T. D. Osselton, M. D., and Moffat, A. C. (1980). Gas liquid chromatographic retention indices of 296 non-drug substances on SE-30 or OV-1 likely to be encountered in toxicological analyses. *J. Chromatogr.* **184**, 185–206.

Raper, S., Crome, P., Vale, J. A., Helliwell, M., and Widdop, B. (1982). Experience with activated carbon-bead haemoperfusion columns in the treatment of severe drug intoxication: a preliminary report. *Arch. Toxicol.* **49**, 303–310.

Ratcliffe, W. A., Fletcher, S. M., Moffat, A. C., Ratcliffe, J. G., Harland, W. A., and Levitt, T. E. (1977). Radioimmunoassay of lysergic acid diethylamide (LSD) in serum and urine by using antisera of different specificities. *Clin. Chem.* **23**, 169–74.

Robinson, C. A., Scott, J. W., and Ketchum, C. (1983). Propylene glycol interference with ethylene glycol procedures. *Clin. Chem.* **29**, 727.

Rogers, D., Tripp, J., Bentovim, A., Robinson, A., Berry, D., and Goulding, R. (1976). Non-accidental poisoning: an extended syndrome of child abuse. *Br. Med. J.* **1**, 793–6.

Rutterford, M. G., and Smith, R. N. (1980). Radioimmunoassay of diazepam in samples of forensic interest. *J. Pharm. Pharmacol.* **32**, 449–52.

Schepers, P., Wijsbeek, J., Franke, J. P., and de Zeeuw, R. A. (1982). Applicability of capillary gas-chromatography to substance identification in toxicology by means of retention indices. *J. Forens. Sci.* **27**, 49–60.

Sohn, D. (1977). The College of American Pathologists Toxicology Program. *J. Analyt. Toxicol.* **1**, 111–7.

Stead, A. H., Gill, R., Wright, T., Gibbs, J. P., and Moffat, A. C. (1982). Standardised thin-layer chromatographic systems for the identification of drugs and poisons. *Analyst (Lond.)* **107**, 1106–68.

Stewart, M. J., Adriaenssens, P. I., Jarvie, D. R., and Prescott, L. F. (1979). Inappropriate methods for the emergency determination of plasma paracetamol. *Ann. Clin. Biochem.* **16**, 89–95.

Sutheimer, C., Hepler, B. R. and Sunshine, I. (1982). Clinical application and evaluation of the EMIT-St TM drug detection system. *Amer. J. Clin. Pathol.* **77**, 731–5.

Taylor, W. T., Finn, A. L., and Gotcher, S. (eds) (1981). *Individualizing Drug Therapy: Clinical Notes on the Application of Drug Monitoring*. Gross, Townsend, Frank; New York (available from Syva).

Teale, J. D., Forman, E. J., King, L. J., and Marks, V. (1974). Radioimmunoassay of cannabinoids in blood and urine. *Lancet* **ii**, 553–5.

Thompson, N., and Henry, J. A. (1983). Carbon monoxide poisoning: Poisons Unit experience over five years. *Human Toxicol.* **2**, 335–8.

Trinder, P. (1954). Rapid determination of salicylate in biological fluids. *Biochem. J.* **57**, 301–3.

Vale, J. A., and Meredith, T. J. (1981). Epidemiology of poisoning in the U.K. In Vale, J. A., and Meredith, T. J. (eds), *Poisoning: Diagnosis and Treatment*. Update Books, London, pp. 1–8.

Vale, J. A., Prior, J. G., O'Hare, J. P., Flanagan, R. J., and Feehally, J. (1982). Treatment of ethylene glycol poisoning with peritoneal dialysis. *Br. Med. J.* **284**, 557.

Vanzeiti, G., Cassani, M., and Valente, D. (1983). Detection of morphine in urine by hemagglutination inhibition, with use of lyophilised reagents. *Clin. Chem.* **29**, 1376–9.

Walberg, C. B. (1981). An ultraviolet spectrophotometric procedure for differentiation and quantitation of barbiturates. *Clin. Toxicol.* **18**, 879–86.

Wheals, B. B. (1980). Isocratic multi-column high performance liquid chromatography as a technique for qualitative analysis and its application to the characterisation of basic drugs using an aqueous methanol solvent. *J. Chromatogr.* **187**, 65–85.

Widdop, B. (1974). Drug analysis in the overdosed patient. In *The Poisoned Patient: The Role of the Laboratory*. Ciba Foundation Symposium 26 (New Series), Associated Scientific Publishers, Amsterdam, pp. 219–38.

Widdop, B. (1976). Detection of paraquat in urine. *Br. Med. J.* **2**, 1135.

Widdop, B. (1980). Screening for drugs of abuse: application of Tox-Elut columns. In A. Kovatsis (ed.), *Toxicological Aspects (Proceedings of the 9th International Congress of the European Association of Poison Control Centres)*. Thessalonika, pp. 231–9.

Widdop, B. (1982). In Kaiser, E. *et al.* (eds), *Applications of Toxicological Analyses in the Diagnosis and Management of Poisoning*. XIth International Congress of Clinical Chemistry. de Gruyter, Berlin and New York, pp. 911–9.

Widdop, B. (1985). Hospital Toxicology. In Moffat, A. C. (ed.), *Clarke's Isolation and Identification of Drugs*, 2nd edn. Pharmaceutical Press, London.

Wilson, J. T., Brown, R. D., Cherek, D. R., Dailey, J. W., Hilman, B., Jobe, P. C., Manno, B. R., Manno, J. E., Redetzki, H. M., and Stewart, J. J. (1980). Drug excretion in human breast milk: Principles, pharmacokinetics and projected consequences. *Clin. Pharmacokinet.* **5**, 1–66.

3
Radioreceptor assays in toxicology

R. F. METCALFE

3.1 INTRODUCTION

Neurotransmitters and many other hormones have long been known to produce their physiological effects by binding to specific receptor proteins on cell surface membranes. More recently, many drugs and toxic compounds have been shown to act both selectively and competitively at these same specific receptor sites. However, it is only with the demonstration of specific receptors in tissues for a wide range of drug classes, with the concomitant stimulation of commercial production of appropriate radioligands of high specific activity, that radioreceptor assays have become possible. Thus the existence of specific receptors for opiate analgesics such as morphine was reported (Pert and Snyder, 1973) before the endogenous peptide transmitters at these sites had been discovered. More recently a specific receptor for benzodiazepines has been reported (Möhler and Okada, 1977; Squires and Braestrup, 1977).

To date, radioreceptor assays have found most application in the monitoring of plasma levels of drugs in clinical pharmacology both so as to optimise therapy and in pharmacokinetic studies. The major advantage of the radioreceptor assay over other assay techniques is that it is capable of measuring the 'total pharmacological activity' of the sample, which may include active metabolites, both known and unknown, as well as the parent-drug molecule. In addition, radioreceptor assays are relatively simple, sensitive and rapid compared with techniques such as gas–liquid chromatography, fluorimetry and radioimmunoassay, which often require extensive technical expertise and usually have to be developed for each individual drug (and metabolite).

3.1.1 Principle of the method

The radioreceptor assay is based on the competitive displacement by an unlabelled drug of a labelled compound which binds with high affinity to a specific receptor protein site. Thus, the radioreceptor assay is analogous to a radioimmunoassay except that ligand binding takes place with a receptor rather than with an antibody. In this lies both the strength and the weakness of the radioreceptor assay, in that receptor proteins typically possess greater pharmacological specificity than antibody proteins, but less chemical specificity.

3.2 METHODS

The basic requirements for a radioreceptor assay are:

1. the sample:
2. a receptor preparation;
3. an appropriate radioligand;
4. a system for separating bound from free ligand;
5. a scintillation spectrometer for counting the bound radiolabel.

3.2.1 Sample preparation

Radioreceptor assays are usually applied to body fluid samples, especially plasma or serum. In many cases, extraction of the drug from biological fluid is not necessary. However, in some cases, the binding of the radioligand to receptors is inhibited by drug-free plasma alone. This has been shown, for instance, for the binding of [^{125}I]hydroxybenzylpindolol and [^{3}H]dihydroalprenolol to β-adrenergic receptors (Bilezikian *et al.*, 1979; Innis *et al.*, 1978), and for the binding of [^{3}H]buprenorphine to opiate receptors (Villiger *et al.*, 1981). Such inhibition appears to be due to binding of radioligand to plasma proteins. The problem may be overcome by subjecting the plasma sample to dialysis or ultrafiltration, or by using standard extraction procedures, where the selection of the appropriate pH and solvent will depend upon the pK_a, the partition coefficient, and the acid–base lability of the drug. Diethyl ether extraction of plasma made basic with ammonium hydroxide solution has been used successfully for a range of basic drugs (Kelly *et al.*, 1981; Villiger *et al.*, 1981). Alternatively, plasma proteins may be precipitated with alcohol and a portion of the supernatant evaporated to dryness in the assay tube under a stream of warm nitrogen. This latter procedure may be preferable for compounds which are acid- or base-labile.

Where plasma proteins do interfere with radioligand binding it may still be possible, especially in toxicological studies, to use unextracted plasma samples.

This is almost certainly the case when volumes of 10 μl plasma or less are sufficient for accurate assay. For such small volumes, blood obtained by fingertip puncture may well be satisfactory and is particularly convenient when dealing with infants.

Analysis of urine samples may be carried out directly (Lund, 1981) or after enzymic hydrolysis of any glucuronide or sulphate conjugates.

Drugs in tissue Conventional procedures may be used to extract drugs from tissues. For compounds that are water-soluble, simple homogenisation of the tissue in water followed by ultracentrifugation may be all that is required. However, for compounds that are tightly bound to tissues more rigorous extraction methods will be required. This may include enzymic digestion of the tissue sample with subtilisin (Osselton *et al.*, 1977). When dealing with samples derived from tissue it is important to be aware of the possibility of interference from endogenous compounds such as neurotransmitters.

3.2.2 Receptor preparation

The receptor preparation usually consists of a crude membrane suspension from a tissue that possesses the desired receptor at an adequate concentration. There is no requirement for the receptor to be purified or solubilised. Indeed for most radioreceptor assays it is advantageous to have the receptor in a membrane-bound form. Also, as specificity is provided by the radioligand, there is no necessity to try to isolate a particular receptor type. Mammalian brain tissue is a rich source for a diverse collection of membrane receptors, including muscarinic, dopaminergic, adrenergic, GABA-ergic, opiate, benzodiazepine and imipramine, and for this reason brain tissue is commonly chosen for the receptor preparation in radioreceptor assays.

Brain material from small laboratory animals, e.g. rat or guinea-pig, may be used as a receptor source, or, as most brain receptors appear to be stable on storage at −20 °C, it may be preferable to use bovine or porcine tissue. The latter has been used by the present author, and has been found to maintain muscarinic-receptor binding activity for at least two years when stored at −20 °C. A further advantage of using brain from calf or pig is that a specific area which has a high density of a particular receptor may be dissected out more easily. The caudate nucleus is especially rich, for example, in dopaminergic receptors and is therefore useful in radioreceptor assays for neuroleptics. The cerebellum on the other hand is relatively rich in β-adrenergic receptors and is therefore useful in radioreceptor assays for β-blocking drugs.

For most radioreceptor assays, however, a receptor preparation from whole brain minus cerebellum will suffice. Brain tissue (10 to 20 g) is homogenised in ice-cold, 0.32M sucrose using a motor-driven teflon pestle in a glass homogeniser to yield a 20 per cent homogenate. This homogenate is then diluted 1 : 1 with

0.32M sucrose and centrifuged at 4° for 10 min at $1000g_{av}$. The pellet is discarded and the supernatant centrifuged at $30\,000g_{av}$ for 30 min. This second pellet is resuspended in either 50 mmol l^{-1} sodium phosphate buffer, pH 7.4, or 50 mmol l^{-1} tris-HCl buffer, pH 7.4, and the suspension centrifuged at 30 000 *g* for 30 min. The crude mitochondrial pellets, containing synaptosomes, thus obtained may be stored at –20 °C until required.

For assay, a pellet is resuspended in the appropriate buffer to a protein concentration of, typically, 2 mg ml^{-1}. The protein assay based on the colour change of the dye Coomassie Blue is perhaps the simplest to use (Bradford, 1976). It is available in kit form. Sodium phosphate buffer may be used for most radioreceptor assays, but in some cases a metal-ion-free buffer may be desirable (see below), in which case tris-HCl or tris-citric acid may be used. The resuspended receptor preparation has been found to maintain binding activity towards muscarinic antagonists for at least one week when stored at 4 °C, and for more than a year when stored at –20 °C.

3.2.3 The radioligand

The ideal radioligand possesses high specificity, high affinity and high specific radioactivity. The purity and stability of the ligand are also important. High specificity and high affinity are by no means the same thing. Acetylcholine does not exhibit high affinity at the muscarinic receptor in antagonising [^{3}H]scopolamine binding, whereas it does exhibit high affinity in competing with [^{3}H]acetylcholine (or other agonist) binding. Also, a muscarinic antagonist such as quinuclidinyl benzilate does not bind quite as specifically to muscarinic receptors as does methyl scopolamine (Hulme *et al.*, 1978), although the former compound possesses higher affinity for the receptor. This is probably because of the lipophilic nature of the quinuclidinyl benzilate molecule, which leads to an increase in nonspecific binding to tissue proteins, including plasma proteins. High-affinity, nonspecific adsorption of ligands may occur to the glass-fibre filter discs used to separate bound from unbound label, and Snyder *et al.* (1975) have demonstrated stereospecific binding of labelled opiates to such filters.

The radioligand must be of sufficiently high affinity or, more strictly, have a low enough dissociation rate constant, to prevent significant loss of bound radioactivity during washing of the filter.

The higher the specific radioactivity of the ligand, the greater the sensitivity of the assay. The most commonly used isotope in receptor binding studies is tritium because (1) a high specific activity is available (typically 30 to 100 Ci $mmol^{-1}$); (2) the radiolabelled molecule behaves chemically and biologically as the unlabelled molecule; (3) the biohazard is low; (4) the half-life is relatively long (12.4 years); (5) the labelled molecule is often stable for months, even years, with proper storage. Some of the commercially available tritiated ligands are shown in Table 3.1.

Table 3.1 Examples of commercially available radioligands

Receptor	Agonist	Antagonist	Example of drug
Adrenergic (α_1)	Noradrenaline	Prazosin HEAT*	Prazosin
Adrenergic (α_2)	Clonidine	Yohimbine Rauwolscine	Yohimbine
Adrenergic (β)	Isoprenaline	Dihydroalprenolol Iodocyanopindolol	Propranolol
Dopaminergic	6,7 ADTN†	Spiroperidol Haloperidol	Chlorpromazine
Muscarinic	Oxotremorine-M	Methylscopolamine	Atropine
Benzodiazepine	Flunitrazepam	DMCM‡	Diazepam
Opiate	Dihydromorphine Lofentanil	Naloxone Diprenorphine	Morphine
Imipramine	Imipramine Desipramine Nitroimipramine		Amitriptyline

* [^{125}I] 2-[β-(4-hydroxy-3-iodophenyl)ethylaminomethyl] -tetralone.
† [5,8-^{3}H] amino-6,7-dihydroxy-1,2,3,4-tetrahydronaphthalene.
‡ [^{3}H] methyl 6,7-dimethoxy-4-ethyl-β-carboline-3-carboxylate.

Radioiodinated ligands are also available, but are usually used only where very high specific radioactivities ($>$ 2000 Ci mmol^{-1}) are required. Radioiodination may offer a very convenient way of labelling molecules which contain an aromatic hydroxyl group. It particularly lends itself to the labelling of tyrosine residues in peptides and proteins. The disadvantages of radioiodinated ligands include (1) possible loss of biological activity; (2) greater susceptibility to radiation-induced damage of molecular structure; (3) increased bio-hazard, (4) relatively short half-life (67 days for ^{125}I).

Manufacturers' estimates of the radiochemical purity and specific radioactivity of tritium-labelled ligands are usually quite accurate. In cases of doubt, the purity of the ligand may be determined by thin-layer chromatography (Stahl, 1969), and the specific radioactivity may be checked in competitive binding studies with unlabelled ligand (Akera and Cheng, 1977; Builder and Segel, 1978).

3.2.4 Separation of bound and free ligand

The choice of separation technique depends upon the rate of dissociation of the receptor–ligand complex and whether the receptor is membrane-bound or soluble. Most radioreceptor assays use particulate receptor preparations and therefore separation by filtration, which is simple, rapid and efficient, may be considered. However, the separation procedure should be completed in less than 0.15 times the half-life of dissociation of the complex to avoid significant (> 10%) loss of bound ligand (Bennett, 1978). Filtration may be carried out most conveniently using an apparatus which permits the filtration of several samples at a time. Manifolds are available which will hold up to a dozen filters (2.5 cm diameter) on individual plastic mesh supports above a large tank to which a vacuum can be applied. Individual samples may then be filtered and washed under partial vacuum. The total separation time (filtration plus washing) with this system is dependent upon the number of washes but is typically 10 to 20 s per sample. This requires the dissociation-rate constant of the bound radioligand to be less than 0.3 min^{-1}. Thus, in practice, K_D values of about 10^{-8} M or less are necessary. Uniform conditions of filtering and washing help to ensure equal dissociation in all samples. Nonspecific binding of the radioligand to the filter material may sometimes occur, in which case either an alternative filter material may be suitable (Klett *et al.*, 1973) or an anti-adsorbent such as albumin (Colquhoun and Rang, 1976) may be included in the incubation and wash buffer. In some cases, siliconisation of the glass-fibre filters may be necessary.

Separation by centrifugation is an alternative procedure when nonspecific adsorption of ligand to the filter material cannot be reduced or where rapid dissociation of the receptor–ligand complex occurs. There should be no apparent dissociation of the complex during centrifugation if equilibrium has been established. Therefore the separation time, if the pellet is not rinsed with buffer, is effectively zero. However, some free radioligand will be trapped in the pellet, thus elevating the apparent nonspecific binding.

Centrifugation may also be used to separate free from bound label when the receptor protein is soluble. In this case, either the receptor–ligand complex may be precipitated (ammonium sulphate) or free ligand may be adsorbed onto an inert particulate material such as charcoal.

3.2.5 Counting of sample

Liquid scintillation counting offers the most versatile technique for counting samples in radioreceptor assays as both β-emitters such as ^{3}H and γ-emitters such as ^{125}I may be counted with equal facility.

When bound and free ligand have been separated by ultracentrifugation, some free ligand will remain trapped with the pellet. The error due to this is usually small but may be reduced by including a second radioisotope to 'label' the supernatant, and hence allow an appropriate correction factor to be applied for the trapped free primary radioligand. The pellet may be solubilised using a preparation such as Hyamine, Soluene or Protosol.

Sample vials containing glass-fibre filters should be shaken vigorously so that the discs are fully dispersed in the scintillation cocktail. Typical scintillation cocktails include Scintillator 299, Picofluor 15 and Dimilume, all of which give counting efficiencies of around forty per cent for tritium. It may be advantageous with some ligands to elute them from the disc by adding a small volume (0.5 to 1 ml) of a polar solvent such as water or ethanol to the filter in the scintillation vial and leaving at room temperature for a few hours before adding the scintillation cocktail. There is room in this area for the individual experimenter to optimise the conditions for both efficient and accurate counting of the sample, as there will be some variation, depending upon the characteristics of the filter, the radioligand and the scintillation cocktail. Sample preparation in liquid scintillation counting has been discussed by several authors (Kobayashi and Maudsley, 1974; Peng, 1977; Peng *et al.*, 1980).

3.3 TYPICAL PROTOCOL FOR A RADIORECEPTOR ASSAY

Radioreceptor assays have been developed for a range of drugs and the assay protocol is broadly similar in each case. Since the identification of benzodiazepine binding sites in brain (Squires and Braestrup, 1977; Möhler and Okada, 1977), a number of radioreceptor assays for benzodiazepines have been reported (Hunt *et al.*, 1979; Skolnick *et al.*, 1979; Lund, 1981; Aaltonen and Scheinin, 1982; Dorow *et al.*, 1982). An example of a protocol (Table 3.2) for the assay of benzodiazepines, a common cause of drug poisoning, will be described to exemplify the procedure.

Assays may be conveniently carried out using 12 x 75 mm glass test-tubes. The receptor preparation, equivalent to 100 to 200 μg protein, is added to the sample in buffer. The radioactive ligands most often used to date are tritiated

Table 3.2 Protocol for the assay of benzodiazepines (all incubations in duplicate or triplicate)

Tube	Volume (μl)					
	Drug-free plasma	Test plasma	Buffer	Diazepam standard	Receptor	2.5×10^{-9} M [^{3}H] Flunitrazepam
1 Standard curve	10	–	300	0	100	100
2 Standard curve	10	–	250	50	100	100
3 Standard curve	10	–	200	100	100	100
4 Standard curve	10	–	100	200	100	100
5 Nonspecific binding	10	–	200	100*	100	100
6 Unknown	–	10	300	–	100	100

*10^{-5} M unlabelled flunitrazepam.

diazepam or flunitrazepam. However, other ligands are becoming commercially available, e.g. methyl clonazepam (NEN). The radioligand is added last, and the assay tubes are incubated in ice for 60 min. Then the samples are filtered through glass-fibre discs (Whatman GF/B or GF/C) under partial vacuum to separate bound from free radioactivity. The incubation tube is rinsed with 3 ml ice-cold buffer, the washings filtered and the discs washed with a further 3 x 5 ml of ice-cold buffer. The filters are placed in vials containing 10 ml of scintillation fluid, and the vials shaken vigorously to suspend the glass-fibre disc.

3.3.1 Analysis of data

The radioactivity bound in tubes containing excess unlabelled benzodiazepine is regarded as being due to nonspecific binding. This value is subtracted from all other counts to give the count due to specific binding. The standard curves are usually plotted so as to give a linear transformation of the inhibition binding curve.

A typical plot is C_0/C_x against concentration of drug (Figure 3.1) where C_0 = cpm of zero standard (e.g. drug-free plasma) and C_x = cpm of standard (or test). Standard curves may also be linearised using logit–log graph paper

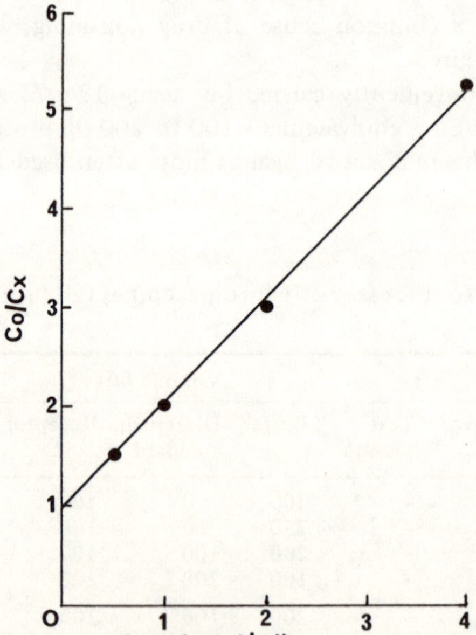

Figure 3.1 Typical plot for a standard curve.

(Rodbard and Lewald, 1970), or a computerised approach may be considered (Munson and Rodbard, 1980). The concentration of unlabelled ligand that reduces the binding of labelled ligand by 50% is termed the IC_{50}.

If the identity of the test benzodiazepine is known, then its concentration may be expressed directly by using the same drug to construct the standard curve. In toxicological studies, however, the identity of the drug is often unknown, in which case its concentration has to be expressed as 'benzodiazepine equivalents'. If diazepam had been used to generate the standard curve, then the unknown would be expressed in 'diazepam equivalents'. The relative potency in binding studies of a number of benzodiazepines is given in Table 3.3.

Table 3.3 Inhibition constants of some benzodiazepine drugs (Möhler and Okada, 1978)

Benzodiazepine	Inhibition of [^{3}H] diazepam* binding to cerebral cortex preparation from	
	Man K_i (nmol l^{-1})	Rat K_i (nmol l^{-1})
Clonazepam	0.87	1.5
Flunitrazepam	2.2	2.8
Lorazepam	2.3	2.7
Triazolam	2.4	2.8
Diazepam	7.4	6.3
Nitrazepam	9.2	6.4
Flurazepam	11	11
Oxazepam	19	14
Chlorazepate	44	41
Chlordiazepoxide	360	220

*Final assay concentration = 1.5 nmol l^{-1}.

3.3.2 Sensitivity

This may be defined in terms of either the minimal detectable dose (MDD) or the minimal detectable concentration (MDC). For a detailed explanation of the statistical estimation of these terms the reader is referred to the paper of Rodbard (1978). The MDD, in radioreceptor assays, is frequently taken to be the amount of drug per assay tube which will produce 20% inhibition of specific radioligand binding. The MDC is the lowest concentration of the drug in blood, urine etc. which can be quantitated at the stated level of statistical significance. The MDC will depend upon the volume of biological fluid taken for assay and on any extraction procedure involved. Thus, for diazepam the MDD is about 1 pmol, which for a 10-μl plasma sample would give an MDC of 100 nmol l^{-1}. This provides more than adequate sensitivity, as plasma levels of benzodiazepines after overdosage are usually well in excess of 1 μmol l^{-1} for several days (Aaltonen and Scheinin, 1982).

If, for any reason, it is desired to extract the benzodiazepines from biological fluid this may be done quite simply, without pH adjustment, using ethyl acetate or diethyl ether (Lund, 1981; Dorow, Seidler and Schneider, 1982). Recoveries of most benzodiazepines are better than 80 per cent with ethyl acetate, but are less than 50 per cent for chlordiazepoxide. However, recoveries of 90 per cent have been found for chlordiazepoxide using diethyl ether (Lund, 1981).

3.3.3 Validity of the assay

The specificity of the radioreceptor assay for benzodiazepines is demonstrated by a study (Braestrup and Squires, 1978) on a wide range of nonbenzodiazepine drugs, representing twenty-two distinct pharmacological classes, none of which possessed any significant affinity for the diazepam binding site ($K_i > 100$ μmol l^{-1}). The radioreceptor assay for benzodiazepines has been validated by several workers using specific chemical assays based on GLC or HPLC techniques. A direct comparison can be made for those drugs which are not metabolised or which produce relatively inactive metabolites, e.g. clonazepam, lorazepam, nitrazepam or triazolam (Aaltonen and Scheinin, 1982; Jochemsen *et al.*, 1982), and in these cases the agreement between the radioreceptor assay and the chemical method is very good (correlation coefficients > 0.95). A comparison of the serum elimination curve obtained by radioreceptor assay and by GLC in a case of lorazepam overdosage is shown in Figure 3.2.

For benzodiazepines such as diazepam that are metabolised to active compounds, the radioreceptor assay measures the total binding activity of the sample. Therefore any attempt to correlate results obtained in a radioreceptor assay with results in a chemical assay must include determinations of both the parent drug and its active metabolites, whose binding activities on a molar basis need to be known. When a comparison was made in this way using drug-free plasma supplemented with diazepam, *N*-desmethyldiazepam and oxazepam (Aaltonen and Scheinin, 1982), the correlation with a GLC method was very good (correlation coefficient = 0.98). When a similar comparison was made with serum samples obtained in cases of diazepam overdosage, the correlation was still reasonable (correlation coefficient = 0.90). As the authors point out, this lower correlation is probably more a reflection of problems associated with the GLC procedure than evidence against the radioreceptor assay.

3.3.4 Neuroleptic radioreceptor assay

The actions of neuroleptic drugs (phenothiazines, thioxanthenes and butyrophenones) are believed to be mediated by blockade of central dopamine receptors

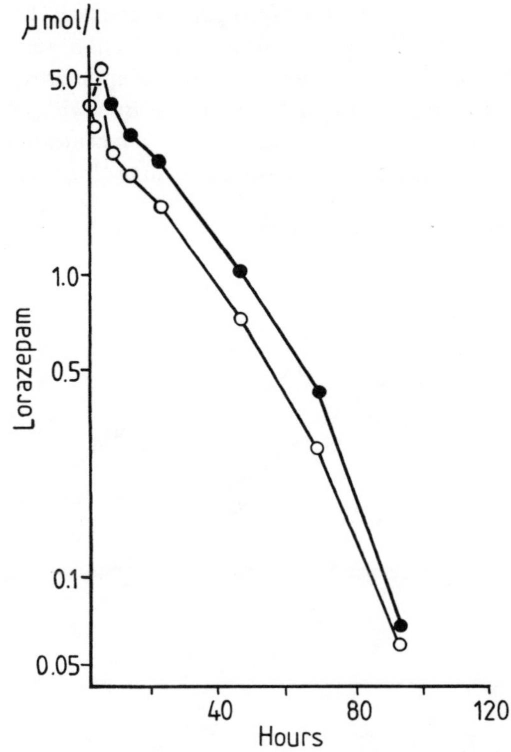

Figure 3.2 Elimination of lorazepam from serum in a female overdose patient (age 64 years, dose 200 mg). Elimination half-life, 19.9 hours; •, radioreceptor assay, ○, gas–liquid chromatography. For lorazepam 1 μg/l = 3.11 nmol l^{-1}. (Courtesy Aaltonen and Scheinin, 1982.)

(Creese *et al.*, 1976; Seeman *et al.*, 1976). The neuroleptic radioreceptor assay of Creese and Snyder (1977) is based on the competitive binding of the dopamine antagonist, [^{3}H] spiroperidol (spiperone), to dopamine receptors from the corpus striatum of calf or rat brain. Again the radioreceptor assay has the advantage of measuring metabolite as well as parent drug activity. This is particularly important in the case of the neuroleptics, which may be given over prolonged periods, and at widely different doses. Chlorpromazine, the most widely used antipsychotic, has been shown to have over 150 metabolites (May and Van Putten, 1978), some of which, for example 7-hydroxychlorpromazine and chlorpromazine sulphoxide, are almost as potent as the parent molecule (Shavit *et al.*, 1980). In some cases, for example thioridazine, the metabolites are more potent than the parent compound.

Samples containing neuroleptic drugs may be stored at or below −20 °C, but repeated freezing and thawing results in reduced neuroleptic levels. Serum or plasma may be assayed without extraction (Creese and Snyder, 1977), although there is some inhibition of both [^{3}H] spiroperidol and [^{3}H] haloperidol binding by control plasma (30% inhibition occuring with 150 μl of serum in a total assay volume of 1 ml). However, the presence of a neuroleptic drug in a serum sample reduces ^{3}H-ligand binding substantially in comparison with control serum, and the degree of inhibition is proportional to the concentration of neuroleptic, which may then be determined from a standard curve (Figure 3.3).

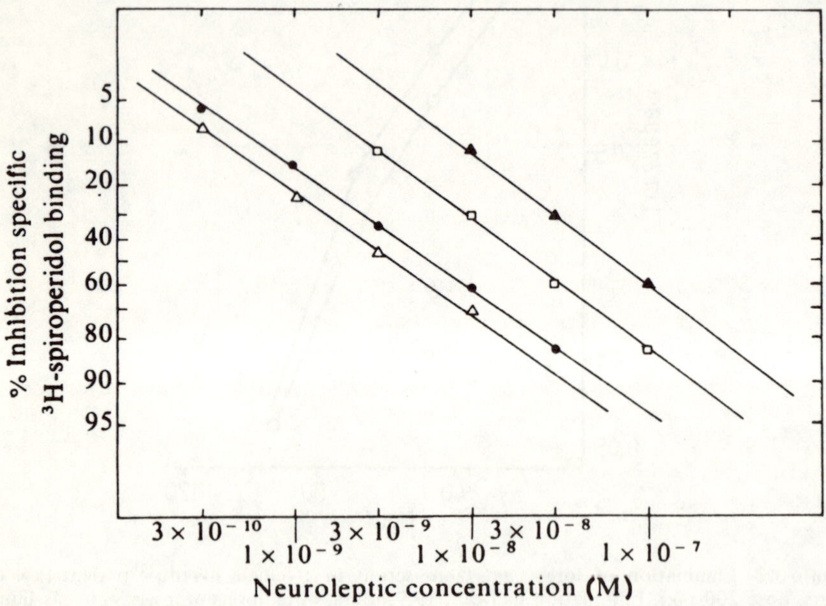

Figure 3.3 Log-probit plots of neuroleptic inhibition of specific [^{3}H] spiroperidol binding to rat striatal membranes. ▲, thioridazine; □, chlorpromazine; ●, haloperidol; △, fluphenazine. (Courtesy Creese and Snyder, 1977.)

The details of the assay have been described by Creese and Snyder (1977). Briefly, plasma or serum is added to incubation buffer (50 mmol l^{-1} tris containing 0.1% ascorbic acid and 10 μmol l^{-1} pargyline, pH 7.1) containing 0.1 nmol-l^{-1} [^{3}H] spiroperidol and a receptor preparation from corpus striatum. After incubation at 37 °C for 15 min, the samples are filtered and the filters washed and counted. As little as 1% of neuroleptic may be free in plasma, with the remainder largely bound to plasma proteins. However, the radioreceptor assay appears to determine total plasma neuroleptic levels, possibly because dilution of the plasma for assay results in dissociation of the bound neuroleptic fraction. The high affinity of the receptor binding site will also disturb the normal plasma-free and bound-drug equilibria. The same authors found that serum neuroleptic levels after haloperidol agreed within a mean of 10% whether samples were estimated directly or were extracted with organic solvent. They also found good agreement between blood haloperidol levels determined by radioreceptor assay and those determined by radioimmunoassay. The lower limits of sensitivity in the radioreceptor assay (15% inhibition of binding) using 150 μl of serum were 1.8 ng ml^{-1}, 2.5 ng ml^{-1} and 8.6 ng ml^{-1} for fluphenazine, haloperidol and chlorpromazine, respectively.

It is usual to express the concentration of neuroleptic in 'chlorpromazine equivalents'. In the case of a neuroleptic like haloperidol with few biologically active metabolites, knowing the IC_{50} of haloperidol with respect to chlorpromazine, the levels of haloperidol may be calculated. In the case of a drug like thioridazine which produces active metabolites, including mesoridazine, sulphoridazine and northioridazine (Cohen *et al.*, 1979), the dopamine blocking activity of the sample may be expressed as 'chlorpromazine equivalents' or 'thioridazine equivalents'. Mesoridazine is about twice as potent as thioridazine at blocking [^{3}H] spiroperidol binding to dopamine receptors (Linnoila *et al.*, 1982). Furthermore, after therapy with thioridazine, serum levels of free mesoridazine are fifty to a hundred times higher than thioridazine levels (Nyberg *et al.*, 1978), so that mesoridazine is the major compound of therapeutic and toxicological importance (Innis and Snyder, 1981). When neuroleptic concentrations were measured in patients treated with thioridazine, there was a good correlation ($r = 0.95$) between results obtained with a radioreceptor assay and those obtained with a spectrophotofluorimetric assay (Javaid *et al.*, 1980). However, there was no obvious correlation when serum thioridazine levels were determined using a radioreceptor assay and HPLC (Linnoila *et al.*, 1982).

The radioreceptor assay is selective in that no drugs other than neuroleptics (and ergot alkaloids) compete significantly for [^{3}H] haloperidol binding (Burt, Creese and Snyder, 1976). This is also true for [^{3}H] spiroperidol if a striatal receptor preparation is used. However, [^{3}H] spiroperidol has been shown to label both dopamine and serotonin receptors in the cerebral cortex of the rat, and there is some evidence that [^{3}H] spiroperidol binds exclusively to serotonin receptors in the hippocampus of rat (Creese and Snyder, 1978).

3.3.5 Opiate radioreceptor assay

The search for compounds possessing potent analgesic activity with minimal addictive qualities has led to the development of a broad range of compounds. These include the benzomorphans, e.g. pentazocine, the oripavine derivatives, e.g. etorphine and the 4-anilino-piperidines such as sufentanil which possesses five thousand times the analgesic potency of morphine. Because of the diverse chemical nature of the opiates and because of their extreme potency and potential for drug abuse, a radioreceptor assay would appear to have wide application in both clinical and forensic toxicology. The presence of opiate receptors in the central nervous system was first reported by two groups of workers (Pert and Snyder, 1973; Simon *et al.*, 1973), and recently an assay, based on the displacement of [^{3}H] buprenorphine from receptor sites on forebrain membranes, has been developed for opiates in human plasma and CSF (Villiger *et al.*, 1981).

Plasma proteins cause significant inhibition of binding of [^{3}H] buprenorphine and therefore extraction of opiates from plasma is necessary. In addition, sodium ions in plasma reduce the binding affinity of opiate agonists, such as morphine (Pert and Snyder, 1974). This phenomenon, the 'sodium shift', may be used to advantage to distinguish between opiate agonists, antagonists and mixed agonist–antagonists, such as nalorphine or pentazocine (Table 3.4). In the procedure of Villiger *et al.* (1981), aliquots of plasma (100 to 300 μl) are made basic with 1 ml of concentrated ammonium hydroxide solution and are extracted three times with 3 ml of diethyl ether. Recoveries are between 80 and 90 per cent. The combined organic phases are evaporated to dryness in the tube or beaker to be used for the binding assay. The final incubation contains 10^{-9}M [^{3}H] buprenorphine and receptor material derived from 20 mg of original brain

Table 3.4 Effect of sodium ions on inhibition of [^{3}H] naloxone binding to rat brain homogenate by opiate agonists and antagonists (Creese, 1978)

	IC_{50} (nmol l^{-1})		
	No NaCl	100 mmol NaCl l^{-1}	Na-shift ratio
Pure antagonists			
Naloxone	1.5	1.5	1
Naltrexone	0.5	0.5	1
Diprenorphine	0.5	0.5	1
Mixed agonists/ antagonists			
Levallorphan	1.0	2.0	2.0
Nalorphine	1.5	4.0	2.7
Pentazocine	15	50	3.3
Pure agonists			
Etorphine	0.5	6	12
Methadone	7.0	200	28
Morphine	3.0	110	37

tissue in 50 mmol l^{-1} tris-HCl buffer, pH 7.4. After incubation at 25 °C for 30 min, bound and free label are separated by filtration through GF/B filters with two washes of ice-cold buffer (5 ml). Nonspecific binding was defined as the binding that occurred in the presence of 1 μmol l^{-1} of unlabelled buprenorphine.

As little as 10 pg of morphine in the assay tube produces twenty per cent inhibition of [^{3}H] buprenorphine binding. The assay was not as sensitive, however, to fentanyl or to the opiate antagonist, naloxone. In view of the potent activity of these two last-named compounds this is somewhat surprising, especially as buprenorphine, morphine and fentanyl have been shown to have very similar activity in displacing [^{3}H] dihydromorphine binding (Wood, 1982). However, dihydromorphine is light-sensitive and is therefore less stable on storage than is buprenorphine. It is possible that other commercially available tritiated ligands possessing high affinity ($K_d \sim 10^{-10}$M) for the μ-receptor, such as diprenorphine (Amersham International), lofentanil (New England Nuclear) or sufentanil (Janssen) may prove useful for radioreceptor assay of opiates. These radioligands have the advantage of possessing very low dissociation-rate constants, so that little dissociation of bound ligand occurs during separation of bound and free radiolabel (Leysen and Gommeren, 1982; Sadee *et al.*, 1982). However, because of the multiple nature of opiate receptors (Wood, 1982), it may well be that no one radioligand is capable of covering the complete spectrum of opiate agonists and antagonists.

It is possible that the phenomenon of the 'sodium shift' mentioned previously could be used to identify a particular opiate agonist (Table 3.4). However, more evidence of the reproducibility of the sodium indices for agonists, under precisely determined assay conditions, would be essential before any reliance could be placed on such an identification.

3.3.6 Tricyclic antidepressant radioreceptor assay

Tricyclic antidepressant drugs (TCA) are widely used and various methods have been described for monitoring blood levels. These include gas–liquid chromatography (Jorgensen, 1975), GLC linked to mass spectrometry (Garland *et al.*, 1979), and radioimmunoassay (Lucek and Dixon, 1977). Such analytical methods are both sensitive and specific, but there does appear to be a need for an alternative method for measuring active metabolites, especially the hydroxy-metabolites which may exist in several isomeric forms (Sjöqvist and Bertilsson, 1981).

A problem in developing a radioreceptor assay for TCA is that the precise mechanism of their action is not known. Unlike the benzodiazepines and neuroleptics there is as yet no receptor interaction of the TCA that can be said unequivocally to be correlated with their antidepressant action. However, specific binding sites with high affinity for [^{3}H] imipramine have been shown to be present in both rat (Raisman *et al.*, 1979) and human (Rehavi *et al.*, 1980) brain, and recently Paul *et al.* (1980) have described a radioreceptor assay for tertiary-amine TCA based on the competitive binding of [^{3}H] imipramine to human platelet membranes.

Briefly, the incubation medium contains crude human-platelet membrane (about 0.6 mg protein, [^{3}H] imipramine (1.5 nmol l^{-1}) and an appropriate volume of diluted plasma, all in a final assay volume of 250 μl of buffer (tris-HCl, 50 mmol l^{-1}; NaCl, 120 mmol l^{-1}; KCl, 5 mmol l^{-1}; pH 7.4). After incubation at 0 to 4 °C for 60 min, 150 μl of the incubate is rapidly diluted in ice-cold buffer (5 ml) and filtered through Whatman GF/F glass-fibre filters. The filters are washed three times with buffer (5 ml) and counted in scintillation vials containing Aquasol.

Inhibition of [^{3}H] imipramine binding occurs at nanomolar concentrations (IC_{50} of imipramine = 7 nmol l^{-1}) for most of the TCA tested, with tertiary amine TCA being more potent than their secondary amine analogues. No inhibition of binding occurs with antimuscarinic, antihistaminic, antiserotonergic or antiadrenergic drugs at concentrations up to 10 μmol l^{-1} and, of the psychotropic drugs tested, only chlorpromazine inhibits binding at concentrations (IC_{50} = 330 nmol l^{-1}) approaching those of the TCA. Normal therapeutic plasma concentrations of chlorpromazine would not be expected to interfere with the assay for tertiary TCA. Analysis of plasma samples from patients maintained on imipramine showed a good correlation (r = 0.95) between values obtained by radioreceptor assay and those obtained by GC–MS (Paul *et al.*, 1980). It is possible that a more general assay for both tertiary and secondary TCA may be developed using [^{3}H] desipramine (Rehavi *et al.*, 1981).

Most TCA are relatively potent muscarinic antagonists (Snyder and Yamamura, 1977) and a radioreceptor assay based upon the competitive inhibition by TCA of the binding of [^{3}H] quinuclidinyl benzilate, a potent muscarinic antagonist, to muscarinic receptors from mammalian brain has been described (Innis *et al.*, 1979). The IC_{50} values for amitriptyline, nortriptyline, imipramine and desipramine were 12, 36, 75 and 150 nmol l^{-1}, respectively. The assay is sensitive and could, for example, detect 2 ng nortriptyline per ml plasma. When plasma samples from patients treated with nortriptyline were determined using both the radioreceptor assay and a gas–liquid chromatographic procedure, results from the two methods were almost identical. However, control plasma produces significant inhibition of [^{3}H] quinuclidinyl benzilate binding to receptor membranes and, unless low volumes of plasma (10 μl) are being used, extraction of blood samples into organic solvent and back-extraction into 0.1M-HCl is necessary. The requirement for solvent extraction could possibly be omitted if [^{3}H] methylscopolamine was used as the ligand (Metcalfe, 1981). This assay could not be used to measure TCA plasma levels in subjects who were also taking classical antimuscarinic drugs or drugs such as phenothiazines or antihistaminics which possess an anti-muscarinic component to their action. However, in cases where TCA overdosage alone was suspected the assay could prove useful.

3.3.7 Radioreceptor assay for β-adrenergic antagonists

Plasma levels of this widely prescribed class of compounds have been measured using a variety of techniques including fluorimetry (Shand *et al.*, 1970), GC–MS (Walle *et al.*, 1975) and radioimmunoassay (Kawashima *et al.*, 1976). These methods tend either to be specific for one compound, for example propranolol, or, in the case of GC–MS, to be technically difficult and costly. Several radioreceptor assays, which have the advantage of general applicability to β-blockers and to their active metabolites, have been reported. Radioligands used include [^{3}H] dihydroalprenolol (Innis *et al.*, 1978; Nahorski *et al.*, 1978) and [^{125}I] hydroxybenzylpindolol (Bilezikian *et al.*, 1979), together with a variety of membrane preparations including mammalian cerebellum and lung (Innis *et al.*, 1978; Nahorski *et al.*, 1978) and turkey erythrocytes (Bilezikian *et al.*, 1979). Control plasma causes significant inhibition of binding of both ligands which may be circumvented by extraction of drug into ethyl acetate or by dialysis. More recent work (Barnett *et al.*, 1982) indicates that the use of a solubilised receptor protein preparation may overcome the problem of plasma inhibition of binding. The limit of sensitivity of the assay is about 1 pmol propranolol per ml plasma. There is no evidence that drugs other than β-adrenergic antagonists occur in plasma in concentrations that would interfere with the assay.

3.3.8 Atropine-like drugs

Accidental overdosage with atropine-like compounds is a not infrequent occurrence. Children are particularly sensitive to anti-muscarinic drugs so that poisoning may occur from an excessive dose of, for instance, an anti-diarrhoeal or a motion-sickness medication, or from ingestion of belladonna alkaloids.

A radioreceptor assay for atropine has been described (Metcalfe, 1981), which is based on the ability of anti-muscarinic drugs to compete with [^{3}H] quinuclidinyl benzilate for muscarinic receptor binding sites from mammalian brain. As stated above, [^{3}H] quinuclidinyl benzilate binding to receptors is significantly inhibited by plasma proteins, and [^{3}H] methylscopolamine has been found to be a more suitable ligand (Muir and Metcalfe, 1983). The assay can reliably detect 300 fmol (about 0.1 ng) of atropine (20% inhibition of binding) using the standard assay volume of 1 ml. Thus 50 μl of neat plasma is adequate to detect therapeutic levels of atropine, and 10 μl plasma would be sufficient when toxic levels ($>$ 50 nmol l^{-1}) were present.

The radioreceptor assay should be equally satisfactory for other anti-muscarinic drugs, and it has been used to determine plasma levels of hyoscine after oral administration (Muir and Metcalfe, 1983), and atropine methyl nitrate levels after inhalation (Metcalfe, unpublished). The same qualifications as to use of the assay, when the presence of other drugs with an anti-muscarinic component to their action is suspected, apply as for the TCA assay using [^{3}H] quinuclidinyl benzilate.

3.4 CONCLUSIONS

Radioreceptor assays for a variety of drug classes have been described. Most of these assays have only recently been developed, and they have been applied, to date, mainly in the area of clinical therapeutics. However, this brief introduction to radioreceptor assays is intended to show the versatility of a method, whose advantages lie in its sensitivity, its simplicity and its applicability not only to the parent drug but also to any active metabolites. In many cases, extraction of drug from the biological sample is not necessary and this helps to make the analysis very rapid–less than one hour for one or two samples, and one day for 50 to 100 samples. The extreme sensitivity of the technique allows determinations to be made on relatively small sample volumes, e.g. 10 to 100 μl plasma. This could prove useful in clinical toxicology to monitor, for example, the effect of a particular treatment on the blood levels of a drug.

Perhaps the greatest value of the radioreceptor assay in toxicology lies in its use for the detection and determination of extremely potent compounds, especially those of novel molecular structure for which a chemical or radioimmunoassay is not yet available. The advantage of a radioreceptor assay over a radioimmunoassay is that only one preparation, for example mammalian brain, is required to detect and quantify a wide variety of drugs in many pharmacological classes using the former technique, whereas a separate antibody preparation is needed for each drug when using a radioimmunoassay (Butler, 1978; Parker, 1981). However, a combination of high-performance liquid chromatography and radioimmunoassay has proved useful in forensic toxicology for the specific and sensitive determination of compounds such as LSD (Twitchett *et al.*, 1978) and the cannabinoids (Williams *et al.*, 1978), for which no radioreceptor assay is available.

A possible future development to facilitate even more rapid and economical screening of biological samples for drugs may be the use of two or more radioligands of different pharmacological class in the same assay tube, each ligand being labelled with a different isotope, e.g. ^{3}H, ^{125}I or ^{35}S. Differential counting of the bound radioligand, with appropriate data analysis, could then indicate the presence of one or more drug classes.

REFERENCES

Aaltonen, L., and Scheinin, M. (1982). Application of radioreceptor assay of benzodiazepines for toxicology. *Acta Pharmacol. Toxicol.* **50**, 206–12.

Akera, T., and Cheng, V.-J. K. (1977). A simple method for the determination of affinity and binding site concentration in receptor binding studies. *Biochim. Biophys. Acta* **470**, 412–23.

Barnett, D. B., Cook, N., Dickinson, K. E. J., and Nahorski, S. R. (1982). Radioreceptor assay for *beta*-adrenoceptor antagonists using solubilised receptor protein. *Br. J. Clin. Pharmacol.* **13**, 284P.

Bennett, J. P., Jun. (1978). In Yamamura, H. I., Enna, S. J., and Kuhar, M. J. (eds), *Neurotransmitter Receptor Binding*, Raven, New York, 57–90.

Bilezikian, J. P., Gammon, D. E., Rochester, C. L., and Shand, D. G. (1979). A radioreceptor assay for propranolol. *Clin. Pharmacol. Therap.* **26**, 173–80.

Bradford, M. M. (1976). A rapid and sensitive method for the quantitation of microgram quantities of protein utilising the principle of protein-dye binding. *Analyt. Biochem.* **72**, 248–54.

Braestrup, C., and Squires, R. F. (1978). Pharmacological characterisation of benzodiazepine receptors in the brain. *Eur. J. Pharmacol.* **48**, 263–70.

Builder, S. E., and Segel, I. H. (1978). Equilibrium ligand binding assays using labelled substrates: nature of the errors introduced by radiochemical impurities. *Analyt. Biochem.* **85**, 413–24.

Burt, D. R., Creese, I., and Snyder, S. H. (1976). Properties of [^{3}H]haloperidol and [^{3}H]dopamine binding associated with dopamine receptors in calf brain membranes. *Mol. Pharmacol.* **12**, 800–12.

Butler, V. P., Jun. (1978). The immunological assay of drugs. *Pharmacol. Rev.* **29**, 103–84.

Cohen, B. M., Herschel, M., and Aoba, A. (1979). Neuroleptic, antimuscarinic, and anti-adrenergic activity of chlorpromazine, thioridazine, and their metabolites. *Psychiatry Res.* **1**, 199–208.

Colquhoun, D., and Rang, H. P. (1976). Effects of inhibitors on the binding of iodinated α-bungarotoxin to acetylcholine receptors in rat muscle. *Mol. Pharmacol.* **12**, 519–35.

Creese, I. (1978). In Yamamura, H. I., Enna, S. J., and Kuhar, M. J. (eds), *Neurotransmitter Receptor Binding*, Raven, New York, 141–70.

Creese, I., and Snyder, S. H. (1977). A simple and sensitive radioreceptor assay for anti-schizophrenic drugs in blood. *Nature, Lond.* **270**, 180–2.

Creese, I., and Snyder, S. H. (1978). ^{3}H-Spiroperidol labels serotonin receptors in rat cerebral cortex and hippocampus. *Eur. J. Pharmacol.* **49**, 201–2.

Creese, I., Burt, D. R., and Snyder, S. H. (1976). Dopamine receptor binding predicts clinical and pharmacological potencies of anti-schizophrenic drugs. *Science* **192**, 481–3.

Dorow, R. G., Seidler, J., and Schneider, H. H. (1982). A radioreceptor assay to study the affinity of benzodiazepines and their receptor binding activity in human plasma including their active metabolites. *Br. J. Clin. Pharmacol.* **13**, 561–5.

Garland, W. A., Muccino, R. R., Cupano, J., and Fann, W. E. (1979). A method for the determination of amitriptyline and its metabolites nortriptyline, 10-hydroxy-amitriptyline and 10-hydroxy-nortriptyline in human plasma using stable isotope dilution and gas chromatography–chemical ionisation mass-spectrometry (GC–CIMS). *Clin. Pharmacol. Therap.* **25**, 844–56.

Hulme, E. C., Birdsall, N. J. M., Burgen, A. S. V., and Mehta, P. (1978). The binding of antagonists to brain muscarinic receptors. *Mol. Pharmacol.* **14**, 737–50.

Hunt, P., Husson, J. M., and Raynaud, J.-P. (1979). A radioreceptor assay for benzodiazepines. *J. Pharm. Pharmacol.* **31**, 448–51.

Innis, R. B., and Snyder, S. H. (1981). In Usdin, E. (ed.), *Clinical Pharmacology in Psychiatry*. Elsevier, New York, 103–20.

Innis, R. B., Bylund, D. B., and Snyder, S. H. (1978). A simple, sensitive and specific radioreceptor assay for β-adrenergic antagonist drugs. *Life Sci.* **23**, 2031–38.

Innis, R. B., Tune, L., Rock, R., Depaulo, R., U'Prichard, D. C., and Snyder, S. H. (1979). Tricyclic antidepressant radioreceptor assay. *Eur. J. Pharmacol.* **58**, 473–7.

Javaid, J. I., Pandey, G. N., Duslak, B., Hu, H.-Y., and Davis, J. M. (1980). Measurement of neuroleptic concentrations by GLC and radioreceptor assay. *Commun. Psychopharm.* **4**, 467–75.

Jochemsen, R., Horbach, G. J. M. J., and Bremer, D. D. (1982). Assay of nitrazepam and triazolam in plasma by a radioreceptor technique and comparison with a gas chromatographic method. *Res. Commun. Chem. Pathol. and Pharmacol.* **35**, 259–73.

Jorgensen, A. (1975). A gas chromatographic method for the determination of amitriptyline and nortriptyline in human sera. *Acta Pharmacol. Toxicol.* **36**, 79–90.

Kawashima, K., Levy, A., and Spector, S. (1976). Stereospecific radioimmunoassay for propranolol isomers. *J. Pharmac. Exper. Ther.* **196**, 517–23.

Kelly, J. G., McGarry, K., O'Malley, K. (1981). Radioreceptor assay for labetalol. *Br. J. Clin. Pharmacol.* **12**, 258–60.

Klett, R. P., Fulpius, B. W., Cooper, D., Smith, M., Reich, E., and Possani, L. D. (1973). The acetylcholine receptor. 1: Purification and characterisation of a macromolecule isolated from Electrophorus electricus. *J. Biol. Chem.* **248**, 6841–53.

Kobayashi, Y., and Maudsley, D. V. (1974). *Biological Applications of Liquid Scintillation Counting.* Academic, New York.

Leysen, J. E., and Gommeren, W. (1982). In vitro binding properties of ^{3}H-Sufentanil, a superior ligand for the μ-opiate receptor. *Archs Int. Pharmacodyn. Ther.* **260**, 287–9.

Linnoila, M., Rosenblatt, J. E., Jeste, D., Skinner, T., Potter, W. Z., and Wyatt, R. J. (1982). Disparate serum thioridazine concentrations: liquid chromatography versus radioreceptor assay. *Acta Pharmacol. Toxicol.* **50**, 25–9.

Lucek, R., and Dixon, R. (1977). Specific radioimmunoassay for amitriptyline and nortriptyline in plasma. *Res. Commun. Chem. Pathol. Pharmacol.* **18**, 125–36.

Lund, J. (1981). Radioreceptor assay for benzodiazepines in biological fluids using a new, dry and stable receptor preparation. *Scand. J. Clin. Lab. Invest.* **41**, 275–80.

May, P. R. A., and Van Putten, T. (1978). Plasma levels of chlorpromazine in schizophrenia. *Arch. Gen. Psychiat.* **35**, 1081–7.

Metcalfe, R. F. (1981). A sensitive radioreceptor assay for atropine in plasma. *Biochem. Pharmac.* **30**, 209–12.

Möhler, H., and Okada, T. (1977). Benzodiazepine receptor: demonstration in the central nervous system. *Science* **198**, 849–51.

Möhler, H., and Okada, T. (1978). Biochemical identification of the site of action of benzodiazepines in human brain by ^{3}H-diazepam binding. *Life Sci.* **22**, 985–96.

Muir, C., and Metcalfe, R. F. (1983). A comparison of plasma levels of hyoscine after oral and transdermal administration. *J. Pharmaceutical and Biomedical Analysis.* **1**, 363–7.

Munson, P. J., and Rodbard, D. (1980). LIGAND: a versatile computerised approach for characterisation of ligand-binding systems. *Analyt. Biochem.* **107**, 220–39.

Nahorski, S. R., Batta, M. I., and Barnett, D. B. (1978). Measurement of β-adrenoreceptor antagonists in biological fluids using a radioreceptor assay. *Eur. J. Pharmacol.* **52**, 393–6.

Nyberg, G., Axelsson, R., and Hartenssen, E. (1978). Binding of thioridazine and thioridazine metabolites to serum proteins in psychiatric patients. *Eur. J. Clin. Pharmacol.* **14**, 341–51.

Osselton, M. D., Hammond, M. D., and Twitchett, P. J. (1977). The extraction and analysis of benzodiazepines in tissues by enzymic digestion and high-performance liquid chromatography. *J. Pharm. Pharmac.* **29**, 460–2.

Parker, C. W. (1981). Radioimmunoassay. *Ann. Rev. Pharmacol. Toxicol.* **21**, 113–32.

Paul, S. M., Rehavi, M., Hulihan, B., Skolnick, P., and Goodwin, F. K. (1980). A rapid and sensitive radioreceptor assay for tertiary amine tricyclic antidepressants. *Commun. Psychopharm.* **4**, 487–94.

Peng, C.-T. (1977). Sample preparation in liquid scintillation counting. Review 17. Amersham International, Amersham.

Peng, C.-T., Horrocks, D. L., and Alpen, E. L. (1980). *Liquid Scintillation Counting. Recent Applications and Development.* Academic, New York.

Pert, C. B., and Snyder, S. H. (1973). Opiate receptor: demonstration in nervous tissue. *Science* **179**, 1011–14.

Pert, C. B., and Snyder, S. H. (1974). Opiate receptor binding of agonists and antagonists affected differentially by sodium. *Mol. Pharmacol.* **10**, 868–79.

Raisman, R., Briley, M., and Langer, S. Z. (1979). Specific tricyclic antidepressant binding sites in rat brain. *Nature, Lond.* **281**, 148–50.

Rehavi, M., Paul, S. M., Skolnick, P., and Goodwin, F. K. (1980). Demonstration of specific high affinity binding sites for [^{3}H]imipramine in human brain. *Life Sci.* **26**, 2273–9.

Rehavi, M., Skolnick, P., Hulihan, B., and Paul, S. M. (1981). 'High Affinity' binding of [^{3}H]desipramine to rat cerebral cortex: relationship to tricyclic antidepressant-induced inhibition of norepinephrine uptake. *Eur. J. Pharmacol.* **70**, 597–9.

Rodbard, D. (1978). Statistical estimation of the minimal detectable concentration ('sensitivity') for radioligand assays. *Analyt. Biochem.* **90**, 1–12.

Rodbard, D., and Lewald, J. E. (1970). Computer analysis of radioligand assay and radioimmunoassay data. *Acta Endocrinol. (suppl.)* **64**, 79–103.

Sadee, W., Perry, D. C., Rosenbaum, J. S., and Herz, A. (1982). [^{3}H]Diprenorphine receptor binding *in vivo* and *in vitro*. *Eur. J. Pharmacol.* **81**, 431–40.

Seeman, P., Lee, T., Chou-Wong, M., Wong, K. (1976). Antipsychotic drug doses and neuroleptic/dopamine receptors. *Nature, Lond.* **261**, 717–9.

Shand, D. G., Nucholls, E. M., and Oates, J. A. (1970). Plasma propranolol levels in adults with observations in four children. *Clin. Pharmacol. Ther.* **11**, 112–20.

Shavit, S., Kutz, I., Korczyn, A. D., and Gitter, S. (1980). Interactions between chlorpromazine and some of its metabolites. *Commun. Psychopharmacol.* **4**, 495–500.

Simon, E. J., Hiller, J. M., and Edelman, I. (1973). Stereospecific binding of the potent narcotic analgesic ^{3}H-etorphine to rat brain homogenate. *Proc. Natl. Acad. Sci. USA* **72**, 4376–80.

Sjöqvist, F., and Bertilsson, L. (1981). In Usdin, E. (ed.), *Clinical Pharmacology in Psychiatry*. Elsevier, New York, pp. 141–153.

Skolnick, P., Goodwin, F. K., and Paul, S. M. (1979). A rapid and sensitive radioreceptor assay for benzodiazepine in plasma. *Arch. Gen. Psychiat.* **36**, 78–80.

Snyder, S. H., and Yamamura, H. I. (1977). Antidepressants and the muscarinic acetylcholine receptor. *Arch. Gen. Psychiat.* **34**, 236–9.

Snyder, S. H., Pasternak, G. W., and Pert, C. B. (1975). In Iversen, L. L., Iversen, S. D., and Snyder, S. H. (eds), *Handbook of Psychopharmacology*. Plenum, New York.

Squires, R. F., and Braestrup, C. (1977). Benzodiazepine receptors in rat brain. *Nature, Lond.* **266**, 732–4.

Stahl, E. (1969). *Thin-Layer Chromatography*. Springer, Berlin.

Twitchett, P. H., Fletcher, S. M., Sullivan, A. T., and Moffatt, A. C. (1978). Analysis of LSD in human body fluids by high-performance liquid chromatography, fluorescence spectroscopy and radioimmunoassay. *J. Chromatogr.* **150**, 73–84.

Villiger, J. W., Boas, R. A., and Taylor, K. M. (1981). A radioreceptor assay for opiate drugs in human cerebrospinal fluid and plasma. *Life Sci.* **29**, 229–33.

Walle, T., Morrison, J., Walle, K., and Conradi, E. (1975). Simultaneous determination of propranolol and 4-hydroxypropranolol in plasma by mass fragmentography. *J. Chromatogr.* **114**, 351–9.

Williams, P. L., Moffatt, A. C., and King, L. F. (1978). Combined high pressure liquid chromatography and radioimmunoassay for the quantitation of Δ-9-tetra-hydrocannabinol and some of its metabolites in human plasma. *J. Chromatogr.* **155**, 273–9.

Wood, P. L. (1982). Multiple opiate receptors: support for uniqe mu, delta and kappa sites. *Neuropharmacology* **21**, 487–97.

4
Solvent abuse

J. S. OLIVER

4.1 INTRODUCTION

In the past decade, solvent abuse, or 'glue sniffing', has become the subject of growing concern in the news media, in Parliament, with parents, with educationalists, with medical workers and with the social services. The concern arises primarily from the fact that the practice appears to be widespread and confined to teenagers with an average age of fifteen years.

Solvent abuse is said to be an import from the United States. The practice was encountered there in the 1950s and has since spread worldwide to Africa, Canada, Japan, Mexico, South America, Sweden and Western Europe (Cohen, 1973). It does not appear to have received much attention in the United Kingdom during the 1960s. However, in Japan, for example, there were reports of 161 solvent-related deaths in 1961 (Alha *et al.*, 1974a), and 100 in 1963 (Cohen, 1973). Bass (1970) reported on 110 sniffing deaths in America in the 1960s. In Sweden, there were 63 deaths related to solvent sniffing during the 1960s. There, the case number appears to have increased from 1 to 2 per year in the early 1960s to 10 to 18 per year in the early 1970s (Edh *et al.*, 1973). In contrast, the annual total of deaths in Denmark between 1959 and 1978 has been almost constant. There were 20 solvent-related deaths in that country in this period (Kringsholm, 1980).

In the United Kingdom, there was in increase from 2 solvent-related deaths in 1971 to 45 in 1981, a total of 140 deaths for the decade (Anderson *et al.*,

1982). Of these, 15 solvent-related deaths were recorded in Scotland in 1981, compared with 8 for the previous three-year period (Oliver, 1983).

4.2 THE PROBLEM

Because of the nature of solvent abuse, it is difficult to get an overall estimate of the scale of the problem. The abusers may be detected by different agencies and for a variety of reasons. The police may detect an individual causing a disturbance, shoplifting, driving under the influence of solvents or committing more serious crimes up to very violent assault. Educational authorities may become involved through behaviour at school, social workers and general practitioners can be involved through requests for help by anxious parents and hospital staff become involved in the treatment of illness or injury subsequent to solvent abuse.

Information on the problem, therefore, tends to relate to the field of interest of the investigator. As a result accurate statistics are not available.

The Chief Constable of Strathclyde's reports in 1981 and 1982 relate to 1560 young persons found inhaling solvents in 1980, 1725 in 1981 and 1139 in 1982. An early study in the West of Scotland, which was limited to children referred to a remand home, revealed that the problem was confined to the 12 to 19 years age group with a mean age of 15 years. The practise was predominantly male and involved impact adhesives containing toluene (Oliver and Watson, 1977). A more balanced study in the same area over a 6-year period involved 400 children referred by various agencies including police, hospital staff, social workers, teachers and parents. Again, those referred were predominantly male (4.8 : 1 male : female) with a peak age incidence of 13 to 15 years. The larger sample confirmed the preference for the abuse of impact adhesives containing toluene (89%). The incidences of other solvents abused were: dry-cleaning substances containing halogenated solvents, 5%; fuel gases, butane and propane, 3%; nail-polish remover, hair lacquer and fire extinguishers 1% each (Watson, 1982).

The order of popularity of abused substances is not reflected in the solvents detected following fatalities. In 12 deaths in Scotland between 1970 and 1977, only 4 involved adhesives (Watson, 1979). In 15 solvent-related fatalities investigated in 1981, 5 involved toluene, 6 involved fuel gases (butane and/or propane), 2 involved trichloroethane (one with dichloromethane), one involved amyl nitrite and one involved nitrous oxide and halothane (Oliver, 1983). Of the 140 deaths recorded in the United Kingdom between 1971 and 1981, 23 involved toluene, 38 involved butane and 59 involved halogenated solvents (Anderson *et al.*, 1982). If the pattern of solvent abuse is similar on a nationwide basis, then the deaths reflect the relative dangers of the abused substances or the means of abusing them.

4.3 METHODS OF ABUSE

The techniques of abusing solvents have been fully documented (Watson, 1982).

Glues are commonly abused with the use of a small polythene or 'crisp' bag. About an inch of substance is decanted into the bag. The abuser places the open end of the bag over the nose and mouth and rebreathes the vapour content of the bag twenty to thirty times until the desired intoxicating effect is achieved. On occasions larger bags have been used over the head to enhance the intoxicating effect. Occasionally cans of glue are heated to increase the solvent yield prior to sniffing.

More-available solvents such as dry cleaning substances and nail-polish removers are inhaled directly from the tops of bottles or caps, or from saturated handkerchiefs or rags formed into a pad and placed over the nose and mouth. Fire-extinguisher fluids are decanted into empty beer-cans and the vapours inhaled directly.

Fuel gases such as butane or propane are abused by spraying directly into the mouth or by inhaling the vapour released into a polythene bag placed over the head and neck.

Aerosol propellants are abused by bubbling the released gas through water to remove the product. The released gas is inhaled directly.

4.4 EFFECTS

The volatile substances are abused to experience some transient effect on the central nervous system. Initially intoxication similar to the effect of alcohol is experienced. Thereafter, euphoria followed by hallucinations may be experienced.

It is at this stage that the authorities become aware of the abuser, generally as a result of antisocial behaviour. The medical profession becomes involved through the more serious effects of the solvents.

4.5 CLINICAL FINDINGS

Apart from the smell of solvent on the breath, adhesive stains on the clothes, the glue sniffer can sometimes be recognised by the appearance of 'glue sniffer's rash'. This consists of a symmetrical distribution of comedones, papules and pustules extending from each nostril up the nasal fold and across the bridge of the nose. This is thought to be caused by the repeated application of the plastic bag (Watson, 1978).

Severely intoxicated children have been admitted to hospital with symptoms of encephalopathy. Euphoria and hallucinations, coma, ataxia, convulsions, behavioural disturbances and diplopia have been described in children under the influence of toluene. One child had persistant cerebellar ataxia when seen after one year (King *et al.*, 1981). The occurrence of status epilepticus in a fifteen-year-old male under the influence of toluene has been reported. This boy had no previous history of epilepsy. Two years after admission, the youth was subject to behavioural disturbances and epilepsy (Allister *et al.*, 1981). Other evidence of neurological damage has been published. These include permanent encephalopathy resulting from toluene inhalation (Knox and Nelson, 1966), prolonged cerebellar dysfunction associated with paint sniffing (Kelly, 1975), permanent cerebellar ataxia after exposure to toluene (Boor and Hurtig, 1977) and cerebellar degeneration resulting from toluene sniffing (Grabski, 1961).

Toxic effects on other organs have been recorded in the literature. These include hepatic and renal damage in a teenager from abuse of a toluene-based cleaner (O'Brien *et al.*, 1971), acute renal failure in a forty-nine-year-old man after acute exposure to toluene (Reisin *et al.*, 1975), and renal damage from toluene sniffing (Will and McLaren, 1981; Venkataraman, 1981).

In contrast to these findings, a study of 132 cases of solvent abuse specifically to investigate the possibility of haematological, hepatic or renal damage failed to reveal any laboratory abnormality directly attributable to solvent abuse. Long-term follow-up of cases is recommended before concluding that solvent abuse is harmless in the above context (Watson, 1978).

Cardiac toxicity due to toluene has not been so clearly documented. In one study it was shown that the inhalation of toluene in mice slows the sinoatrial rate, prolongs the p.r. interval and sensitises the heart to asphyxia-induced atrioventricular block. The authors postulate that this may be the mechanism of sudden sniffing deaths in humans (Taylor and Harris, 1970).

The results of a series of experiments on animals which were exposed to a variety of solvents including aerosol propellants, fire extinguishants and halogenated solvents have been published. They revealed that if death was caused by the solvent, it occurred during exposure, never afterwards. In fact, recovery from nonlethal exposure was rapid. Additionally, all chemicals tested caused cardiac sensitisation in dogs. The authors conclude that dizziness in man should act as an early warning, indicating that a dangerous concentration of solvent was being reached. Since intoxication is the aim of the solvent abuser, he will be at risk from cardiac sensitisation and sudden death (Clark and Tinston, 1982).

4.6 ANALYSIS

The detection, identification and measurement of solvents in blood and tissue samples can be accomplished readily using gas–liquid chromatography. At the levels likely to be encountered resulting from solvent abuse, the necessary preparation of samples is minimal. An ether extraction of a blood sample prior to gas chromatography to detect and measure toluene has been used (O'Brien *et al.*, 1971).

A simple headspace analysis to measure paraldehyde, toluene and methylene chloride in blood, plasma and urine samples has been described (Anthony *et al.*, 1978). The technique employed a column packed with Carbowax 1500 on Carbopack C. This technique, using Carbowax 20M on Carbopack C, was used for the detection and identification of organic solvents in blood samples from solvent abusers (Ramsay and Flanagan, 1982). Carbowax 400 on Chromosorb W (Oliver and Watson, 1977; Oliver, 1982), Tenax GC and an Emulphor WCOT column (Lush *et al.*, 1980) are all suitable gas-chromatography columns for the detection, identification and measurement of volatile substances in biological materials. This technique is outlined in Figure 4.1.

Sample: lung tied at main bronchus → 250 μl trapped air → Gas chromatography analysis

Sample: tissue specimen: 1 g tissue + 20 ml glass distilled water

↓

Homogenise

Sample: blood, urine, tissue homogenate, standard solution 500 μl + 1 μg ml^{-1} ethyl benzene in glass distilled water 500 μl

↓

Seal in 6 ml hypovial; warm at 60 °C 45 min

↓

250 μl headspace sample

↓

Gas chromatography analysis

Figure 4.1 The analysis of biological samples for solvents.

Following death from solvent abuse, a lung, tied at the main bronchus, should be submitted to the laboratory, together with specimens of blood, urine, liver, kidney and brain. All specimens should be in glass containers with aluminium foil inserts in the sealing caps. An aliquot of the air trapped in the bronchus can be sampled and, within a few minutes, the lung returned to the pathologist for full investigation. This air sample, when analysed by gas chromatography, will reveal rapidly the identities of the solvents to which the deceased has been exposed.

Prior to analysis, the purity of solvents should be checked by headspace gas chromatography. Many commercial solvents contain appreciable amounts of impurities in the form of breakdown products, other solvents and stabilising agents. These materials can readily be identified by gas chromatography-mass spectrometry. This preliminary investigation can assist with the identification of unexpected peaks found in the gas-chromatography trace of a blood sample taken from a solvent abuser. Ethyl benzene is a suitable reference solvent for most solvent-abuse analyses. Commercially available ethyl benzene contains an appreciable amount of toluene. This can be removed by distillation using a fractionating column.

Standard reference solutions are prepared by dissolving 1 g of solvent in 500 ml of methanol and making up to 1 l with distilled water. Working solutions are prepared by diluting 1 ml of this stock solution to 1 l with distilled water.

Tissue samples (1 g) should be homogenised with 20 ml of glass-distilled water. The homogenate can then be treated as a blood sample.

Blood, urine or tissue homogenate (500 μl) is placed in a 6-ml hypovial with ethyl benzene internal standard (500 μl of a 1 μg ml^{-1} solution). This and a hypovial containing a standard solution of a sought-for solvent (500 μl of a 1 μg ml^{-1} solution) with the ethyl benzene internal standard (500 μl) are warmed at 60 °C for 45 minutes. 250 μl aliquots of headspace vapour are injected directly onto the gas chromatography column.

Tenax GC polymer columns are best used at a preselected temperature for the required analysis. Methane, ethane, propane and butane can be separated at 80 °C, ethanol and methanol at 105 °C, chloroform, trichloroethane and trichloroethylene at 140 °C and trichloroethanol at 180 °C.

The use of Carbowax 400 or Chromosorb W at 90 °C permits the separation and identification of a wide range of solvents. Retention times relative to ethanol are listed in Table 4.1.

If required, the sensitivity of the simple headspace procedure can be increased by degassing the blood sample using helium. A simple procedure similar to that

Table 4.1 Retention times relative to ethanol of solvents using a Carbowax 400 column at 90 °C

Solvent	Retention time relative to ETOH	Solvent	Retention time relative to ETOH
methyl bromide	0.39	trichloroethylene	0.96
cyclohexane	0.40	ethanol	1.00
methyl acetate	0.56	chloroform	1.05
acetone	0.60	perchloroethylene	1.13
carbon tetrachloride	0.61	toluene	1.24
trichloroethane	0.64	1,2-dichloroethane	1.35
ethyl acetate	0.68	butan-2-ol	1.44
methylene chloride	0.73	*n*-butyl acetate	1.52
methyl ethyl ketone	0.80	*n*-propanol	1.59
benzene	0.82	paraldehyde	1.61
methyl alcohol	0.91	1,4-dioxan	1.66
iso-propanol	0.94	*n*-butanol	2.73
formaldehyde	0.94	*n*-amyl alcohol	3.82

described by Blackmore (1970) for the release of carbon monoxide from blood can be used. This is illustrated in Figure 4.2. A syringe containing 1 ml blood is attached to one containing 4 ml helium. The gas is transferred to the blood syringe and rolled gently for a few minutes and then an aliquot is gently transferred to a sample loop prior to analysis by gas chromatography.

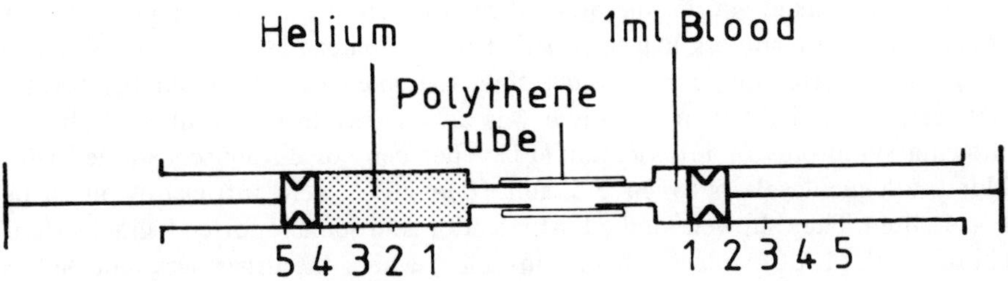

Figure 4.2 Syringe arrangement for the degassing of blood.

An approximate quantitation of fuel gases released from blood following simple degassing with helium can be obtained by comparison with commercially available standard calibration gas mixtures (Phase Separations Ltd, Deeside Industrial Estate, Queensferry, Clwyd). Using a sample loop, an aliquot of the headspace gas can be compared with the gas-chromatography trace of the standard gas mixture.

An alternative procedure when Tenax GC is used as the gas-chromatography column packing material with a helium carrier gas is as follows. The column temperature is lowered to about 20 °C. A 1-ml sample of blood placed in a 6-ml hypovial is warmed to 60 °C for 45 min. Three or four 500-μl aliquots of headspace gas can be injected sequentially on to the column. The start of the column will trap volatile materials and allow air to be carried through, so concentrating the volatile components. By ballistically programming the gas chromatograph to 80 °C and then increasing the column temperature at 5 °C per minute, a profile of the organic volatile components in the blood sample will be obtained. This technique is useful for the identification of low levels of solvents by the use of a gas chromatograph linked to a mass spectrometer.

A rigorous degassing procedure for the detection of low levels of volatiles in blood samples prior to mass spectrometry using a cold trap has been described (Anderson *et al.*, 1979). This method is described in full in the chapter entitled 'Fire Death Investigation'.

At the levels of solvents found in abusers, it is seldom necessary to resort to detection techniques other than simple headspace analysis.

4.7 INTERPRETATION

In a study of workmen exposed to toluene in the factory environment where the maximum allowable concentration in the atmosphere in 200 p.p.m., the blood concentrations of the solvent ranged up to 0.25 $\mu g\ ml^{-1}$ except in two cases where exposure was known to have exceeded the threshold limit value. In both instances, the blood concentrations were below 0.4 $\mu g\ ml^{-1}$. In all cases, blood samples were taken within one hour of removal from the contaminated area. A study of solvent abusers has shown that blood toluene levels between 0.4 and 1.0 $\mu g\ ml^{-1}$ gave rise to little more than the smell of solvent on the breath. Between 1.0 and 2.5 $\mu g\ ml^{-1}$ there was an increase in the number of abusers showing symptoms of intoxication. Fifty per cent of all abusers studied with blood toluene levels between 2.5 and 10 $\mu g\ ml^{-1}$ were sufficiently ill to be hospitalised. They showed marked intoxication and some reported hallucinations (Lush *et al.*, 1980). Except in one instance, where the driver was reported in court by the police surgeon to be asymptomatic, with a blood toluene level of 10.5 $\mu g\ ml^{-1}$, all abusers with blood toluene levels above 10 $\mu g\ ml^{-1}$ were either unconscious or deceased at the time of sampling.

The latter statement requires to be put into perspective. Death is more likely to occur as a result of being intoxicated by toluene than from direct poisoning by the solvent. This is shown in Table 4.2, which lists toluene levels measured in fatalities involving abusers.

Table 4.2 Toluene-related fatalities

Case No.	Solvent	Concentration in blood ($\mu g\ ml^{-1}$)	Cause of death
1	toluene	0.14	inhalation of gastric contents
2	toluene	0.13	multiple injuries (fall)
3	toluene	2.1	multiple injuries (walked into a train)
4	toluene	14.3	drowning
5	toluene	15.0	drowning
6	toluene	52.0	hanging
7	toluene	39.6	hanging
8	toluene	0.53	myocytolysis

The toluene levels show that the deceased in cases 1 and 2 were unlikely to be impaired at the time of their deaths. In both instances, exposure to toluene within forty-eight hours prior to their deaths was confirmed by witnesses. Cases 3, 4 and 5 are examples of death occurring while the individual was under the influence of toluene. In one of the drowning cases, fellow glue-sniffers attempted to lead the police away from the scene of possible rescue in the belief that the deceased would get into trouble for glue sniffing.

Cases 6 and 7 were solvent abusers who, under the influence of very high levels of toluene, were still capable of placing ligatures round their necks. In case 7, this was known to have happened following the sniffing session. In either case, death may have been accidental or suicidal. It is possible that unconsciousness or loss of foothold occurred while trying to achieve a partial anoxia to enhance the effect of the solvent. Alternatively, death may have been suicidal as a result of a depressant effect on the individual following a 'buzz' with the solvent.

Case 8 presented in hospital following collapse into unconsciousness. The patient did not regain consciousness and died within a few hours of admission. He was a known solvent abuser. At post-mortem the major finding was a giant cell myocarditis. Although there is no known link with his solvent abuse, the possibility remains.

Table 4.3 lists the causes of death and the blood levels found following exposure to halogenated solvents.

Table 4.3 Halogenated-solvent-related fatalities

Case No.	Solvent	Concentration in blood ($\mu g\ ml^{-1}$)	Cause of death
1	nitrous oxide halothane	2.1 73.9	abuse of anaesthetic gases
2	trichloroethane dichloromethane	1.02 2.3	solvent abuse (glue)
3	trichloroethane	1.3	aspiration of vomit
4	trichloroethane	0.24	solvent abuse (cleaning fluid)
5	trichloroethylene	3.1	industrial accident
6	trichloroethylene	5.9	industrial accident

Case 1 was a straightforward one of the medical technician abusing anaesthetic gases.

The toxicology of 1,1,1-trichloroethane has been reviewed in detail (Torkelson, 1958; Stewart, 1963 and 1968). On the basis of anaesthetic data it has been estimated that a trichloroethane blood level of 10-15 $\mu g\ ml^{-1}$ is required before a person will be overcome. However, a report of six fatal cases includes one with a trichloroethane blood level as low as 1.5 $\mu g\ ml^{-1}$. From the high lactic-acid concentration in the brain, it was concluded that this man died mainly from oxygen deprivation (Stahl *et al.*, 1969).

Case 2 involved the misuse of an impact adhesive which used trichoroethane and dichloromethane as solvents. The levels are of similar magnitude to those found in the above case. In addition there are similar levels of dichloromethane.

The deceased was found slumped in the corner of a room; there was no evidence of violence. Two tins of glue found near the locus were found to contain 1,1,1-trichloroethane and dichloromethane as the major solvents. Since no polythene bag was involved, it was concluded that death occurred as a direct result of poisoning by the solvent.

Case 3 involved the misuse of a proprietary brand of cleaning fluid containing 1,1,1-trichloroethane. The deceased was found head-down on his bed with a solvent-impregnated pad of cloth over his nose and mouth. The only significant post-mortem finding was the aspiration of vomit.

In Case 4 the trichloroethane blood level was even lower at 0.24 μg ml^{-1}. This young man was in the open together with a bottle of 1,1,1-trichloroethane dry-cleaning fluid. No information was given as to whether or not a polythene bag was involved. Death may have occurred as a result of asphyxia or ventricular fibrillation.

Cases 5 and 6 were industrial accidents where two workmen with high blood alcohol contents were in charge of a drum of degreasing fluid. In an already intoxicated state, they exposed themselves to trichloroethylene, a powerful narcotic and anaesthetic (Mitchell and Parsons-Smith, 1969). The levels found are similar to those recorded in the literature for other fatalities (Alha *et al.*, 1974b; Bell, 1951).

Table 4.4 records fuel-gas levels measured following abuse. Cases 1 and 2 were deaths from the direct inhalation of lighter fuel causing freezing injuries which produced laryngeal oedema. At the post-mortem, both lungs showed severe oedema. Cases 3, 4, 5 and 6 were simple asphyxial deaths. Cases 7 and 8 were deaths immediately following sniffing sessions. Both are possible cases of death

Table 4.4 Fuel-gas-related fatalities

Case No.	Solvent	Concentration in blood (μg ml^{-1})	Cause of death
1	butane	present	asphyxia
2	butane	present	asphyxia
3	propane	14.5	asphyxia (industrial cylinder and plastic bag)
4	butane propane	1.12 0.86	asphyxia (lighter fuel and plastic bag)
5	butane propane	3.2 1.0	asphyxia (lighter fuel and plastic bag)
6	butane propane	53.0 44.2	asphyxia (plastic bag and lighter fuel)
7	butane	3.5	see text
8	butane	1.0	see text

resulting from cardiac arrhythmia since both were engaged in strenuous activity at the time of death. One fled from the scene, collapsed, and was dead on admission to hospital.

REFERENCES

Alha, A., Korte, T., and Naeminen, R. (1974a). Personal communication, reported in Watson, J. M. (1979).

Alha, A., Korte, T., and Naeminen, R. (1974b). Personal communication. *Bull. Int. Assn Forens. Toxicol.* **10.1**, 14-15.

Allister, C., Lush, M., Oliver, J. S., and Watson, J. M. (1981). Status epilepticus caused by solvent abuse. *Br. Med. J.* **283**, 1156.

Anderson, H. R., Dick, D., Macnair, R. S., Palmer, J. C., and Ramsey, J. D. (1982). An investigation of 140 deaths associated with volatile substance abuse in the United Kingdom (1971-1981). *Human Toxicol.* **1**, 207-21.

Anderson, R. A., Thomson, I., and Harland, W. A. (1979). The importance of cyanide and organic nitriles in fire fatalities. *Fire Mater.* **32**, 91-9.

Anthony, R. M., Bost, R. O., Thompson, W. L., and Sunshine, I. (1978). Paraldehyde, toluene and methylene chloride analysis by headspace gas chromatography. *J. Analyt. Toxicol.* **2**, 262-4.

Bass, M. (1970). Sudden sniffing death. *J. Amer. Med. Assn* **212**, 2075-80.

Bell, A., (1951). Death from trichloroethylene in a drycleaning establishment. *New Zeal. Med. J.* **50**, 119-26.

Blackmore, D. J. (1970). The determination of carbon monoxide in blood and tissue. *Analyst* **95**, 439-58.

Boor, J. W., and Hurtig. H. I. (1977). Permanent cerebellar atoxia after exposure to toluene. *Ann. Neurol.* **2**, 440-2.

Clark, D. G., and Tinston, (1982). Acute inhalation toxicity of some halogenated and non-halogenated hydrocarbons. *Human Toxicol.* **1**, 239-47.

Cohen, S. The volatile solvents. *Publ. Hlth Rev.* **2**, 185-214.

Edh, M., Selerud, A., and Sjoberg, C. (1973). Death and sniffing. A report on 63 cases. *Lakartidningen* **70**, 3949-59.

Grabski, D. A. (1961). Toluene sniffing producing cerebellar degeneration. *Amer. J. Psychiatry* **118**, 461-2.

Kelly, T. W. (1975). Prolonged cerebellar dysfunction associated with paint sniffing. *Paediatrics* **56**, 605-6.

King, M. D., Day, R. E., Oliver, J. S., Lush, M., and Watson, J. M. (1981). Solvent encephalopathy. *Br. Med. J.* **283**, 663-5.

Knox, J. W., and Nelson, J. R. (1966). Permanent encephalopathy from toluene inhalation. *New Engl. J. Med.* **275**, 1494-6.

Kringsholm, B. (1980). Sniffing–associated deaths in Denmark. *Forens. Sci. Internat.* **15**, 215-25.

Lush, M., Oliver, J. S., and Watson, J. M. (1980). The analysis of blood in cases of solvent or suspected solvent abuse, with a review of results during the period of October 1977 to July 1979. In Oliver J. S. (ed.), *Forensic Toxicology*. Croom Helm, London, pp. 304-23.

Mitchell, A. B. S., and Parsons-Smith, B. G. (1969). Trichloroethylene neuropathy. *Br. Med. J.* i, 422-3.

O'Brien, E. T., Yeoman, W. B., and Hobby, J. A. E. (1971). Hepatorenal damage from toluene in a glue-sniffer. *Ibid.*, **ii**, 29-30.

Oliver, J. S. (1982). The analytical diagnosis of solvent abuse. *Human Toxicol.* **1**, 293-7.

Oliver, J. S. (1983). The investigation of solvent abuse deaths. *J. Foren. Sci. Soc.* **23.3**, 247-9.

Oliver, J. S., and Watson, J. M. (1977). Abuse of solvents 'for kicks'. *The Lancet* 8.1.77, 84-86.

Ramsey, J. D. and Flanagan, R. J. (1982). The role of the laboratory in the investigation of solvent abuse. *Human Toxicol.* **1**, 299–11.

Reisen, E., Teicher, A., Jaffe, R., and Eliahou, H. E. (1975). Myoglobinuria and renal failure in toluene poisoning. *Br. J. Industr. Med.* **32**, 163–4.

Stahl, C. J., Fatteh, A. V. , and Dominguez A. N. (1969). Trichloroethane poisoning: Observations on the pathology and toxicology in six fatal cases. *J. Forens. Sci.* **14.3**, 393–7.

Stewart, R. D. (1963). The toxicology of methyl chloroform. *J. Occup. Hyg. Med.* **5**, 259–62.

Stewart, R. D. (1968). The toxicology of 111-trichloroethane. *Ann. Occup. Hyg.* **11**, 71–9.

Taylor, G. J., and Harris, W. S. (1970). Glue-sniffing causes heart block in mice. *Science* **170**, 866–8.

Torkelson, S. O., Oyen, S., McCollister, D. D., and Rowe, V. K. (1958). Toxicity of 111-trichloroethane as determined on laboratory animals and human subjects. *Amer. Industr. Hyg. Assn J.* **19**, 353–62.

Venkataraman, G. (1981). Renal damage and glue sniffing. *Br. Med. J.* **283**, 1467.

Watson, J. M. (1978). Clinical and laboratory investigations in 132 cases of solvent abuse. *Med. Sci. Law* **18.1**, 40–3.

Watson, J. M. (1979). Morbidity and mortality statistics on solvent abuse. *Ibid.* **19.4**, 246–52.

Watson, J. M. (1982). Solvent abuse: presentation and clinical diagnosis. *Human Toxicol.* **1**, 249–56.

Will, A. M., and McLaren, E. H. (1981). Reversible renal damage due to glue sniffing. *Br. Med. J.* **283**, 525–6.

5
Mass spectrometry

L. V. JONES

5.1 INTRODUCTION

As long ago as 1913 Sir J. J. Thomson had proposed the use of mass spectrometry for chemical analysis (Thomson, 1913). While much of the development of that application has been financed by the oil industry, developments over the last two decades have meant that it has been in the biomedical fields that the greater benefits have been reaped. The single most important development has been the production of viable interfaces to connect gas chromatographs to mass spectrometers but developments in methods of ionisation, high-pressure liquid-chromatography interfacing and sophisticated use of double-focusing instruments have broadened the scope of the technique considerably.

Mass spectrometry involves the production of ions from a compound and the subsequent measurement of the mass/charge ratios and relative abundances of those ions. The resulting spectrum is usually presented as the familiar bar-graph of relative abundances (% int) plotted against mass/charge ratio (*m/e*) (Figure 5.1). The spectrum can provide a characteristic 'fingerprint' of a molecule and can also be understood and predicted with a knowledge of a compound's structure. Organic toxicology is usually concerned with aromatic molecules of very varied structures which can be expected to yield distinctive spectra. Thus mass spectrometry offers the toxicologist a technique of invaluable specificity and sensitivity.

The early work of Aston (1933) showed that the various isotopes of elements do not have integral mass—they are not simple multiples of a fundamental unit; thus accurate measurement of mass/charge ratios can yield unambiguous elemental formulae for an ion.

The essential elements of any mass spectrometer system are shown in Figure 5.2. Each element of that system is discussed separately below.

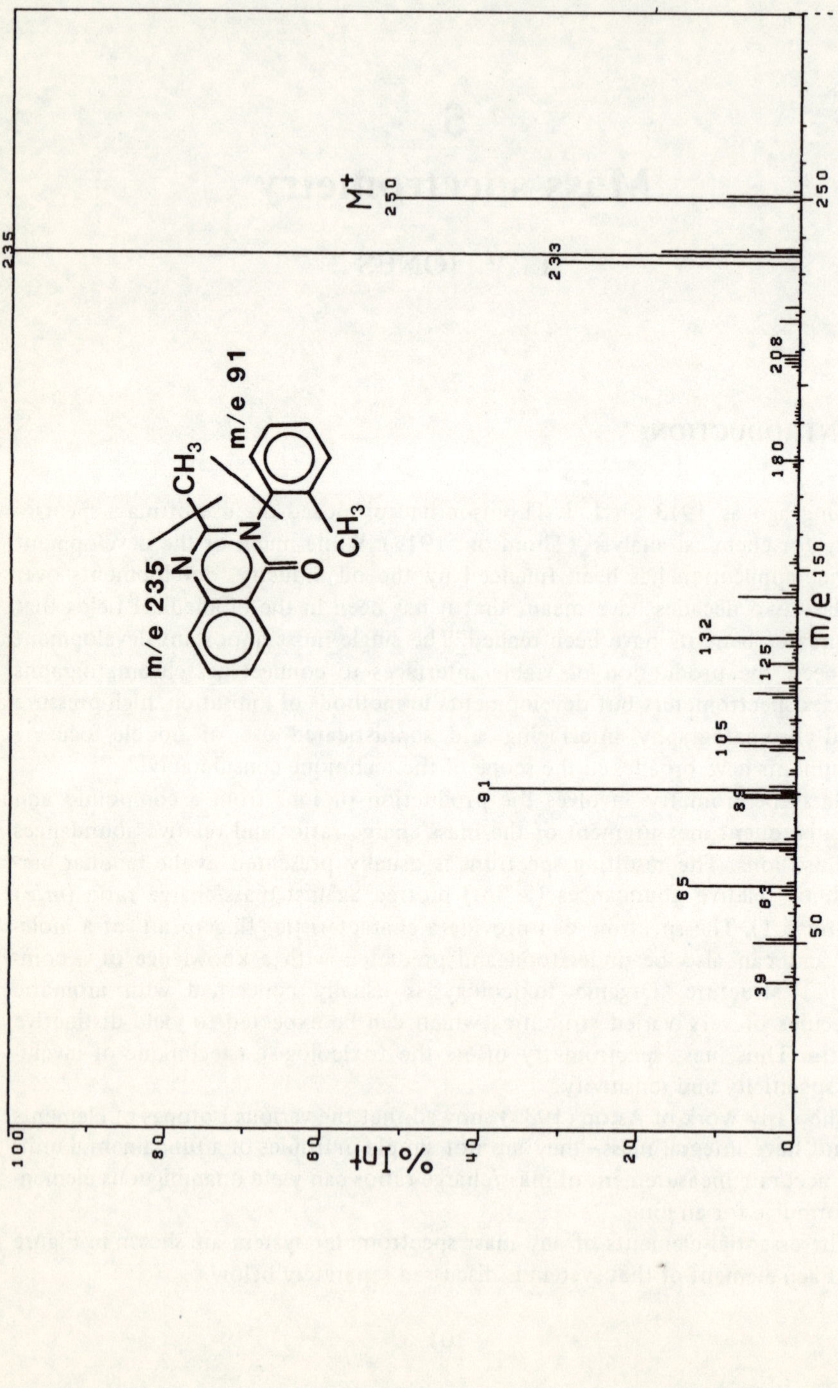

Figure 5.1 GC–EI mass spectrum of methaqualone.

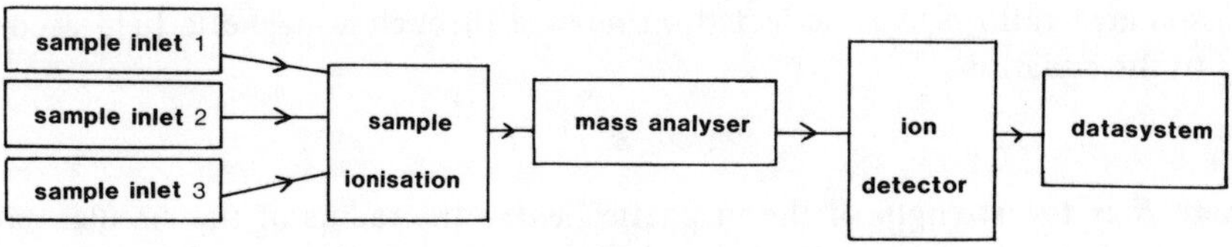

Figure 5.2 Schematic of mass spectrometer.

5.2 MASS ANALYSER

5.2.1 Types of instruments

Mass spectrometers may be grouped according to the method of mass analysis that they use. Many designs, operating on a wide range of principles, have been adopted for the analyses of mass spectra (Knewstubb, 1969). The three used most commonly in toxicology are both magnetic-sector and quadrupole low-resolution instruments, and high-resolution double-focusing instruments.

Low-resolution spectrometers yield spectra calibrated to the nearest whole mass, or mass ranges of 1000 or 2000 a.m.u., requiring a resolution of up to 2000 to achieve this. The resolution of an instrument is defined somewhat differently for different types of instrument, but basically measures the ability to resolve ions differing by unit mass and an instrument operating at a resolution of 1000 would resolve ions of masses up to 1000 a.m.u. to a predefined standard.

5.2.2 Magnetic-sector instruments

A beam of ions is accelerated from an ion source through several kilovolts and thence through a magnetic field to a detector (Figure 5.3). A beam of ions of

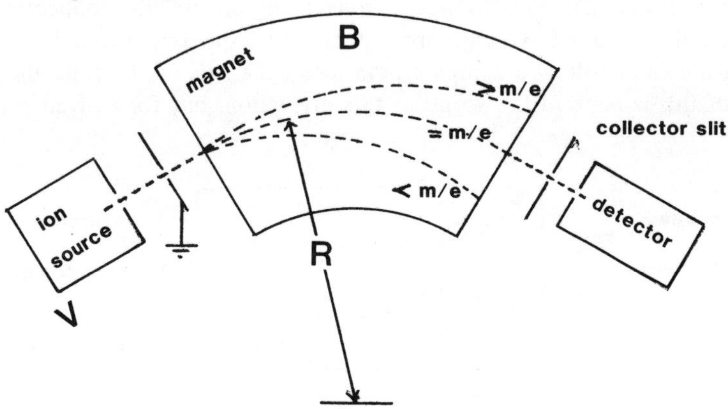

Figure 5.3 Schematic of magnetic-sector single-focusing mass spectrometer.

mass/charge ratio m/e is deflected on passage through a magnetic field according to the equation

$$m/e = B^2r^2/2V$$

where B is the strength of the magnetic field, r the radius of the circular path into which the ions are deflected and V the voltage in volts used to accelerate the ions out of the ion source. Ions are usually detected in a device such as an electron-multiplier tube, placed behind a narrow slit through which the ions must pass. A spectrum is produced by scanning the magnetic field so that ions of successive m/e value achieve the correct path through the collector slit, the accelerating voltage being kept constant. Alternatively, the magnetic field can be held constant and the accelerating voltage scanned, but this method is not commonly used, as sensitivity decreases with decreasing accelerating voltage and the important high-mass end of a spectrum would be recorded at considerably reduced sensitivity. The resulting spectra are of the form of intensity plotted against m/e value and not mass–and while most ions detected will be singly charged, low-intensity doubly charged ions are often seen appearing at half the expected mass of the ion. In fact, magnetic sector instruments analyse on the basis of momentum/charge rather than mass/charge; the result only approximates to a mass analysis in so far as all the ions are given the same kinetic energy on acceleration, the extent to which this is the case being a major limitation of the resolution of the instrument. The common electron-impact source (see below) yields a sufficiently monoenergetic beam of ions for moderate resolution, but other sources such as field-desorption and fast-atom-bombardment sources may not.

5.2.3 Quadrupole mass filter

This is truly a mass analyser (Figure 5.4; Dawson, 1976). The filter takes the form of four parallel rods–opposite rods being electrically connected and a combined d.c. and r.f. voltage applied between the two pairs. Ions passing through the filter follow a complex path along the axis of the rods; the mathematics of this is beyond the scope of this discussion, but for a given combined

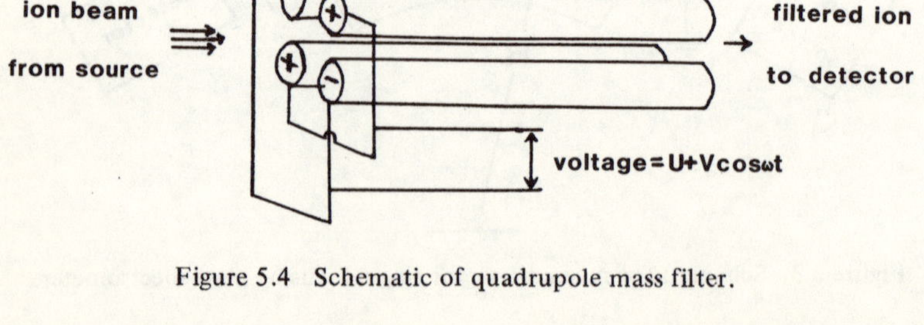

Figure 5.4 Schematic of quadrupole mass filter.

voltage only ions in a small-mass window have a stable path between the rods. A mass spectrum is obtained by sweeping the voltages at a constant r.f.–d.c. ratio.

Until recently quadrupoles gave rather poorer performance in terms of resolution and sensitivity than did magnetic-sector instruments, but now this deficiency has been remedied they are finding increasing application, offering as they do some advantages over magnetic-sector instruments. Because they are mass analysers they tolerate a spread of energy in the ion beam. They are also tolerant of higher source-pressures because high accelerating voltages are not needed; however, pressures must still be low enough to preclude collision between species in the analyser. They have the potential to scan spectra at very high rate, but in practice are limited to scanning just a little faster than magnetic instruments, by the rate at which the data system can operate. Perhaps their greatest advantage lies in the ability to switch quickly and easily from monitoring one particular chosen ion to another in selected-ion monitoring—a technique used to provide selective and sensitive detection of a particular compound (see below). This can be achieved easily over the whole mass range, as only voltages have to be changed. Similar experiments are usually performed on magnetic instruments by keeping the magnetic field constant and switching between precalculated accelerating voltages to bring different ions to detection; however, it is not recommended to scan more than 10 to 20% away from the highest mass, otherwise serious loss of sensitivity at high mass will be experienced. It is possible to change the magnetic field keeping the accelerating voltage constant, but hysteresis effects in the magnet preclude fast cycling times and make accurate detection of a mass difficult to achieve.

Both magnetic-sector and quadrupole mass spectrometers are in widespread and routine use in toxicological laboratories. Spectra calibrated to nominal mass are used to fingerprint compounds of interest to a high degree of specificity.

5.2.4 Double-focusing instruments

These use two analysing fields to measure m/e ratios to a high precision (Figure 5.5). An energy-focusing electrostatic analyser is used to provide a more nearly monoenergetic beam of ions for analysis in a magnetic sector, resolutions of over 100 000 being thus attainable. At such resolutions, the deviation of atomic and molecular masses from integral values are accurately measurable, peaks which appear simple under low resolution may be revealed as multiplets, and unambiguous assignments of elemental formulae are possible. This facility can be used as an aid to the interpretation of unknown spectra where no reference material is available (Ehrenthal and Pfleger, 1977), or to detect ions of specific elemental composition in complex mixtures (Facchetti *et al.*, 1979).

The higher resolution gained over a single-focusing magnetic-sector instrument is made at the expense of sensitivity, because only a limited number of

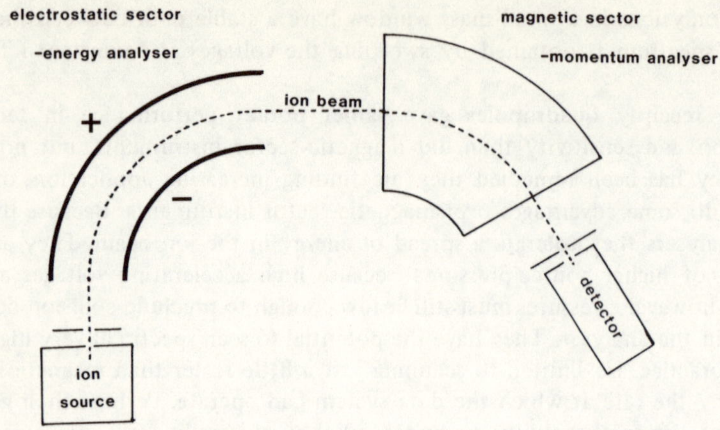

Figure 5.5 Schematic of double-focusing mass spectrometer (Nier–Johnson geometry).

ions in a narrower energy-band are analysed. However, double-focusing instruments can be detuned to a required extent, compromising resolution and sensitivity for a given application.

Reversed-geometry instruments are constructed such that the magnetic sector analyses the ion beam before the electrostatic sector. Such an instrument can be used to perform MIKES (*m*ass-*a*nalysed *k*inetic-*e*nergy *s*pectra) experiments. An ion is selected for continuous monitoring by the magnetic sector and thus isolated from all other ions produced in the source. In the field-free region between the two analysers that ion may fragment or be induced to fragment by passing it through a collisional activation chamber containing an inert reagent gas. The resulting fragments will have the same velocity as the parent ion, so that their kinetic energies relative to the parent ion will be in proportion to their masses. Subsequent scanning of electrostatic analyser will scan kinetic energy and yield a mass spectrum of the selected ion. In this way the fragmentation pattern of a fragment may be observed, enabling identification of that species as an aid to identification of the whole molecule (Bozorgzadeh *et al*., 1978). Alternatively, possible molecular species may be observed from a mixture to yield a simple spectrum of one component. This technique has been applied to the direct analyses of drugs in mixtures such as opiates in crude plant material (Kondrat and Cooks, 1978).

Equivalent experiments are possible on instruments of conventional geometry, and are termed linked-scan experiments (Boyd and Beynon, 1977; Millington and Smith, 1977). In this technique, fragments of a selected ion are collected by scanning both the magnetic (***B***) and electrostatic (***E***) field strengths simultaneously so that the ratio $\boldsymbol{B/E}$ is kept constant. Similarly a scan with $\boldsymbol{B^2/E}$ kept constant yields all precursor ions giving rise to a selected fragment ion.

Interest in techniques such as these, which essentially use mass spectrometry as the separation technique as well as the analytical technique, has prompted manufacturers to offer tandem spectrometers with such combinations of analysers as electrostatic-magnetic-quadrupole and quadrupole-quadrupole (McLafferty and Lory, 1981).

5.3 DATA SYSTEM

A computerised data system (Chapman, 1978) is now considered an essential part of any GC–MS setup. A basic data system provides for the collection, storage and calibration of spectra. The calibration process involves establishing a scan law relating mass to a variable, measuring peak position. The scan law is derived by running the spectrum of a calibration compound and relating the known masses of the ions to the measured peak-position data. The peak-position data may be time of arrival of ion in a reproducible scan, or Hall probe measurement of magnetic field for a magnetic-sector instrument, or it may be a measure of rod voltage for a quadrupole instrument. Subsequent unknown spectra are then calibrated by reference to the derived scan law. Spectra may be collected and calibrated at rates as fast as a fraction of a second per spectrum—this facility permits complicated capillary GC runs to be readily dealt with and may permit mass-spectral resolution of poorly resolved peaks for a packed-column GC. A data system will then permit various manipulations of previously acquired data, including the following.

1. Textual or graphical output of individual spectra, usually with ion intensities normalised to that of the strongest ion in the spectrum.
2. Subtraction of spectra, permitting removal of background ions or the spectra of interfering compounds.
3. Plotting of total-ion currents. That is, plotting the number of ions produced in the source, which is a measure of the amount of material in the source, against time. The resulting plot is usually closely similar to a GC flame-ionisation detector plot.
4. Plotting of individual ion intensities through a GC run, which may prove the presence of an expected component at low level at the expected retention time, or may help in the resolution of GC components.
5. Provision for the comparison of unknown spectra with a library of spectra held on the computer. That library may be a commercially available general library such as the National Bureau of Standards (NBS) Library in the USA, which currently contains over thirty thousand entries, or it may be a specialised library compiled by the user to suit his own needs, such as the library compiled for use in the British Home Office Forensic Science Service (Allan *et al.*, 1982) which contains over three thousand spectra, mainly of drugs and pesticides.
6. Heuristic interpretation. Computer programs have been developed by which

the computer interprets spectra from first principles as a trained spectroscopist might, taking into account such aspects of the spectrum as isotope patterns, neutral losses, previous experience of similar compounds and also other available chemical data (McLafferty and Venkataraghavan, 1979).

7. Computer methods for accurate mass-determination at low resolution have developed. (Powers *et al*., 1978). These methods rely on reproducibility been of peak shape at low resolution to accurately centroid unknown peaks with reference to peaks from a calibration compound. The methods were developed for use on detuned double-focusing instruments for capillary-column GC–MS where fast scan rates employed are incompatible with high-resolution techniques, but they can also be used with success on low-resolution magnetic-sector and quadrupole instruments.

5.4 INLET

In order that mass/charge ratios be measured, mass separation must be achieved in the spectrometer without collision between species. To prevent such collisions, mass spectrometers are kept at low pressure by vacuum pumping systems. Any sample inlet system must then allow introduction of a sample without loss of this vacuum. If the inlet system incorporates a separation technique such as gas or liquid chromatography then the integrity of that system should also be maintained.

5.4.1 Direct

Samples may be introduced directly into the ion source of the spectrometer. Liquids can be injected into a heated reservoir where they evaporate, the vapour being leaked slowly into the ion source for analysis. For solids a direct-insertion probe may be used. Micrograms or less of the solid are deposited directly, or evaporated from solution into a disposable glass probe-tip. The probe is introduced into the mass spectrometer via a system of vacuum locks with seals against the probe shaft. The tip is pushed home into the ion source, where the sample vaporises–heated either by the source itself or by a heater built into the probe.

Direct probe-insertion of samples has several advantages. Sample throughput is quick and there is little opportunity for breakdown to occur; involatile, polar and thermally labile compounds which are not suitable for GC introduction can be dealt with. Figure 5.6 shows the structures of didesethylflurazepam, a metabolite of flurazepam, and its dehydration product (Clatworthy *et al.*, 1977). Spectra of the metabolite obtained by probe insertion and GC introduction differed markedly, the probe spectrum being consistent with the structure of the metabolite. It was seen that while a well-shaped peak was obtained for the compound by GC, it had undergone degradation on column and the spectrum

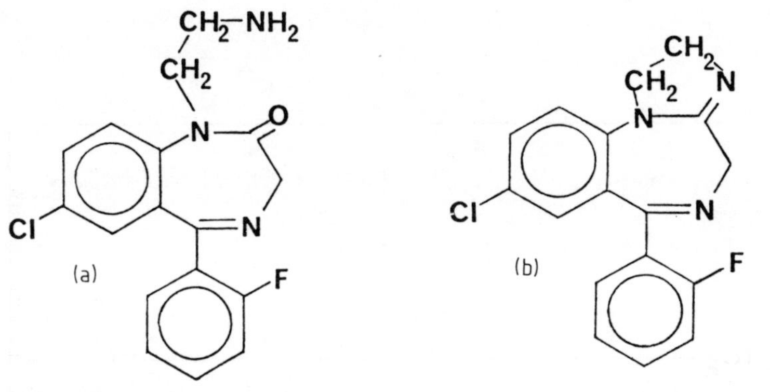

Figure 5.6 (a) Structure of didesethylfluorazepam and (b) structure of didesethylflurazepam GC dehydration product.

obtained was that not of the original compound but of its dehydration product. Of course the limitation of probe insertion is that mixtures are not resolved and so it is difficult to deal with samples of more than one or two components. Chemical ionisation (see below) has been used in conjunction with probe insertion to simplify the spectra of mixtures–ideally only a quasimolecular ion for each component present is seen. This approach is useful where only a limited range of known compounds is expected, so that molecular weight information is adequate for identification and has been used to identify five major alkaloids in opium (Zitrin and Yinon, 1977). Figure 5.7 shows such a chemical ionisation probe spectrum of a crude opium. Protonated molecular ions are seen for: papaverine (*m/e* 340), thebaine (*m/e* 312), codeine (*m/e* 300), a weak morphine (*m/e* 286) and meconine (*m/e*195). However, the spectrum still shows fragmentation, the ion *m/e* 220 being from narcotine and the two ions *m/e* 268 and 282 being formed by loss of water from the protonated molecular species of morphine and codeine respectively.

As mentioned above, MIKES and linked-scan experiments on double-focusing instruments can be used to yield full spectra of each component in a complex mixture inserted by probe.

5.4.2 Gas chromatography (GC)

The pressure difference between the outlet of a gas chromatograph (1 atm) and the mass-spectrometer ion source (10^{-6} torr) requires a pressure reduction system, which transfers the effluent from the gas chromatograph to the ionisation chamber. Three basic systems are used in GC-MS: direct connection, effluent split and molecular separation. (McFadden, 1973 and 1979.)

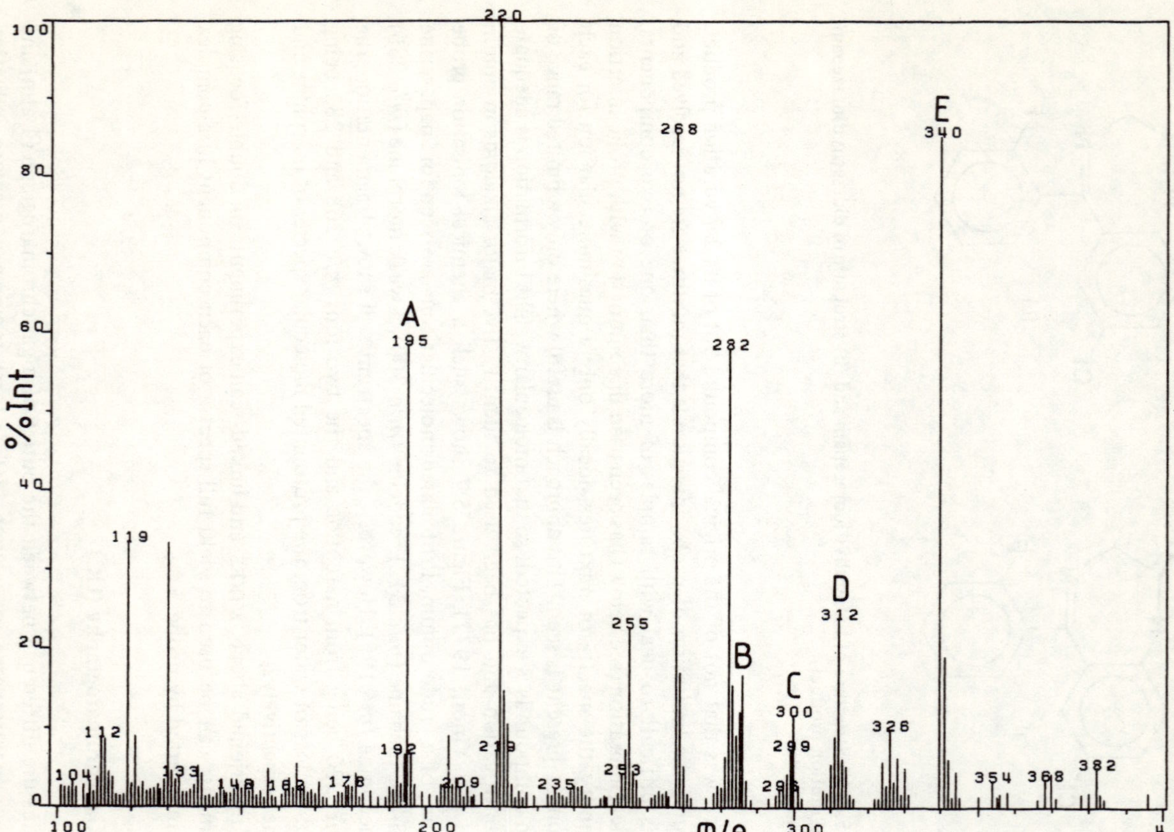

Figure 5.7 Probe/CI (isobutane) mass spectrum of a crude-opium sample showing $(M + H)^+$ ions for A, meconine; B, morphine, C, codeine, D, thebaine; E, papaverine.

5.4.2.1 Direct connection

Modern mass spectrometers have efficient differentially pumped systems—which maintain the analyser at a lower pressure than the ion source by use of two independent pumps. Such a pumping system can cope with flows into the source of at least 2 std cm^3 min^{-1}, which allows the direct connection of capillary columns.

5.4.2.2 Effluent split

Reduction of gas flow can easily be achieved by a split of the GC effluent. An open split system has the advantage that the outlet of the chromatographic column is at atmospheric pressure, maintaining chromatographic integrity but with the consequent loss of over 90% of the sample. This loss of sensitivity makes the device unsuitable for toxicology.

5.4.2.3 Molecule separators

Several types of separator suitable for interfacing a packed-column chromatograph to a mass spectrometer have deen devised. That most commonly made available by spectrometer manufacturers is the Ryhage jet separator (Figure 5.8). In this device helium is pumped away from heavier sample molecules as

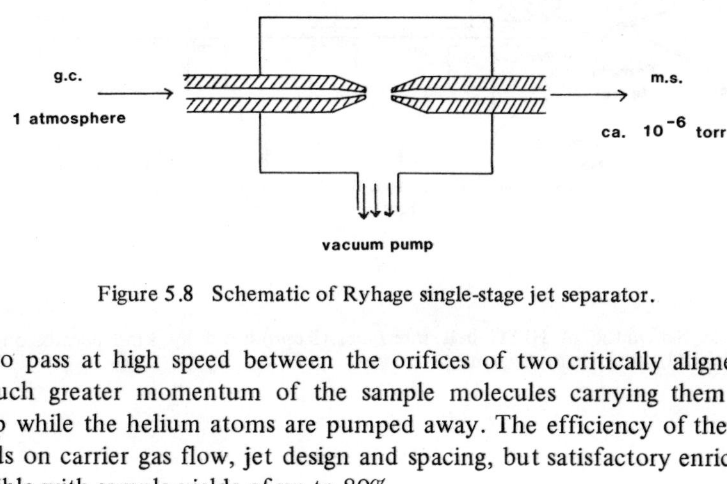

Figure 5.8 Schematic of Ryhage single-stage jet separator.

the two pass at high speed between the orifices of two critically aligned jets, the much greater momentum of the sample molecules carrying them across the gap while the helium atoms are pumped away. The efficiency of the device depends on carrier gas flow, jet design and spacing, but satisfactory enrichment is possible with sample yields of up to 80%.

5.4.3 Liquid chromatography (HPLC)

Since the establishment of GC–MS as a powerful analytical tool, much effort has been applied to the linking of liquid chromatographs to mass spectrometers

(McFadden, 1979). The combination appeals to the toxicologist and/or the spectroscopist who seeks a separation and inlet system for polar and thermally labile compounds—liquid chromatography would be ideal—while the liquid chromatographer has yet to find a universal detector. However, the problems to be overcome are considerably greater than for GC-MS. Liquid chromatography flows of 1 $cm^3\ min^{-1}$ of solvent would yield up to 1000 std $cm^3\ min^{-1}$ of vapour to be disposed of. To date several devices have been developed, two of which are available commercially.

5.4.3.1 Moving-belt interface

The moving-belt interface offered by Finnegan and VG Analytical (Figure 5.9) was developed (McFadden *et al*., 1976) from the moving-wire interface of Scott

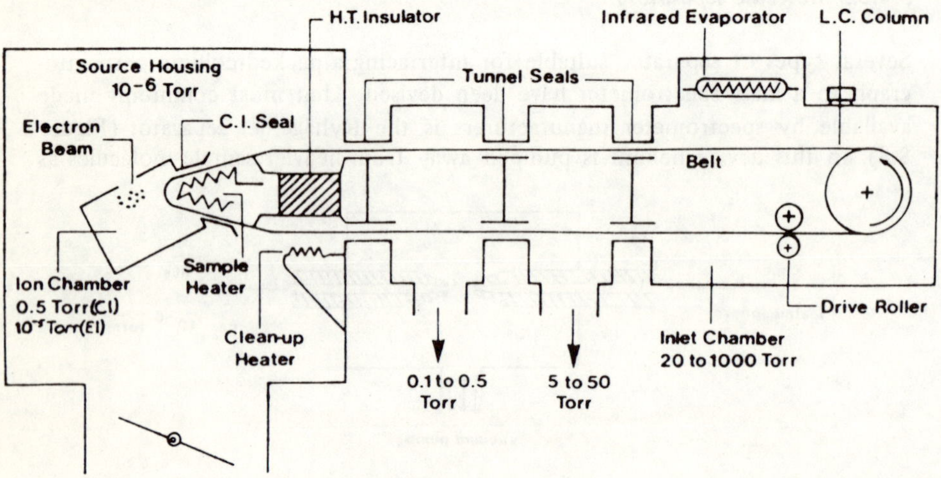

Figure 5.9 Schematic of HPLC belt interface. (Reproduced by kind permission of VG Analytical Ltd, Altrincham, England.)

(Scott *et al*., 1974). The HPLC eluent is fed onto a looped belt. The belt passes first under the infrared heater which evaporates the solvent and then through a series of vacuum chambers at decreasing pressures via tunnel seals around the belt. The belt passes into the mass-spectrometer source housing, where the sample residue is flash-heated off the belt and ionised in the ion source. The belt continues back through the vacuum chambers and over a clean-up heater to repeat the cycle. The system works well for some compounds and can provide a useful alternative to direct probe insertion: solutions of a sample can be injected onto the belt, and the flash heating of the sample into the ion source introduces the sample as a concentrated slug of vapour, giving greater sensitivity than conventional probe analysis. Polar solvents are difficult to deal with; it may be necessary to reduce belt speed or increase heating to facilitate evaporation of the solvent, which may result in decomposition of thermally labile compounds. Solvents of high water-content and gradient-eluted solvents are not easily dealt with. The method has been applied to the analysis of several drugs and pesticides with some success (Games, 1981).

5.4.3.2 Direct liquid introduction

The system offered by Hewlett Packard and Ribermag was developed from one devised by McLafferty and co-workers (Dawkins *et al.*, 1978). A fraction of the HPLC eluent is evaporated directly into the source through a fine-bore capillary. Chemical-ionisation (see below) spectra of the sample are observed with the solvent vapour acting as a reagent gas. The system will work well even for polar solvents, but does require adjustment of the capillary length with change in solvent; the interface can also block.

Neither system is ideal. The belt system is limiting on the HPLC system as to solvent used and can also show decomposition of thermally labile compounds, while direct liquid introduction gives only the molecular weight information available by chemical ionisation. This information, without fragmentation, is not always sufficient to make identifications in a general screen. The two systems complement each other and future instrumentation could include both as options, but development of these interfaces and others is still in its early stages; the next decade could see refinement of one of these or the emergence of some new device. Meanwhile, the development of microbore HPLC systems will ease the difficulties of interfacing liquid chromatographs and mass spectrometers.

While great difficulties are encountered in interfacing liquid chromatographs and mass spectrometers, sample collection is very easy for HPLC and many applications have appeared of 'off-line' collection of HPLC peaks for subsequent mass-spectral analysis. This approach has been used to analyse nonvolatile organic compounds in water using fraction collection and probe analysis (Crathorne *et al.*, 1979), and barbiturates from various biological samples using sample collection followed by field desorption ionisation (see below) (Schulten and Kummler, 1980). Good electron-impact spectra can readily be obtained from 200 ng of sample or less. Figure 5.10 shows the probe electron-impact spectrum of 200 ng of lorazepam. The sample was an HPLC eluent fraction, collected, freeze dried and redissolved in ethanol for evaporation into an MS probe tip, and was extracted from the blood of a man alleged to have been driving under the influence of lorazepam (Entwistle *et al.*, 1982).

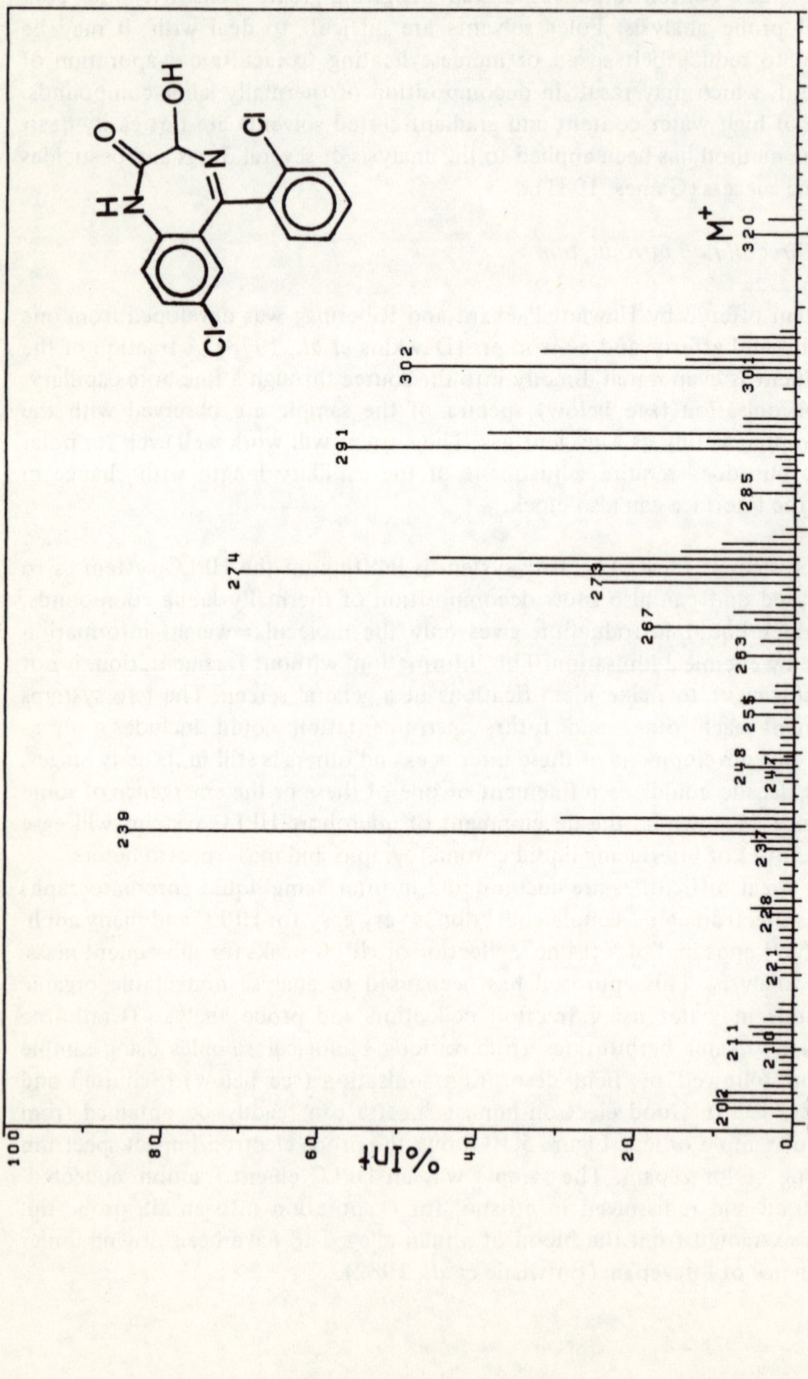

Figure 5.10 Probe/EI mass spectrum of lorazepam collected from HPLC.

5.5 IONISATION

In 1965 the only widely used method of ionising organic molecules in a mass spectrometer was electron impact. Now other ionisation methods are in common use and several are being developed (Jennings, 1980). Electron impact is still the mode most commonly used; the obtaining and interpretation of an electron-impact spectrum is usually the first approach to analysing a sample by mass spectrometry. Many authoritative works have been written on the interpretation of electron-impact spectra (McLafferty, 1973; Beynon *et al.*, 1968) and as mentioned elsewhere comprehensive libraries of electron-impact spectra are readily available. The uses and limitations of this and other modes are discussed below.

5.5.1 Electron-impact (EI)

Figure 5.11 shows a typical electron-impact source. A beam of electrons is drawn from a heated filament, F, into the ion source by a voltage, usually

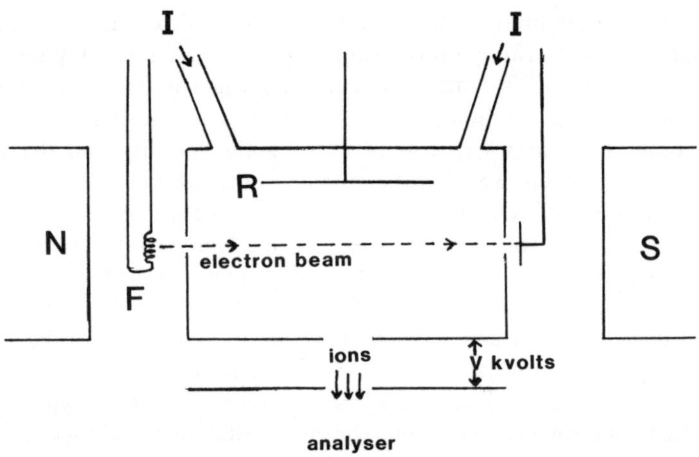

Figure 5.11 Schematic of electron-impact ion source.

70 V. Such an electron beam has an energy of 70 eV, which is in excess of the ionisation potentials of organic molecules, these lying typically between 10 and 20 eV. Sample vapour is admitted to the source from one of the inlet systems, I. Small source magnets, N, S, produce a field which causes the electrons to follow a tight helical path through the source. Collision between sample molecules and electrons in the beam result in ionisation of the sample in a well-defined region of the source. A small voltage on the repeller plate, R, causes

the produced ions to drift out of the source. Once through the source exit slit, the ions are accelerated through a strong electrostatic field into the mass analyser.

Radical anions, the molecular ion of the compound, are formed according to the process:

$$M + e \rightarrow M^{+\bullet} + 2e.$$

The excess of beam energy over ionisation potential will appear in the molecular ion as internal energy, which may fuel fragmentation of the molecular ion to produce positively charged and neutral fragments:

$$M^{+\bullet} \rightarrow A^{+} + B^{\bullet}$$

$$M^{+\bullet} \rightarrow A^{\bullet} + B^{+}$$

$$M^{+\bullet} \rightarrow C^{+} + D^{\bullet}$$

etc.

Further fragmentation of the fragments themselves also occurs in the source, prior to separation in the analyser.

The abundance of the fragments formed will depend on many factors, including the relative stabilities of the species formed, which may be stabilised by delocalisation. The resulting electron-input spectra are remarkably reproducible even between machines of different types, the fragmentation pattern obtained being characteristic of the molecule. For highly aromatic molecules the molecular ion and other high-mass ions are often of good intensity and the spectrum affords easy and conclusive identification, e.g. methaqualone (Figure 5.1). In some cases, however, fragmentation is so extensive that no molecular ion is seen. In the example of amitriptyline (Figure 5.12a), cleavage of the bond beta to the nitrogen group is highly favoured and yields a low-mass-base peak at *m/e* 58. The spectrum contains little other information to differentiate this spectrum from that of many other amines. Sometimes weak minor ions in the spectrum, or other analytical information such as GC retention time, can conclude the necessary differentiation, otherwise a 'softer' mode of ionisation which gives rise to less fragmentation may be used. The most established of these is chemical ionisation (Figure 5.12b).

5.5.2 Chemical ionisation (CI)

Chemical ionisation (Munson, 1977) uses a reagent gas; methane, isobutane, ammonia and water have all been used. The gas is introduced into the source at a pressure of about 1 torr ($\approx$ 133 Pa). The reagent gas is ionised by an electron beam to produce positive ions. When a sample is introduced into the source its molecules are ionised by reaction with the reagent gas ions. This ionisation occurs by transfer of either a positive charge or a charged fragment from the

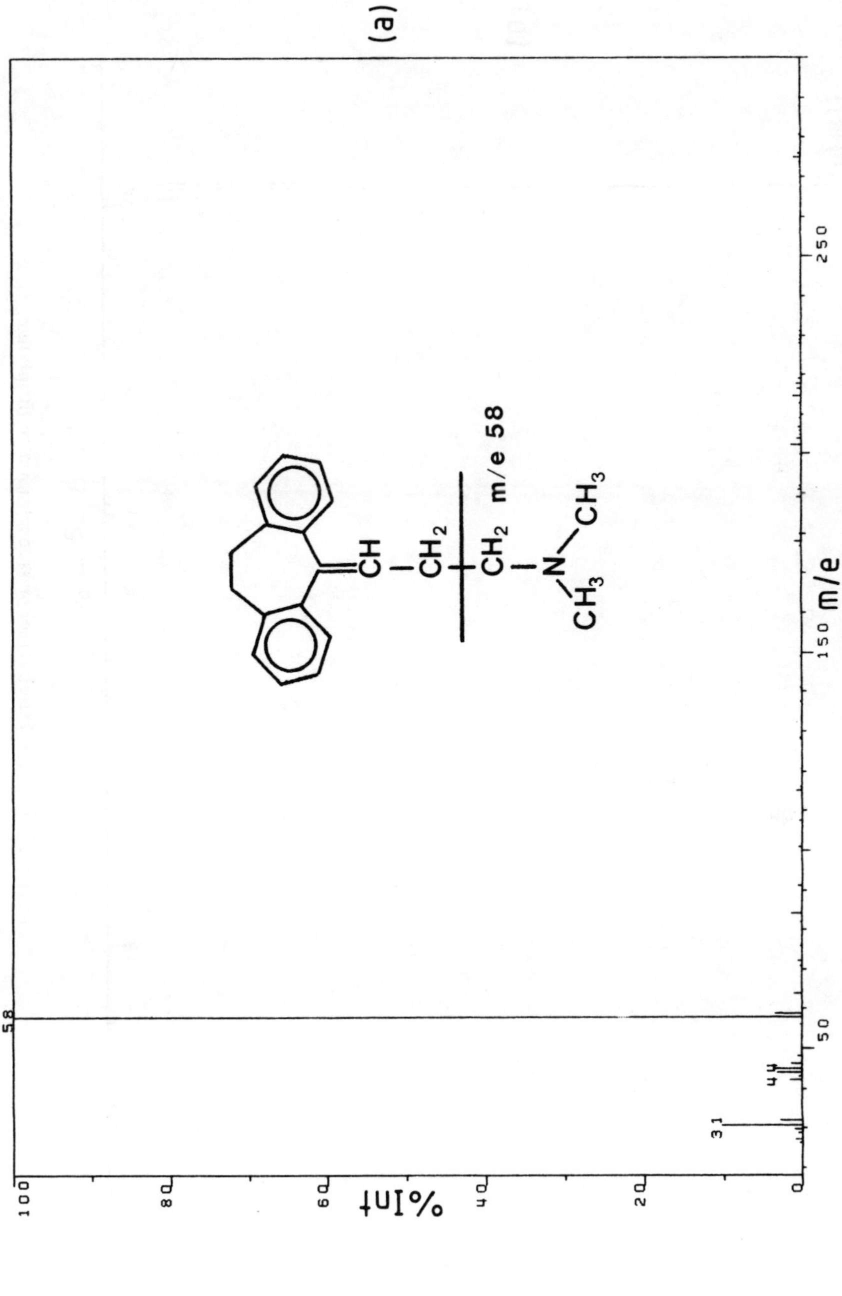

Figure 5.12(a) GC–EI mass spectrum of amitriptyline.

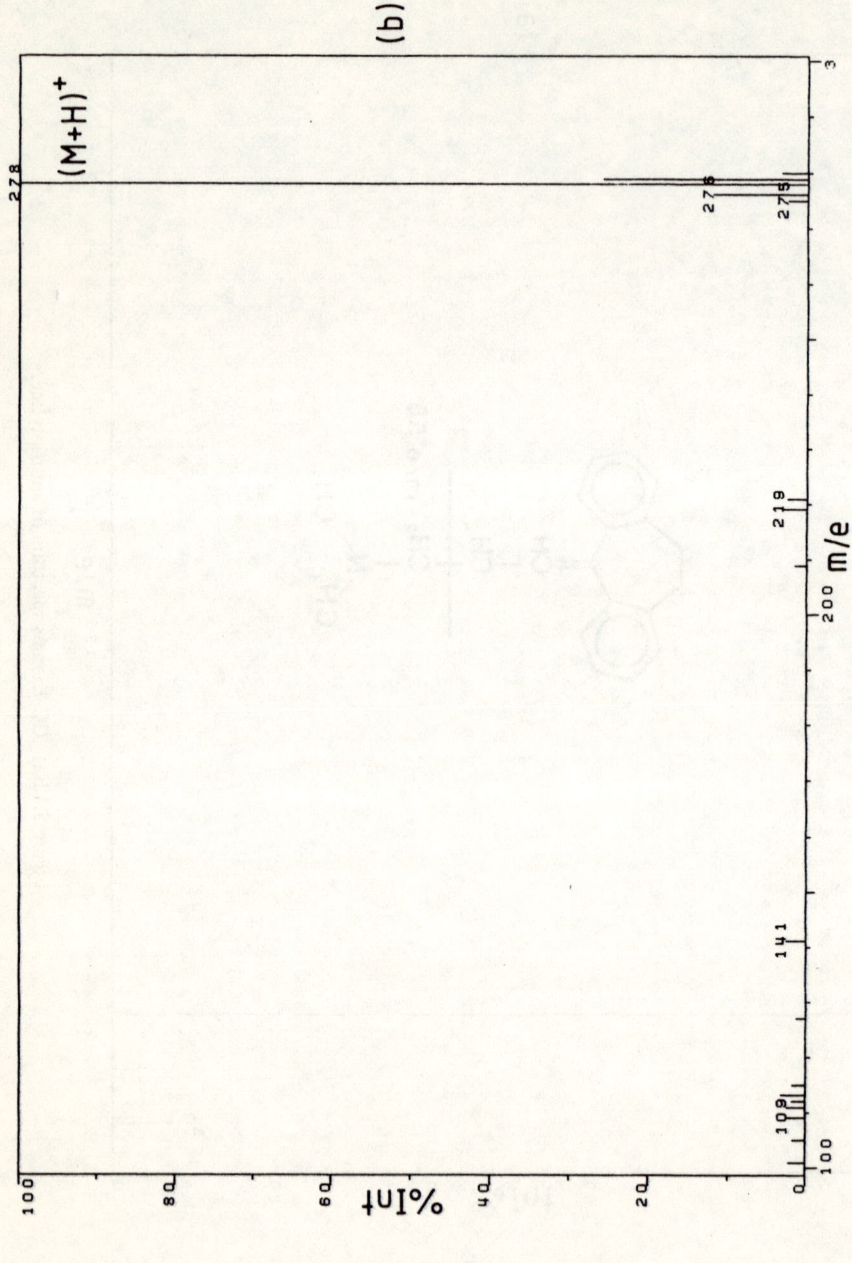

Figure 5.12(b) GC–CI (isobutane) mass spectrum of amitriptyline.

reagent gas ions to the unknown molecule. Because less energy is transferred to the sample molecule during ionisation, less fragmentation occurs and the resulting chemical ionisation spectrum is much simpler than the electron impact spectrum. Often only a 'quasimolecular ion' is seen; for methane or isobutane CI this would be the protonated molecule $(M + H)^+$. Care should be taken in interpreting CI spectra, however, as loss of neutral species can occur to yield an intense high-mass ion, which is not a quasimolecular ion. Hydroxy metabolites of drugs for example may lose water after protonation to show a strong $(M + H - H_2O)^+$ ion.

CI is used to yield information on the molecular weights of unknowns and to remove the ambiguity of identification based on EI alone. It has been used to simplify spectra so that mixtures can be analysed by probe (see Figure 5.7) and to provide high-mass ions to monitor and quantitate compounds giving less characteristic EI spectra. For the last two applications some prior knowledge is needed of the compounds expected. For general screening purposes, molecular weight information is not sufficient for identification and EI and CI spectra complement each other. Spectrometers are now available which will automatically switch from EI to CI operation quickly enough to enable alternate EI and CI spectra to be collected, both spectra being obtained for a packed-column GC peak.

The added facility of CI operation requires a modified mass-spectrometer. A less-open ion source is used so that high reagent-gas pressures are maintained in the ion source, while differential pumping of the source and analyser housings ensures that low pressures are maintained in the analyser and resolution is unimpaired. Plumbing to conduct the reagent gas into the source is also required and may be computer-controlled through solenoid valves to give the facility to scan alternate spectra in different modes.

5.5.3 Desorption chemical ionisation (DCI)

A variation of CI, desorption chemical ionisation uses a probe which introduces a sample, coated onto a filament, directly into the plasma contained in a chemical ionisation source. By this means, labile materials may be evaporated as molecular species before decomposition processes occur (Hunt *et al.*, 1977).

5.5.4 Field desorption

This also is a mode of soft ionisation (Reynolds, 1979), yielding simple spectra often showing only a molecular ion. The sample is ionised in the solid state on a special probe and desorbed as an ion, making the technique useful for thermally labile and involatile samples. The sample is coated onto an activated emitter by evaporation from solution. The emitter is introduced into the ion source at the end of a probe and a high potential ($\approx$ 10 kV) is applied between the emitter and a second electrode a few millimetres away. The intense electrostatic field causes ionisation of sample molecules which then desorb and are accelerated into the analyser for mass determination. A variety of emitters ranging from razor blades to needles or wires have been used, but the most widely used at the present time consist of 10-μm tungsten wires coated with a dense deposit of carbon-fibre microneedles (dendrites) formed by pyrolysis of acetone or benzonitrile vapour. The precise mechanism of ionisation is not fully understood—electron tunnelling has been proposed, as has been the involvement of species in the matrix or the emitter. The presence of small amounts of alkali metals in a matrix can enhance ionisation, but can also be a problem; sodium and potassium present in biological extracts can severely interfere with and confuse ionisation.

Field desorption has been proposed for rapid detection of drugs from biological materials in cases of acute poisoning (Goenechea and Goebel, 1978); here crude extracts containing less than 10 μg of drugs were coated onto a nonactivated tungsten wire and molecular species observed. Field desorption of collected LC fraction has been used to identify unequivocally barbiturates in biological samples with detection limits of between 1 ng g^{-1} and 10 ng g^{-1} (Schulten and Kummler, 1980).

Field ionisation is a closely related soft-ionisation method. The sample is introduced into the source as a vapour, perhaps from a GC inlet, and ionised in a high electrostatic field, often using a probe electrode which is also used for field desorption.

5.5.5 Fast-atom bombardment (FAB)

Fast-atom bombardment (Barber *et al.*, 1981a and b) is a recent development which has aroused a great deal of interest. The sample in the solid state is made the target for a beam of atoms, usually argon, from a fast-atom gun. Collisions result in ionisation of the sample molecules in the solid phase, so that the technique is useful in the analysis of fragile and involatile molecules. Fragmentation is seen in the spectra so that some structural as well as molecular formula information is obtained. The mode has been used mainly for large biological molecules, but could also be used to ionise samples directly from TLC plates, or from the belt of a moving-belt LC interface, although this would not overcome the problem of evaporating polar and involatile eluents on to the belt, or that of decomposition of labile compounds during the evaporation stage.

5.5.6 Negative chemical ionisation (NCI)

Until recently analytical mass spectrometry has concentrated on the study of positive-ion spectra. Under normal electron-impact conditions the yield of positive ions is several orders of magnitude greater than the yield of negative ions. Efficient negative ionisation requires electrons of thermal energy; 70-eV electrons are of too high an energy for electron capture to take place. It has been found that under chemical-ionisation conditions thermal electrons are available (Jennings, 1980), as a by-product of the ionisation process:

$$M + e \rightarrow M^{+\bullet} + 2e$$

As colliding and ejected electrons carry on to more collisions, more and more electrons are produced with lower and lower energies, until a cloud of electrons of thermal energy is present in the source. Molecules with positive-electron affinities will under such circumstances produce negative ions. The usage 'negative chemical ionisation' may be a misnomer if ionisation occurs by electron capture rather than by chemical mediation, however it is rarely clear whether ionisation involves electrons or anion species produced from the reagent gas—often both are involved.

Spectrometers capable of CI operation can be cheaply and easily modified for anion studies. Magnetic-sector instruments require the reversing of magnetic field and accelerating voltage, while quadrupole instruments require the reversal of voltages only and have been adapted to yield alternate positive and negative spectra (Hunt *et al.*, 1976). A growing number of studies have now been made applying anion mass-spectrometry to chemical analyses. The technique may offer one of three advantages over cation mass-spectrometry:

5.5.6.1 Sensitivity

Some compounds of high electron affinity have been detected at very low concentrations by NCI—notably highly halogenated pesticides (Hass *et al.*, 1978; Kuehl *et al.*, 1980) and organophosphorus pesticides (Busch *et al.*, 1978).

5.5.6.2 Selectivity

Many drugs and pesticides have much higher electron affinities than fatty compounds present as unwanted background in biological extracts and so can be detected without interference in samples too dirty for normal study. Indeed, for this reason lower detection limits may be achieved in NCI compared with EI, even though the latter shows higher absolute sensitivity and comparison of practical detection limits may be the most useful comparison of sensitivities to be made between the two modes. Useful analyses have been developed (Garland *et al.*, 1979, 1980, 1981) for several of the potent benzodiazepine group of drugs, which have excellent electron-capture properties.

5.5.6.3 Fragmentation

Fragmentation patterns in NCI are generally simpler than in EI and, as the processes are necessarily different, NCI spectra contain different information. Use of this has been made in the study of barbiturates (Jones and Whitehouse, 1981). Differentiation of barbiturates by probe NCI was achieved, which otherwise would require lengthier EI and CI runs together with measurement of GC retention times (Figure 5.13).

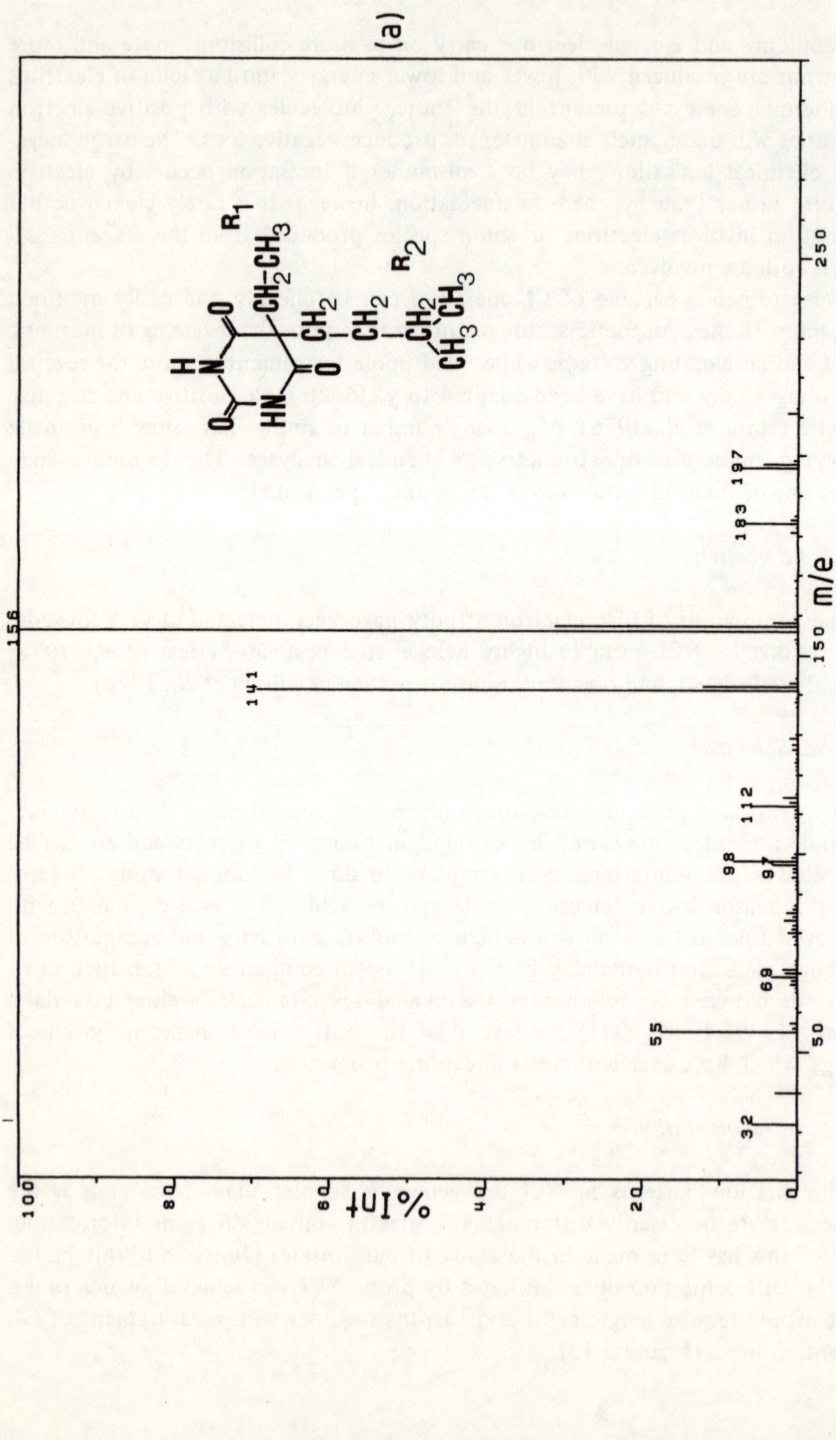

Figure 5.13(a) GC–EI mass spectrum of amobarbital.

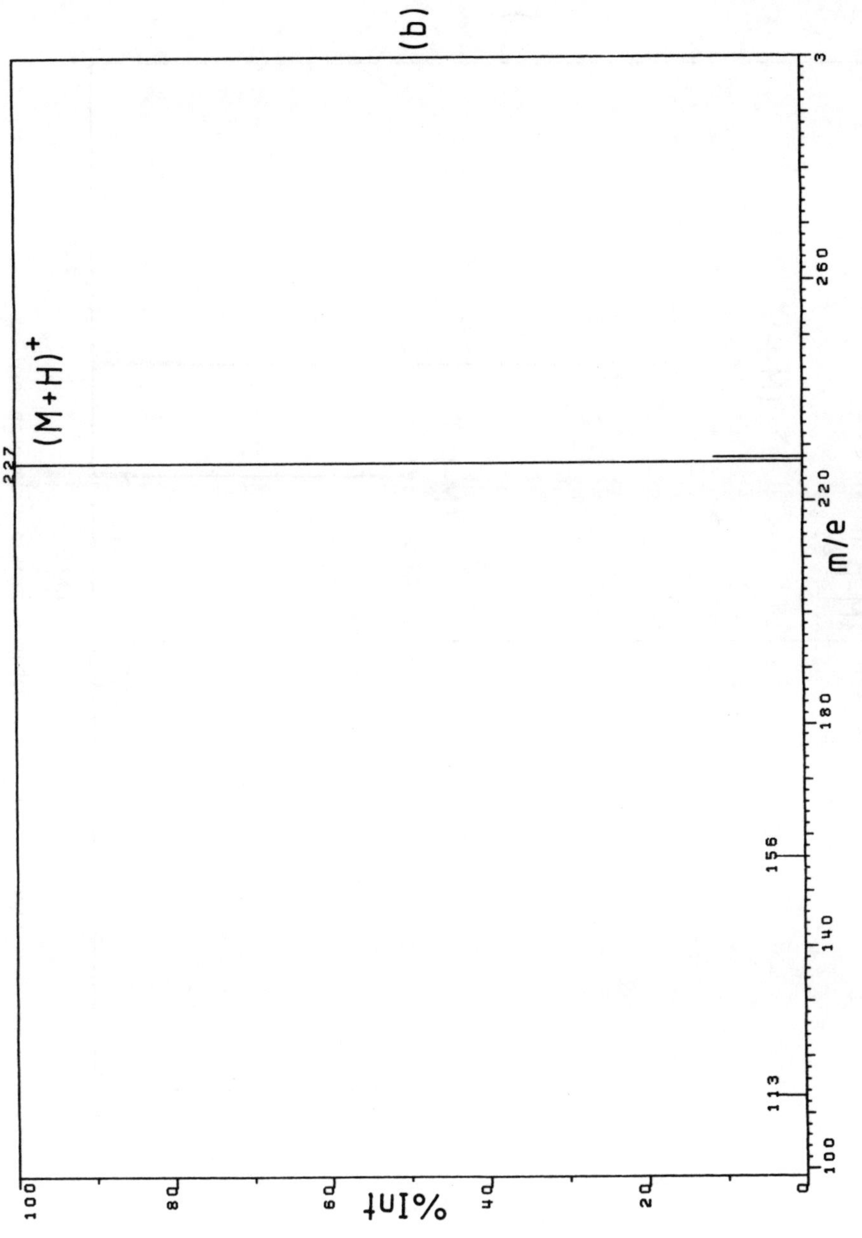

Figure 5.13(b) GC–CI (isobutane) mass spectrum of amobarbital.

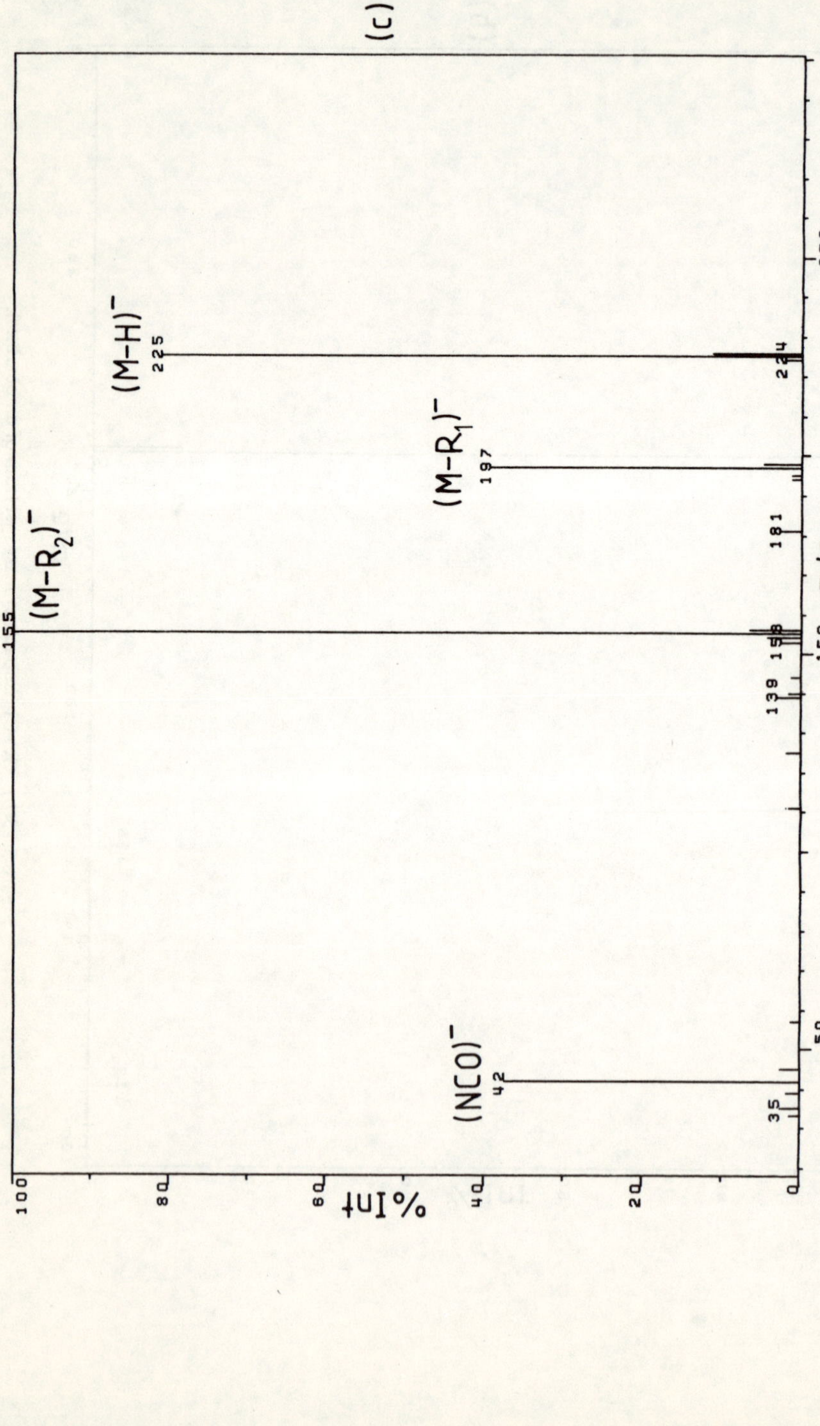

Figure 5.13(c) GC–CI (isobutane) mass spectrum of amobarbital.

5.6 GENERAL

5.6.1 Screening

Gas chromatography–mass spectrometry using electron-impact ionisation has become an invaluable technique for screening biological samples for drugs and pesticides. Most drugs and pesticides give EI spectra which contain sufficient information to characterise the compound. In other cases an EI spectrum will suggest a limited number of possibilities, which may be further resolved using other information available such as GC retention time, or a determination of molecular weight by a soft-ionisation technique–usually CI. A simple temperature-programmed run on a suitable GC column can cover an enormous number of possibilities and such a GC/EI screen can be used on samples with very little previous knowledge of the compounds expected. Identification of spectra obtained is facilitated by the availability of many reference collections of spectra which may be resident in a computer and accessed by the computer's library matching programs, or may be in book form. Figure 5.14 shows part of a page of such an index of spectra of compounds of forensic interest (Allan *et al.*, 1982). The index uses the common eight-peak format, spectra being indexed by the mass of the most intense ion (the base peak) in the spectra, followed by other ions in decreasing order of intensity. The index is also cross-referenced in other sections by molecular weight and alphabetic listing of name. From this extract the spectrum of methaqualone (see Figure 5.1) is readily identified. Often metabolites can be provisionally identified in such a screen, if they are consistently seen as unknowns in extracts containing the parent compound, share ions in common with the parent, or show ions shifted by a certain mass from those in the spectrum of the parent. As an example of the latter, many drugs have desmethyl metabolites which show appropriate ions shifted by 14 a.m.u. (equivalent to a methylene group) from those in the spectrum of the parent. If the spectrum entered as methaqualone metabolite in Figure 5.14 were seen with methaqualone in a urine extract, a metabolite might be suggested even without an index match. The ions in common with methaqualone and the possible molecular ion at m/e 266, which is 16 a.m.u. higher than the molecular ion in methaqualone, and equivalent to an oxygen atom, would indicate a hydroxy metabolite of that drug. Confirmation of the molecular weight by chemical ionisation could be used to support the provisional identification.

Unfortunately not all organic compounds of interest are amenable to GC study, by virtue of thermal lability, volatility, or polarity. Many of these can be studied by HPLC–MS but on-line HPLC is so far not flexible enough for general screens, and off-line collection of samples may still be the method of preference. In other cases samples may need preparation for direct introduction into the mass spectrometer for probe, field-desorption or FAB analysis.

IMIPRAMINE	235*	58	234	85	280	195	193	35	MWT: 280
3-METHYLHEXOBARBITONE	235*	81	169	171	79	236	170	91	MWT: 250
METHYLHEXOBARBITONE	235*	81	171	79	169	80	77	53	MWT: 250
2-METHYLHEXOBARBITONE (OR 4-METHYL-)	235*	150	165	236	79	137	250	164	MWT: 250
METHAQUALONE METABOLITE	235*	160	266	77	235	251	146	0	MWT: 266
METHYSERGIDE	235*	210	195	221	0	0	0	0	MWT: 353
ETHYL PHENYLMALONDIAMIDE (PRIMIDONE DERIVATIVE) DI TMS DERIVATIVE	235*	220	73	75	204	145	236	130	MWT: 350
DDT(P,P'-)	235*	237	165	75	50	51	352	0	MWT: 352
DDT(O,P-)	235*	237	165	75	199	246	352	0	MWT: 352
DDT	235*	237	165	212	246	75	176	36	MWT: 352
TDE (P,P'-)	235*	237	165	236	199	239	82	238	MWT: 318
AROMATISED 2-OXO-LSD	235*	237	337	236	221	338	209	238	MWT: 337
METHAQUALONE	235*	250	233	91	236	65	132	76	MWT: 250
IMIPRAMINE	235	58*	85	234	195	194	193	0	MWT: 280
DESIPRAMINE	235	195*	234	193	208	266	194	84	MWT: 266

*** ASTERISK INDICATES TRUE BASE PEAK ***

Figure 5.14 Page from "*An Eight-peak Index of Mass Spectra Compiled Specifically for Use in Forensic Science*" (Allan *et al.*, 1982; reproduced by kind permission of HMSO).

5.6.2 Derivatisation

Polar compounds are often rendered suitable for GC–MS study by derivatisation. Methylation of extracts containing acid compounds is used to reduce the polarity of drugs such as barbiturates (Brochmann-Hansen and Oke, 1969) or of acid pesticides (Fysh and Jones, 1980) to improve their gas chromatography. Likewise, silyl derivatives have been used for morphine (Nakamura and Noguchi, 1974) and cannabinoids (Harvey, 1978).

Derivatisation can also be used to change fragmentation to provide more structural information. In the case of amphetamine, for instance, the EI spectrum (Figure 5.15a) shows a very strong fragment at *m/e* 44 ($C_2NH_6^+$) with an extremely weak molecular ion. However, addition of carbon disulphide to an amphetamine solution yields the condensation product amphetamine thiocyanate (Worthington, 1974) which shows an EI spectrum (Figure 5.15b) with three intense ions of *m/e* 86, 91 and 177, the latter being the molecular ion; further, the derivative being less polar than amphetamine shows much better GC peak shape. Electron-impact analysis of this derivative yields then a more rigorous identification of amphetamine. Derivatives may also be made to improve the electron-capturing properties of a compound and so render it amenable to a more sensitive and selective NCI analysis (Bergner and Dougherty, 1981).

5.6.3 Specific analyses

Not only are general screens possible using mass spectrometry but also highly specific and sensitive analyses.

Selected-ion monitoring techniques yield this higher sensitivity and selectivity. Instead of scanning full spectra, during which only a very small part of the time is spent observing ions characteristic of a compound, the mass spectrometer is set to monitor a small number of selected characteristic ions, with several orders of magnitude improvement in detection limits. Greatest sensitivity is achieved if only the strongest ion expected for a compound is monitored, but usually some of this sensitivity will be traded off for specificity and a number of characteristic ions (four would be typical) monitored. The compound of interest is detected when responses for the monitored ions are observed at the appropriate GC retention time. Specificity can be further improved for some compounds by monitoring quasimolecular ions in chemical ionisation mode, an approach successfully used for the tricyclic antidepressant class of drugs which show predominantly low-mass common fragments in electron-impact mode (Lapin, 1980; Wilson *et al.*, 1977). With double-focusing instruments, accurate masses can be monitored, greatly increasing selectivity as a specific elemental formula is then monitored. In reaction monitoring, a double-focusing instrument is used first to monitor an expected parent ion and then, using a MIKES or linked-scan

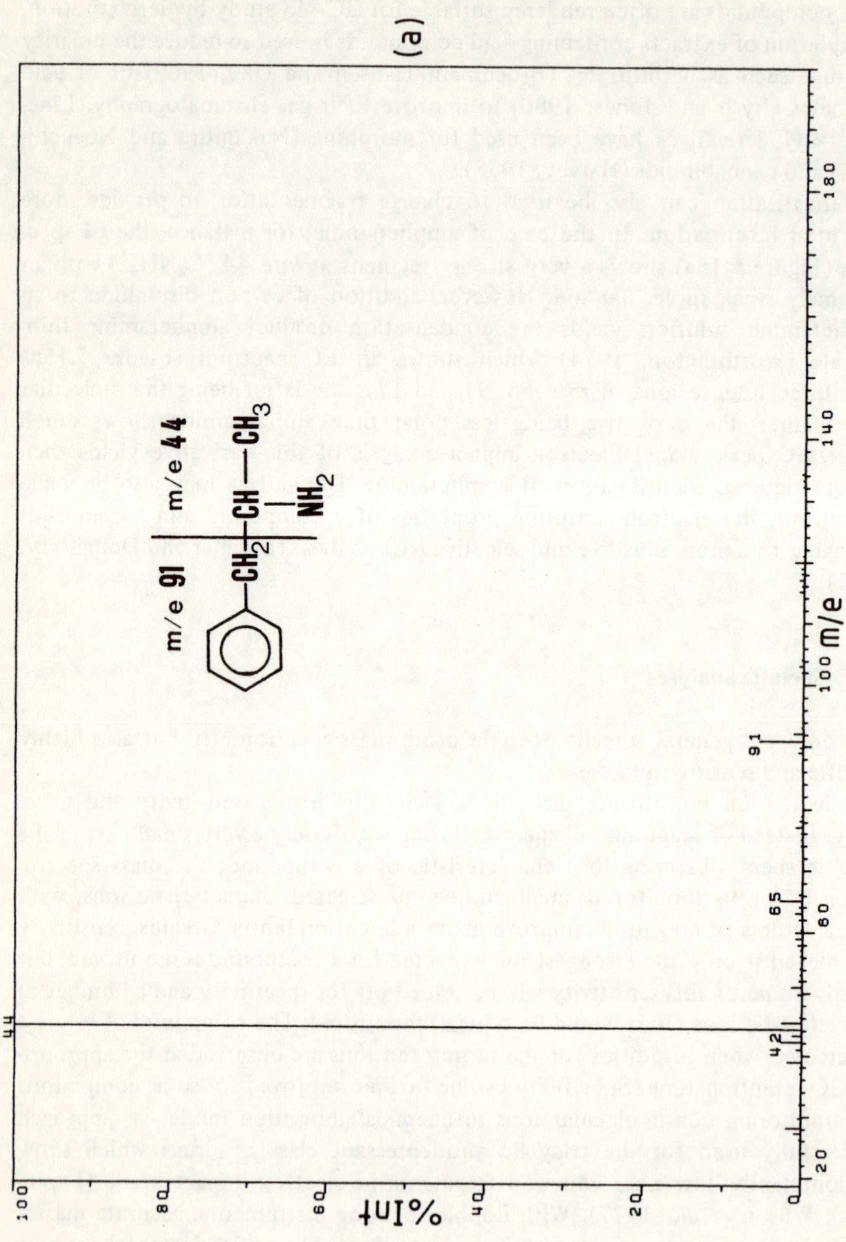

Figure 5.15(a) GC/EI mass spectrum of amphetamine.

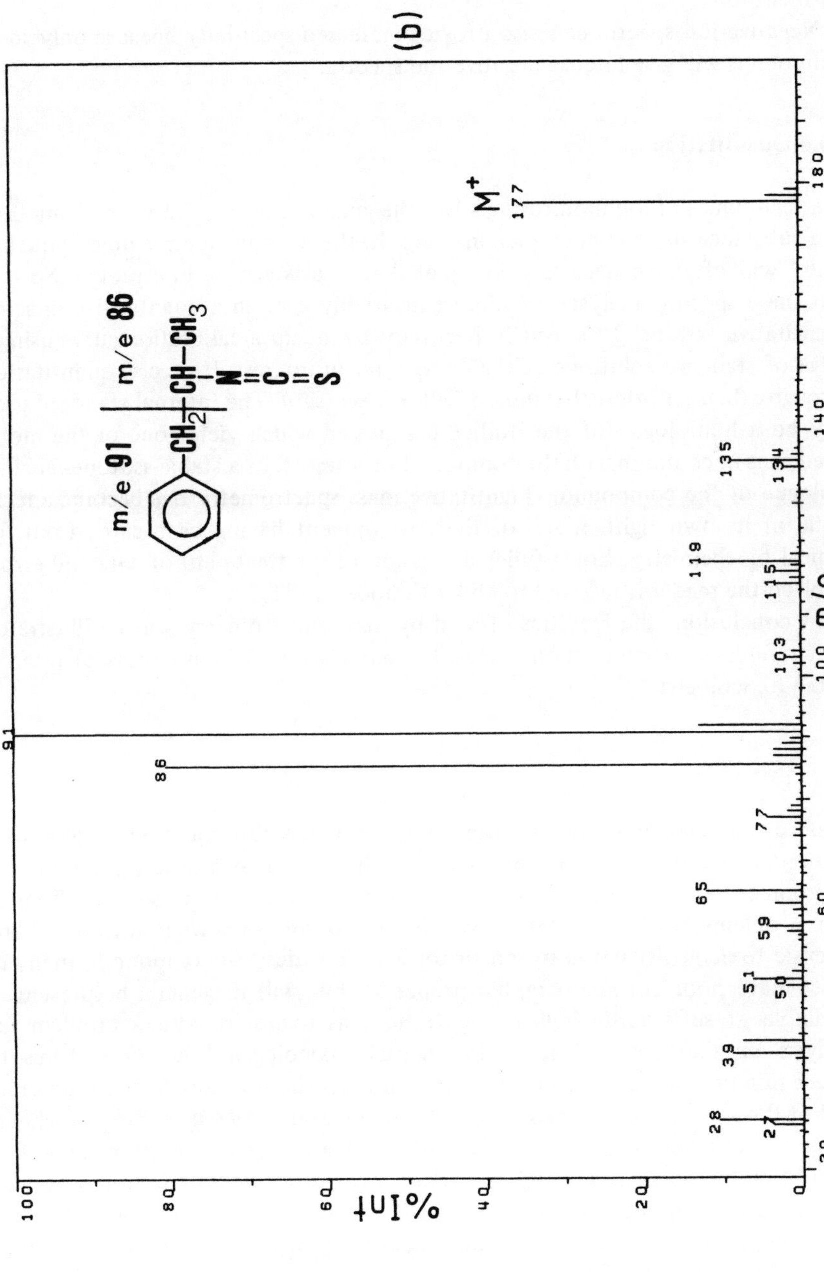

Figure 5.15(b) GC/EI mass spectrum of amphetamine thiocyanate.

mode, to monitor a daughter ion; thus a response is only given by a compound which yields the selected parent ion which fragments directly to the selected fragment ion.

Negative-ion spectra can also provide increased specificity because only some compounds will give intense negative-ion spectra.

5.6.4 Quantitation

The techniques of ion monitoring allow the analyst to detect very small amounts of a substance in a very complex mixture. In these circumstances precise quantitation will often be necessary in order that results can be interpreted. So it is that these specific analyses are almost invariably used in a quantitative or semiquantitative fashion. It is usually necessary to set up a calibration curve using a range of standard solutions of the compound of interest. If precise quantitation is sought then an internal standard will be necessary. The internal standard used may be a homologue of the studied compound which yields one of the monitored ions in common with the compound of interest, or a stable-isotope-labelled analogue of the compound. Quantitative mass spectrometry has become a technique in its own right, much of the development having been carried out for clinical biochemistry. For a fuller discussion of the treatment of data and errors involved the reader is referred to Millard's book (1981).

In conclusion, the facilities offered by mass spectrometry will be illustrated with reference to applications made to four classes of compounds of interest to the toxicologist.

5.6.5 Pesticides

These are a class of particular interest to both the forensic toxicologist, who encounters them as poisons employed by the would-be murderer, and to the environmental toxicologist, who is interested in them as possible pollutants. The problems posed for these two specialists are somewhat different. The forensic toxicologist needs to screen for a wide variety of compounds, many of which have poor chromatographic properties but will in general be present in a sample at sufficiently high concentrations as to not present a problem for analysis on that count. The environmental toxicologist however requires to detect minute traces, of often specific pollutants, in large amounts of material.

For the forensic toxicologist, Fysh (Fysh and Jones, 1980) proposes a scheme using gas chromatography with dual nitrogen and flame-ionisation detection, with methylation of acid extracts to screen for possible pesticides in a sample. Any positive response is then confirmed by GC/EI. There is a wealth of EI information for the pesticides, much appearing in a book on the subject by Safe and Hutzinger (1973).

Schulten (1976) applies the techniques of field desorption to the qualitative and semiqualitative analyses of commercially available pesticides and mixtures of pesticides. The technique is admirably suited to polar compounds and the simple spectra with high molecular-ion intensity allow mixtures to be dealt with. Further, with careful control of technique the analysis can be made semi-quantitative and has also been applied to the analysis of pesticides extracted from soil (Suzuki *et al.*, 1978).

Extensive use has been made in environmental toxicology of negative-ion mass spectrometry. Many halogenated and organophosphorus pesticides show intense negative-ion spectra while other background components in the studied matrices are transparent to NCI mass spectrometry. So it is that detection limits may be several orders of magnitude better than those for EI (Hass *et al.*, 1978), and GC/NCI screens for organochlorine pesticides have been proposed with minimal prior clean-up (Dougherty and Piotrowska, 1976; Dougherty *et al.*, 1976).

5.6.6 Tricyclic antidepressants

These have been widely prescribed in the treatment of depression and as such are often encountered in overdose cases; they have also been the subject of much clinical analysis. The drugs themselves are metabolised to pharmacologically active desmethyl metabolites, and so effective analysis requires characterisation and quantitation of closely related compounds. Mass spectrometry has been extensively employed for this analysis. However the compounds are all secondary and tertiary amines and their EI spectra are dominated by low-mass fragment ions formed by cleavage of the bond beta to the nitrogen of the side-chain amine group with generally only very weak high-mass ions to characterise the rest of the molecule, e.g. amitriptyline (Figure 5.12a). Thus soft-ionisation techniques have been extensively used. Many assays are reported using chemical ionisation coupled with selected-ion monitoring of the protonated molecular ions to give selective and quantitative analyses. Lapin (1980), Wilson *et al.* (1977) and Heck *et al.* (1978) report an analysis for imipramine which involves collection of a sample from HPLC for MS probe analysis using field ionisation. They report an order-of-magnitude increase in sensitivity over analyses using GC–MS with EI and CI ionisation with selected-ion monitoring.

Ryhage and Brandenberger (1978) report the negative-ion mass spectra of several phenothiazines. The spectra show $(M - 1)^-$ ions of moderate intensity, with strong base peaks corresponding to the condensed ring systems. These spectra complement the EI spectra which show strong ions produced by beta cleavage to the side-chain nitrogen (Figure 5.16). A negative-ion approach may be useful in the cases of other tricyclic antidepressants where the EI spectra carry even less information; the selectivity of negative-ion mass spectrometry may also improve detection limits in ion-monitoring experiments on these drugs.

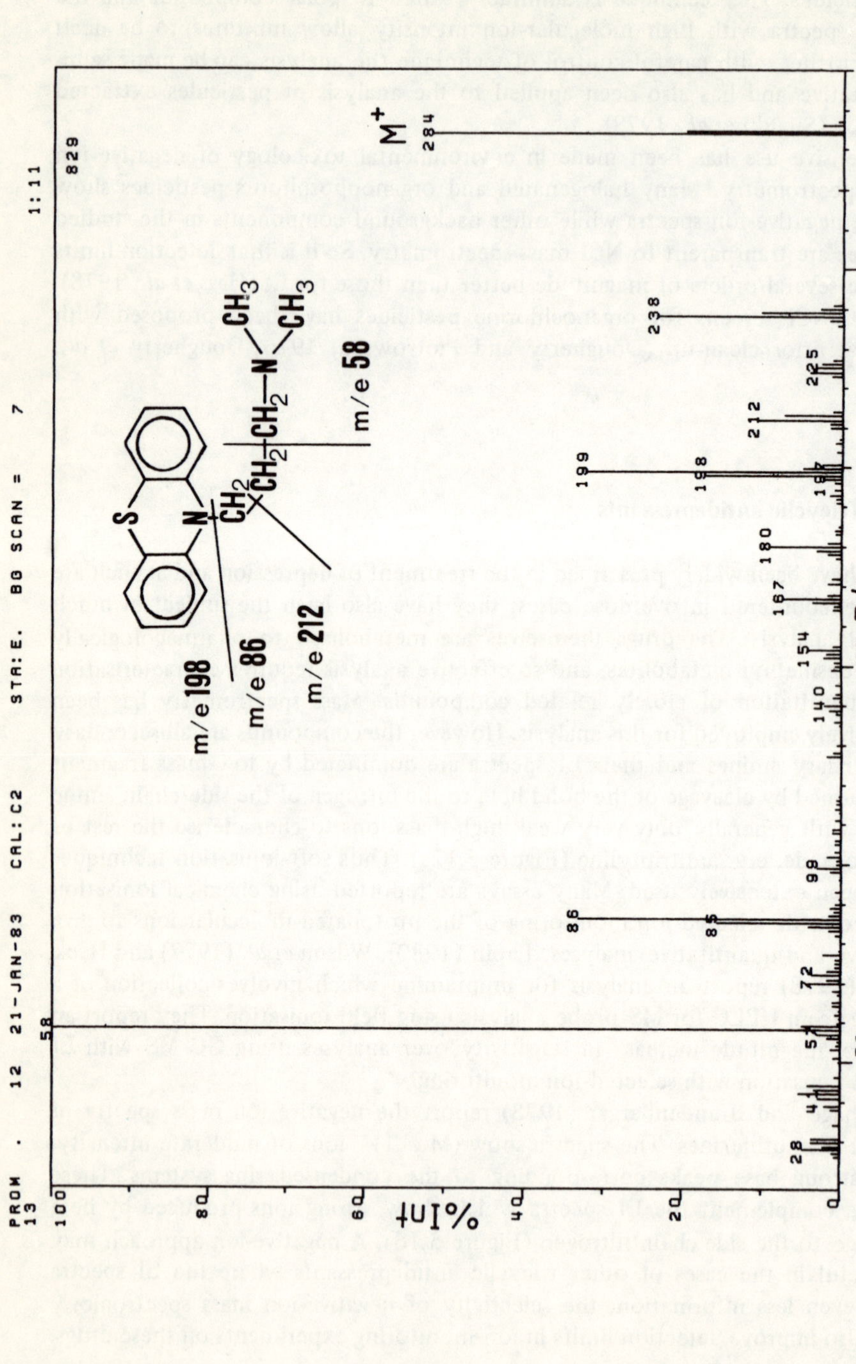

Figure 5.16 GC/EI mass spectrum of promazine.

5.6.7 Benzodiazepines

These are a very widely prescribed group of hypnotics/sedatives and as such are frequently encountered in clinical and forensic toxicology. Further, the drugs are very potent, requiring sensitive analyses for their detection and quantitation in body fluids. Sensitive methods of analysis have been devised, such as gas chromatography using an electron-capture detector (De Silva *et al.*, 1976) or acid hydrolysis to the corresponding benzophenone followed by spectrofluorimetry and thin-layer chromatography (De Silva *et al.*, 1971, 1974). In forensic cases, particularly where low levels of the drug or metabolites are involved, further confirmation may be obtained by GC-MS. In general the electron-impact spectra of the benzodiazepines are highly characteristic and screens for drugs and their metabolites can be made (Clatworthy *et al.*, 1977). However many of the compounds are unsuitable for GC. Methods involving acid hydrolysis of the benzodiazepine to the corresponding amino-benzophenones have been suggested (Maurer and Pfleger, 1981) but here ambiguity may arise where two or more drugs or metabolites give rise to the same hydrolysis product. The drugs oxazepam and lorazepam have been determined as the N_1, O_3-bistrimethylsilyl derivatives by GC–MS with ion monitoring of a common fragment (Higuchi *et al.*, 1979).

Many laboratories now use HPLC for determination of the benzodiazepines and successful confirmation of peak identities can be made by probe electron-impact mass spectrometry (see above) on collected HPLC fractions containing of the order of 100 ng of benzodiazepine (Figure 5.10). Analysis by NCI may improve detection limits in these cases by reducing the background spectra seen from such probe samples. Indeed, GC–NCI with selected-ion monitoring has been shown to be a useful mode for the quantitation of some benzodiazepines (Garland *et al.*, 1979, 1980, 1981) showing less background interference than positive electron-impact methods.

5.6.8 Barbiturates

Barbiturates have long been of interest to the toxicologist, first as widely prescribed sedatives, often used by the suicide and occasionally the murderer, and more recently because the drugs have been increasingly and dangerously abused. In response to the latter trend it has been proposed to restrict some or even all of the barbiturates and the implementation of the resulting legislation could require specific identification of barbiturates. The general structure of the barbiturates is shown in Figure 5.17.

EI mass spectrometry may be used to identify the barbiturates, but molecular ions are generally absent or of very low intensity. The major ions in the EI spectra in most cases only serve to identify one of the two 5-substituents to the ring, typically an ethyl or allyl group. Figure 5.13a shows the EI spectrum of

Table 5.1 The major ions in the anion mass spectra of 5-ethyl-substituted barbiturates

barbiturate	mol. wt	*R*	*R'*	*R''*	Major ions (M – H)⁻ *m/e*	(%*I*)	(M – *R'*)⁻ *m/e*	(%*I*)	(M – *R*)⁻ *m/e*	(%*I*)	(M – *R* – *R'* + H)⁻ *m/e*	(%*I*)	(N CO)⁻ *m/e*	(%*I*)
amobarbital	226	C_2H_5	$CH_2{-}CH_2{-}CH(CH_3)_2$	H	225	(65)	155	(100)	197	(49)	127	(8)	42	(30 to 200)
pentobarbital	226	C_2H_5	$-CH(CH_3){-}CH_2{-}CH_2{-}CH_3$	H	225	(9)	155	(100)	197	(13)	127	(3)	42	(20 to 70)
butethal	212	C_2H_5	$-CH_2{-}CH_2{-}CH_2{-}CH_3$	H	211	(65)	155	(100)	183	(45)	127	(8)	42	(30 to 400)
butabarbital	212	C_2H_5	$CH(CH_3){-}CH_2{-}CH_3$	H	211	(14)	155	(100)	183	(5)	127	(2)	42	(20 to 30)
barbital	184	C_2H_5	C_2H_5	H	183	(82)	155	(100)	–	(–)	127	(12)	42	(50 to 120)
cyclobarbital	236	C_2H_5	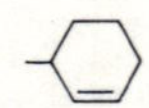	H	235	(11)	155	(100)	207	(11)	127	(4)	42	(30 to 130)
heptabarbital	250	C_2H_5	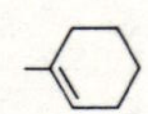	H	249	(17)	155	(100)	221	(12)	127	(14)	42	(3)
phenobarbital	232	C_2H_5	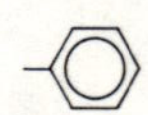	H	231	(6)	155	(100)	203	(43)	127	(7)	42	(11 to 60)
probarbital	198	C_2H_5	$-CH(CH_3)_2$	H	197	(33)	155	(100)	169	(9)	127	(1)	42	(20 to 40)
vinbarbital	224	C_2H_5	$-C(CH_3){=}CH{-}CH_2{-}CH_3$	H	223	(16)	155	(100)	195	(8)	127	(11)	42	(30)
5-ethyl-5-*p*-tolyl barbituric acid	246	C_2H_5	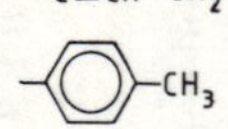	H	245	(10)	155	(100)	217	(38)	127	(13)	42	(25)

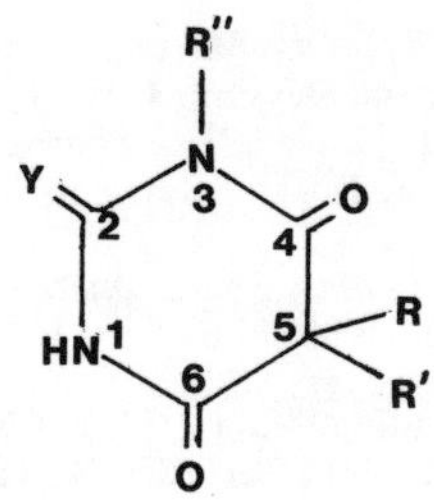

Figure 5.17 The general structure of the barbiturates (Y = O except for thiobarbiturates, when Y = S).

amobarbital but is typical of many 5-ethyl-substituted barbiturates. CI determination of molecular weight can complement the information of an EI spectrum (Figure 5.13b) but ambiguity remains for several barbiturates differing only in isomeric side chains. Jones and Whitehouse (1981) show that NCI of probe samples can provide quick and easy identification. The spectra are comparatively simple (Figure 5.13c), ions arising from proton and side-chain elimination clearly indicating molecular weight and the masses of the substituents. Further, as relative fragment intensity was strongly influenced by side-chain branching, all but two of thirty barbiturates analysed were readily differentiated. Table 5.1 summarises the NCI spectra of eleven 5-ethyl-substituted barbiturates and shows complete differentiation of all these. The technique was applied to pure probe samples, but can also be used with GC separation: unfortunately, the alkylated derivatives often used for GC analysis show somewhat less intense NCI spectra than do the parent drugs.

Schulten and Kummler (1980) use the off-line combination of HPLC and field-desorption MS to identify barbiturates from body fluids, allowing definite identification at levels down to $\approx 10 \text{ ng g}^{-1}$ of body fluid. The spectra obtained by field desorption (Games *et al.*, 1976) give intense molecular or quasimolecular ions and some fragmentation, giving information similar to that available from electron-impact spectra.

REFERENCES

Allan, A. R., Ardrey, R. E., Bal, T. S., Brown, C., and Moffat, A. C. (1982). An eight peak index of mass spectra compiled specifically for use in forensic science. *Home Office Central Research Establishment Rept* No. 448 (to be published).

Aston, F. W. (1933). *Mass Spectra and Isotopes.* Edward Arnold, London.

Barber, M., Bordoli, R. S., Sedgwick, R. D., and Tyler, A. N. (1981a). *J. Chem. Comm.* 325.

Barber, M., Bordoli, R. S., Sedgwick, R. D., Tyler, A. N., and Walley, E. T. (1981b). *Biomed. Mass Spectrom.* 8, 337–42.

Bergner, E. A., and Dougherty, R. C. (1981). *Ibid.*, 204–10.

Beynon, J. H., Saunders, R. A., and Williams, A. E. (1968). *The Mass Spectra of Organic Molecules*. Elsevier, Amsterdam.

Boyd, R. K., and Beynon, J. H. (1977). *Org. Mass Spectrom.* **12**, 163.

Bozorgzadeh, M. H., Morgan, R. P., and Beynon, J. H. (1978). *Analyst* **103**, 613-22.

Brochmann-Hanssen, E., and Oke, T. O. (1969). *J. Pharm. Sci.* **58**, 370.

Busch, K. L., Bursey, M. M., Hass, J. R., and Sovocool, G. W. (1978). *Appl. Spectrosc.* **32**, 388-99.

Chapman, J. R. (1978). *Computers in Mass Spectrometry*. Academic, London.

Clatworthy, A. J., Jones, L. V., and Whitehouse, M. J. (1977). *Biomed. Mass Spectrom* **4**, 248-54.

Crathorne, B., Watts, C. D., and Fielding, M. (1979). *J. Chomatogr.* **185**, 671-90.

Dawkins, B. G., Arpino, P. J., and McLafferty, F. W. (1978). *Biomed. Mass Spectrom.* **5**, 1.

Dawson, P. H. (ed.) (1976). *Quadrupole Mass Spectrometry*. Elsevier, Amsterdam.

De Silva, J. A. F., and Strojny, N. (1971). *J. Pharm. Sci.* **60**, 1303.

De Silva, J. A. F., Bekersky, I., and Puglisi, C. V. (1974). *J. Pharm. Sci.* **63**, 1837.

De Silva, J. A. F., Bekersky, I., Puglisi, C. V., Brooks, M. A., and Weinfeld, R. E. (1976). *Analyt. Chem.* **48**, 10.

Dougherty, R. C., and Piotrowska, K. (1976). *Proc. Natl Acad. Sci. USA* **73**, 1777-81.

Dougherty, C., Bergner, A., Levonowich, P., and Roberts, J. D. (1976). *Adv. Mass Spectrom. Biochem. Med.* **1**, 181-92.

Ehrenthal, W., and Pfleger, K. (1977). *Acta. Pharmacol. Toxicol.* **41**, Suppl. II, 199-211.

Entwistle, N., Jones, L. V., and Owen, P. (1982). Private communication.

Facchetti, S., Fornari, A., and Montagna, M. (1979). Abstracts of the 8th International Mass Spectrometry Conference, Oslo.

Fysh, R. R., and Jones, L. V. (1980). In Oliver, J. S. (ed.), *Forensic Toxicology*. Croom Helm, London, pp. 189-204.

Games, D. E. (1981). *Biomed. Mass Spectrom.* **8**, 454-62.

Games, D. E., Jackson, A. H., Taylor, K. T. and Haskins, N. J. (1976). *Adv. Mass Spectrom. Biochem. Med.* **1**, 383-90.

Garland, W. A., and Min, B. H. (1979). *J. Chromatogr.* **172**, 279-86.

Garland, W. A., and Miwa, B. J. (1980). *Environm. Hlth Persp.* **36**, 69-76.

Garland, W. A., Miwa, B. J., and Blumenthal, P. (1981). *Analyt. Chem.* **53**, 793-97.

Goenechea, S., and Goebel, K. J. (1978). *Freznius Z. Analyt. Chem.* **290**, 110-1.

Harvey, D. J. (1978). *J. Chromatogr.* **147**, 291-8.

Hass, J. R., Friesen, M. D., Harvan, D. J., and Parker, C. E. (1978). *Analyt. Chem.* **50**, 1474-9.

Heck, H. d'A., Flynn, N. W., Buttrill, S. E., Jun., Dyer, R. L., and Anbar, M. (1978). *Biomed. Mass Spectrom.* **5**, 250-7.

Higuchi, S., Urabe, H., and Shiobara, Y. (1979). *J. Chromatogr.* **164**, 55-61.

Hunt, D. F., Shabonowitz, J., Botz, F. K., and Brent, D. A. (1977). *Analyt. Chem.* **49**, 1160.

Hunt, D. F., Stafford, G. C., Jun., Crow, F. W., and Russel, J. W. (1976). *Ibid.* **48**, 2098.

Jennings, K. R. (1980). *Analyt. Proc.* **17**, 320-2.

Jones, L. V., and Whitehouse, M. J. (1981). *Biomed. Mass Spectrom.* **8**, 231-6.

Knewstubb, P. F. (1969). *Mass Spectometry and Ion-Molecule Reactions*. Cambridge University Press, Cambridge.

Kondrat, R. W., and Cooks, R. G. (1978). *Analyt. Chem.* **50**, 81-89A.

Kuehl, D. W., Whitaker, M. J., and Dougherty, R. C. (1980). *Ibid.* **52**, 935-40.

Lapin, A. (1980). *Eur. J. Mass Spectrom. Biomed. Med. Environm. Res.* **1**, 121-7.

Maurer, H., and Pfleger, K. (1981). *J. Chromatogr.* **222**, 409-19.

McFadden, W. H. (1973). *Techniques of Combined Gas Chromatography/Mass Spectrometry: Applications in Organic Analysis*. Wiley-Interscience, New York.

McFadden, W. H. (1979). *J. Chromatogr. Sci.*, **17**, 2-17.

McFadden, W. H., Schwartz, H. L., and Evans, S. (1976). *J. Chromatogr.* **122**, 389.

McLafferty, F. W. (1973). *Interpretation of Mass Spectra.* Benjamin, Reading, Mass.

McLafferty, F. W., and Lory, E. R. (1981). *J. Chromatogr.* **203**, 109-16.

McLafferty, F. W., and Venkataraghavan, R. (1979). *J. Chromatogr. Sci.* **17**, 24-9.

Millard, B. J. (1978). *Quantitative Mass Spectrometry*. Heyden, London.

Millington, D. S., and Smith, J. A. (1977). *Org. Mass Spectrom.* **12**, 264.

Munson, B. (1977). *Analyt. Chem.* **49**, 772–8A.
Nakamura, G. R., and Noguchi, T. T. J. (1974). *J. Forensic Sci. Soc.* **14**, 347–53.
Powers, D., D'Arcy, P. H., Bill, J. C., and Wallington, M. J. (1978). *26th Annual Conference on Mass Spectromety and Allied Topics, St Louis, Mo.* p. 480.
Reynolds, W. D. (1979). *Analyt. Chem.*, **51**, 283–93A.
Ryhage, R., and Brandenberger, H. (1978). *Biomed. Mass Spectrom.* **5**, 615–20.
Safe, S., and Hutzinger, O. (1973). *Mass Spectometry of Pesticides and Pollutants*. CRC Press, Cleveland, Ohio.
Schulten, H. R. (1976). *J. Agric. Food Chem.* **24**, 743–9.
Schulten, H. R., and Kummler, D. (1980). *Analyt. Chim. Acta* **113**, 253–67.
Scott, R. P. W., Scott, C. G., Monroe, M., and Hess, J. (1974). *J. Chromatogr.* **99**, 395–405.
Suzuki, M., Yamoto, Y., and Koga, M. (1978). *Biomed. Mass Spectrom.* **5**, 518–23.
Thomson, J. J. (1913). *Rays of Positive Electricity and Their Application to Chemical Analysis*. Longmans, London.
Wilson, J. M., Williamson, L. J., and Vidmantas, A. R. (1977). *Clin. Chem.* **23**, 1012–7.
Worthington, J. V. (1974). Home Office Central Research Establishment, Report No. 121.
Zitrin, S., and Yinon, J. (1977). *Analyt. Lett.* **10**, 235–41.

6
Tricyclic antidepressants and neuroleptics

R. WHELPTON

6.1 INTRODUCTION

Although the compounds discussed in this chapter may be grouped in different classes according to their pharmacological properties, similarities in their structures and chemistry make it convenient to consider them together. Compounds given the generic name 'tricyclic antidepressants' are thought to exert their major effects by blocking the neuronal uptake of central-nervous-system transmitters—principally, noradrenaline and 5-hydroxytryptamine (serotonin). Neuroleptic phenothiazines and thioxanthenes have marked anti-dopaminergic properties but other phenothiazines may be used for their anti-histaminic (H_1-receptor block) or anti-cholinergic properties.

6.1.1 Chemistry

The basic ring-structures are shown in Figure 6.1. The early tricyclic antidepressants are derivatives of dibenzazepine (also known as iminodibenzyl) or dibenzcycloheptadiene, but compounds with more diverse structures are marketed now. In protriptyline the two-carbon bridge is unsaturated. Doxepin and dothiepin have -CH_2-O- and -CH_2-S- bridges respectively. Maprotiline, mianserin, nomifensine, tandamine and zimelidine do not have the typical structure but are generally included in any discussion of tricyclic antidepressants. The side-chain structure

-C-C-C-N<

is common to most of the antidepressants. Tertiary (imipramine, clomipramine, trimipramine, amitriptyline, doxepin and dothiepin) and secondary amines (desipramine, nortriptyline, protriptyline and maprotiline) are marketed.

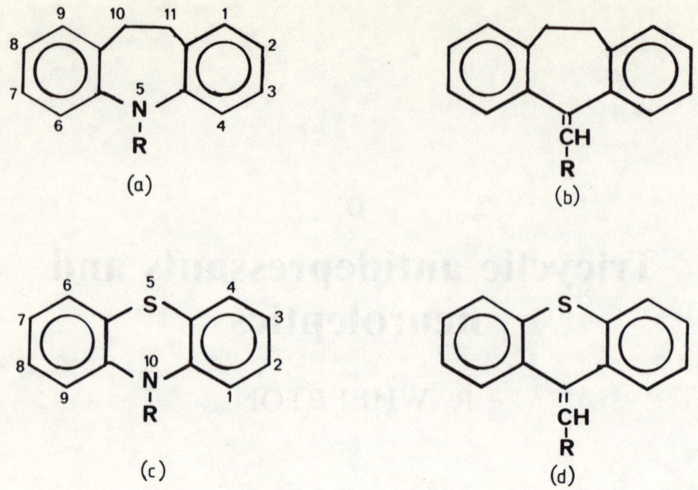

Figure 6.1 (a, b) Basic ring structures of tricyclic antidepressant derivatives: (a) iminodibenzyl; (b) dibenzocycloheptadiene. (c, d) Basic ring structures of neuroleptics: (c) phenothiazine, (d) thioxanthene. Note the different conventions in numbering.

The substitution of a sulphur bridge in place of the C_{10}–C_{11} bridge produces a more planar ring-system in phenothiazines and thioxanthenes. As a result of a large number of different side chains plus various ring substituents, there are a large number of commercially available phenothiazines. Phenothiazines with side chains

$$-C-C-N<$$

have marked anti-histaminic or anti-cholinergic properties. Promethazine (Figure 6.2) is primarily used for its anti-histamine, anti-motion sickness or sedative properties.

The *NN*-diethyl analogue, ethopropazine, has been used for its anti-cholinergic properties to treat Parkinsonian-like symptoms.

Neuroleptic phenothiazines and thioxanthenes have a three-carbon-atom chain between the ring and side-chain nitrogens. Compounds with piperazine side

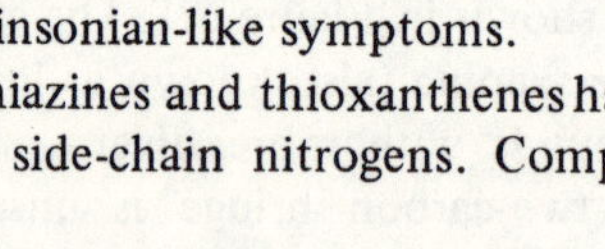

Figure 6.2 Structure of promethazine

chains are particularly potent (e.g. fluphenazine and flupenthixol). Potency is also increased by ring substitution at the two position in the order H$<$Cl$<$$CF_3$. It is not clear whether these effects are pharmacodynamic, or arise chiefly from differences in distribution. Some compounds, such as fluphenazine, pipothiazine and flupenthixol, which have terminal alcohol groups, have been esterified and the esters used as depot injections to give a long duration of effect. Up to four weeks duration of action has been claimed.

6.1.1.1 Stereochemistry

Ring-substituted thioxanthenes, e.g. chlorprothixene, flupenthixol, exist as *cis–trans* isomers. The *cis*-isomers are about twenty times more potent. Likewise, doxepin and dothiepin, being unsymmetrical, can take *cis*- or *trans*-forms. As *cis*-doxepin is metabolised to the *trans*-isomer (Rosseel *et al.*, 1978) it is difficult to assign biological activity to one isomer.

Several of the compounds (trimipramine, butriptyline, promethazine, ethopropazine, thioridazine) contain asymmetric carbon atoms, but this fact appears to have been largely ignored. The analgesic phenothiazine, levomepromazine, as its name implies, is marketed as the more active (–)-isomer.

6.1.1.2 Ionisation constants

All the compounds contain basic nitrogen atoms. A selection of pKa values are given in Table 6.1. The majority of the compounds show only a very small spectral shift on protonation and the low aqueous solubilities mean that the pKa values are usually determined by nonaqueous titration (Chatten and Harris, 1962) or by limiting solubility experiments (Green, 1967). Phenothiazine sulphoxides show sufficient change in ultraviolet extinction with changing pH to allow spectroscopic determination (Beckett *et al.*, 1974; Whelpton, 1978). Amine oxides can be titrated in aqueous solution (Bickel and Weder, 1969; Becket *et al.*, 1974).

Table 6.1 Ionisation constants

Compound	pKa	Compound	pKa
chlorpromazine N-oxide	4.7	promazine	9.4
imipramine N-oxide	4.7	amitriptyline	9.5
perphenazine	7.8	imipramine	9.5
prochlorperazine	8.1	nor_1chlorpromazine sulphoxide	9.5
trifluoperazine	8.1	thioridazine	9.5
chlorprothixene	8.4	ethopromazine	9.6
chlorpromazine sulphoxide	9.0	nor_2chlorpromazine sulphoxide	9.7
promethazine	9.1	nor_1chlorpromazine	9.9
triflupromazine	9.2	nortriptyline	10.0
methotrimeprazine	9.2	nor_2chlorpromazine	10.2
chlorpromazine	9.3	desipramine	10.2

The dimethylamine and piperidine derivatives have pKa values between approximately 9 and 9.5. The secondary and primary amines have correspondingly higher values. The piperazine derivatives have two pKa values of approximately 8 and 4. Naturally, the amine oxides are much weaker bases.

6.1.1.3 Metabolism

Imipramine and chlorpromazine serve as useful model compounds when discussing metabolic fate (Crammer *et al.*, 1968; Crammer *et al.*, 1969, Crammer and Rolfe, 1970, Fishman and Goldenberg, 1960; Fishman *et al.*, 1962; Fishman and Goldenberg, 1963). Not surprisingly, several pathways appear to be common and inhibition of tricyclic antidepressant metabolism by phenothiazines has been reported (Gram and Overφ, 1972). Both compounds are oxidatively demethylated to give secondary and then primary amines. The tertiary amines form amine oxides. Aromatic hydroxylation leads to 2-hydroxyimipramine or 7-hydroxychlorpromazine; the site of hydroxylation is para to the ring nitrogen in both cases and one should not be misled by the different conventions of numbering.

The C_{10}–C_{11} bridge is oxidised with the formation of 10-hydroxyimipramine. Oxidation of sulphur gives chlorpromazine sulphoxide. Side-chain cleavage giving iminodibenzyl and 2-hydroxyiminodibenzyl appears to be relatively important in imipramine metabolism, whereas 2-chlorphenothiazine is a minor component in the urine of patients treated with chlorpromazine. Chlorpromazine is deaminated to give proprionic-acid derivatives. Conjugates, mainly glucuronides, of phenolic metabolites form a major proportion of the urinary metabolites. Fluphenazine glucuronide, as well as 7-hydroxyfluphenazine glucuronide, is found in human urine (Curry *et al.*, 1979). Piperazine derivatives may be ring-opened to ethylenediamine derivatives (Gaertner and Breyer, 1972) and, at least, two amine oxides are possible (Spirtes, 1974). Thioridazine is metabolised to side-chain (2-) sulphoxides and sulphones as well as ring (5-) sulphoxides (Zehnder *et al.*, 1962). As a result of a combination of reactions, biological samples are likely to contain complex mixtures of drug and metabolites. Chlorpromazine could have over 160 metabolites and more complex molecules even more.

6.2 ANALYSIS

6.2.1 Sample preparation

A combination of extensive metabolism and high apparent volumes of distribution means that plasma concentrations are expected to be in the ng ml^{-1} range. For the more potent compounds, plasma concentrations below 1 ng ml^{-1}

may be encountered. Consequently, preliminary separation and concentration steps are usually required. For most techniques, concentration by 10 to 100 times will be required. The compounds are very lipophilic and are readily extracted from dilute alkaline solutions into organic solvents. If phenolic metabolites are to be determined, the pH of the aqueous phase must be optimised to ensure maximum recovery (Figure 6.3). Alternatively, solutions of

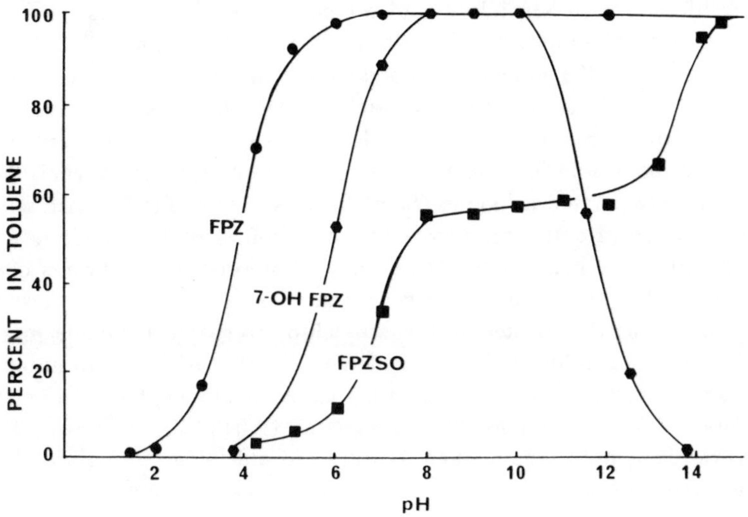

Figure 6.3 pH-partition characteristics of fluphenazine (FPZ), fluphenazine sulphoxide (FPZSO) and 7-hydroxyfluphenazine (7-OHFPZ) distributed between toluene and aqueous buffers.

higher pH values may be used to separate a 'phenolic fraction'. The least-polar solvent that will extract the compound(s) of interest should be used to effect the maximum separation from unwanted metabolites and endogenous contaminants. Generally, the parent compounds can be extracted into aliphatic hydrocarbons such as pentane, hexane, heptane etc. Small quantities of suitable alcohols are sometimes included to reduce adsorptive losses onto the glassware. When an evaporation step is to be included, low-boiling-point solvents may be an advantage but the possibility of unwanted evaporation during handling procedures should be considered. The extraction of metabolites may require solvents of higher polarity. Some analytical techniques, particularly gas chromatography with electron-capture detection (ECD), need 'cleaner' samples than those produced by a single extraction and the compounds, being basic, can be backwashed into dilute mineral-acids to leave unwanted lipids etc. in the organic phase. A further extraction into fresh organic solvent, after suitable adjustment of the pH of the aqueous phase, is required for most techniques. High-purity solvents are essential and it may be necessary to purify commercially available solvents before use, particularly if the sample is concentrated by evaporation. Back extraction into a small volume of organic phase alleviates the need to evaporate (Curry, 1968) and reduces the problems of solvent impurities and reconstitution of the dry residue.

Derivatisation has been used to separate metabolites prior to analysis. This is a separate approach from producing derivatives to improve chromatographic peak shapes or as part of the detection techniques which are discussed in the appropriate sections below. Secondary- and primary-amine metabolites can be separated from tertiary amines by acetylation. The tertiary amine will extract into dilute acid, leaving the amides in the organic solvent. Brunswick *et al.* (1978 and 1979) used succinic anhydride to separate tertiary and secondary amines. The derivative, containing a carboxylic acid, was extracted from heptane into sodium hydroxide solution and the parent compound into dilute acid. Primary amines can be separated as imines (Schiff's bases). Overø (1972) used salicyclic aldehyde to separate the primary amine metabolites of nortriptyline and Lu 5-079 before radiochemical derivatisation. In his original gas-chromatographic method for chlorpromazine and its heptane extractable metabolites, Curry (1968) fortuitously separated didesmethylchlorpromazine from the monodesmethyl metabolite as the imine formed with iso-valeraldehyde, an impurity in the iso-amyl alcohol (3-methylbutan-1-ol) added to the heptane. The effect of other aldehydes and ketones was investigated (Whelpton and Curry, 1976a). Aldehydes react more readily than ketones but aldehydes with alpha-H atoms are best avoided as they may form enamines with secondary amines.

6.2.2 Radioderivatives, radioimmunoassay and radioreceptor assays

In 1967 Hammer and Brodie described their isotope-derivative technique for the estimation of desipramine. Their success appears to be based on (1) the careful purification of [^{3}H]acetic anhydride before use, (2) the stability of the [^{3}H]acetamide to NaOH solutions at 95 °C, thus allowing a further purification, and (3) the negligible amounts of primary-amine metabolites present. The method had a lower limit of detection of 5 ng ml^{-1} and a relative standard deviation of 4% at 100 ng ml^{-1}. Preventing the interference of primary-amine metabolites in the radioacetylation of nortiptyline by imine formation (Overø, 1972) was discussed above. Further modifications to the original technique have involved isotope dilution with ^{14}C-labelled tricyclic to improve the precision and thin-layer chromatography to improve the specificity, e.g. the assay of maprotiline (Riess, 1974). Radioacetylation has even been applied to the tertiary amine, clomipramine, which was demethylated by hydrolysing the carbamate formed with trichloroethylchloroformate (Cornis *et al.*, 1976). Quaternisation of imipramine (Harris *et al.*, 1970) and chlorpromazine (Efron *et al.*, 1971) with ^{14}C-iodomethane have been described as methods for analysis.

Spector's group were the first to describe radioimmunoassays for desipramine

(Spector *et al.*, 1975) and chlorpromazine (Kawashima *et al.*, 1975). Ten published methods for tricyclic antidepressants are described in the review by Scoggins *et al.* (1980). High sensitivities, low sample-volumes and ease and speed of assay are obvious advantages, but problems of specificity are common. Some methods include a separation step such as solvent extraction and/or derivatisation before assay (Brunswick *et al.*, 1978; Brunswick *et al.*, 1979). When plasma concentrations below 10 ng ml^{-1} are to be determined then radioimmunoassay is an obvious choice and has been applied to the more potent drugs: flupenthixol (Robinson and Risby, 1977; Jørgensen, 1978), fluphenazine (Wiles and Franklin, 1978; Midha *et al.*, 1980), perphenazine (Midha *et al.*, 1981c) and trifluoperazine (Midha *et al.*, 1981b).

A radioreceptor assay method for neuroleptics has been described by Creese and Snyder (1977). It is a saturation assay based on the displacement of [^{3}H]haloperidol or [^{3}H]spiroperidol from dopamine receptors prepared from rat-brain striatum. The sensitivities vary depending upon the compound being assayed, e.g. fluphenazine, 1.8 ng ml^{-1}; trifluoperazine, 2.2 ng ml^{-1}; chlorpromazine, 8.6 ng ml^{-1}, and thioridazine, 30 ng ml^{-1}, and are more than those expected of radioimmunoassay. The specificity is poor but it has been argued that this is an advantage when the method is used to assess the clinical situation.

6.2.3 Thin-layer chromatography

The thin-layer chromatographic properties of 45 psychotropic drugs in 5 solvent systems were described by Zingales (1967). Most of the tricyclic antidepressants have too little u.v. absorbance or native fluorescence for direct quantification on thin-layer plates. An exception is protriptyline, which has been determined by fluorescence scanning (Gupta and Molnar, 1980). Amitriptyline, nortriptyline and nomifensine fluoresce after exposing the plate to perchloric acid (Faber *et al.*, 1974). Thioridazine and its metabolites are highly fluorescent after oxidation with H_2O_2 (Muusze, 1975). Kaul *et al.* (1970) dansylated and chromatographed eleven desmethyl and/or hydroxylated metabolites of chlorpromazine. The spots were eluted for fluorescence measurements. The tertiary amines, chlorpromazine (Lehr and Kaul, 1975) and amitriptyline (Kaul *et al.*, 1978) were reacted with 9-bromomethylacridine and the quaternary-ammonium salts separated by thin-layer. Fluorescent products were obtained by exposing the plates to ultraviolet light. Because of the greater u.v. extinctions several phenothiazines may be quantified by direct densitometric scanning without prior treatment (Breyer and Schmalzing, 1977; Kresse *et al.*, 1980). Imipramine and despiramine have been determined as yellow spots after the plate had been exposed to nitrous acid vapours (Nagy and Treiber, 1973).

6.2.4 Gas chromatography (GC)

An inspection of the literature (Scoggins *et al.*, 1980; Gupta and Molnar, 1980) shows 50% phenylmethylsilicone (OV-17 or SP 2250) stationary phase to be the most common choice for the gas chromatography of these compounds. Occasionally, less-polar methylsilicone (OV-101, SE-30) is used (Alfredsson *et al.*, 1976) and on other occasions OV-225 has been shown to be useful (Whelpton and Curry, 1975). In our laboratory 3% OV-17 on 80–100 or 100–120 mesh Chromosorb W HP is the choice for preliminary investigations into the chromatographic behaviour of centrally acting drugs.

Although chlorpromazine and some ot its metabolites in urine had been chromatographed by Driscoll *et al.* in 1964 using flame-ionisation detection (FID), the breakthrough in measuring plasma concentrations came when Curry (1968) used a ^{63}Ni electron-capture detector (ECD). The sensitivity was $\approx$ 10 ng ml^{-1} for a 1-ml plasma sample, or lower if larger samples were used. The extraction and chromatographic characteristics of five metabolites were also described. The requirement for compounds to be electron-capturing limits the applicability of this detector, particularly for the tertiary-amine phenothiazines which are not amenable to derivatisation. A method for fluphenazine and perphenazine as heptafluorobutyryl (HFB) esters has been described (Larsen and Naestoft, 1973) but never applied. In later work, perphenazine assays relied on the electron-capturing properties imparted by the 2-chlorosubstituent (Hansen and Larsen, 1974; 1977). Fluphenazine pentafluorobenzoate has been prepared using pentafluorobenzoylimidazole but, although it was stable to thin-layer chromatography, it was heat-labile and decomposed on gas chromatography (this laboratory, unpublished). Zimelidine, containing an aromatic bromine, has been determined by GC–ECD without derivatisation (Larsen and Marinelli, 1978) but other tricyclics must be suitably derivatised to make them electron-capturing. The secondary amines are chromatographed as trifluoroacetyl (TFA) or heptafluorobutyryl derivatives (Scoggins *et al.*, 1980). An interesting approach is the formation of trichloroethyl carbamates for determining tertiary-amine tricyclics (Hartvig and Naslund, 1977). The secondary-amine metabolites are separated before derivatisation.

Flame-ionisation detection has been used successfully for tricyclic antidepressants, but large sample volumes are generally required and the sensitivity is relatively poor. The first such assay was applied to the tertiary amine, amitriptyline (Braithwaite and Widdop, 1971). Nortriptyline was separated as the trifluoroacetamide. With 5 ml of plasma the sensitivity was $\approx$ 20 ng ml^{-1}. The GC–FID of seven tricyclics has been described in a single paper (Nyberg and Martensson, 1977). The FID determination of thioridazine was described by Curry and Mould (1969) but it was shown later that poor resolution from desmethylthioridazine could be a problem. Treatment with trifluoroacetic anhydride should resolve any desmethyl metabolite (Ng and Crammer, 1977).

The introduction of the nitrogen–phosphorus detector (NPD) made a major contribution to the GC of this class of compounds. Its use avoids the need to derivatise to make the compounds detectable and sensitivities below 1 ng ml^{-1} are possible. Gifford *et al.* (1975) described the chromatographic properties and sensitivities for eleven tricyclic antidepressants using NPD. The potential for plasma assay was exemplified using plasma samples 'spiked' with imipramine. A single extraction into heptane was employed and a column back-flushing technique used to avoid detector contamination. Scoggins *et al.* (1980) list twelve papers describing plasma tricyclic determinations using GC–NPD. Volin (1981) expressed a preference for SP-2250 rather than OV-17 in a method describing the GC–NPD of nine tricyclic antidepressants. Nitrogen detectors based on electrically heated rubidium silicate are suitable for determining trimethylsilyl derivatives (TMS) (see Figure 6.4 and Whelpton and Curry, 1976b). Nitrogen detection was an obvious choice for quantifying the phenothiazines that are not readily amenable to ECD. Franklin *et al.* (1978) described the GC–NPD of plasma fluphenazine chromatographed as the TMS-ether. The sensitivity was 2 ng ml^{-1}. Dekirmenjian and co-workers increased the sensitivity to 0.5 ng ml^{-1} using a 5-ml plasma sample and chromatographing the acetate ester (Dekirmenjian *et al.*, 1978; Jarvaid *et al.*, 1981). NPD can be substituted for ECD in the original chlorpromazine method as the sensitivities are similar—the advantage being improved linearity and less problems from detector contamination. The Hall conductivity detector (Risk and Hall, 1977) appears to have no advantage over NPD for quantifying phenothiazines.

A gas-chromatographic–mass-fragmentographic (GC–MF) method for chlorpromazine was described as early as 1968 (Hammer *et al.*, 1968). The same group (Borga *et al.*) reported a GC–MF method for nortriptyline and desmethylnortriptyline in 1971. The GC–MF of seven tricyclic antidepressants was reported by Biggs *et al.* in 1976. The use of GC–MF enabled Alfredsson *et al.* (1976) to detect concentrations of chlorpromazine, desmethylchlorpromazine and 7-hydroxychlorpromazine as low as $\approx$ 1 ng ml^{-1} in plasma and chlorpromazine to $\approx$ 0.2 ng ml^{-1} in CSF. The use of deuterium-labelled internal standards is useful when handling sub-nanogram quantities. Alfredsson (1976) used d_3-labelled materials and, similarly, Whelpton *et al.* (1982) used [methyl-^{2}H] trifluoperazine in a GC–MF method that was sensitive to $\approx$ 200 pg ml^{-1} of plasma. Midha *et al.* (1982) labelled the piperidine ring to give a d_4-trifluoperazine internal standard. The sensitivity of their method was approximately 78 pg ml^{-1}.

6.2.5 Liquid chromatography (LC)

The use of microparticulate packing materials has revolutionised liquid chromatography. Separations can be achieved in minutes rather than taking several hours or days. The price paid for the vast increase in column efficiencies is very much higher back-pressures, so that pumps, columns, injection ports, etc., have to withstand pressures of several thousands of pounds per square inch—hence the term 'high-pressure' liquid chromatography. The term 'high-performance', particularly favoured by instrument manufacturers, is also used, although this seems to prejudge the results. 'High-speed' is a third choice. A range of packing materials is available. Most are 'straight' silica or silica that has been surface-modified to give dimethyl (C_2), octyl (C_8), octadecyl (C_{18}, ODS), aminopropyl (NH_2) or cyanopropyl (CN) columns. To prevent excessive back-pressures the particle sizes have to be rigidly controlled. Popular packings have mean particle sizes of 10, 5 or 3 μm.

Early methods for phenothiazines and tricyclic antidepressants were based on liquid–solid adsorption or ion-pair methods. Muusze and Huber (1974) described an LC determination of thioridazine and several metabolites. The eluent was a rather complex mixture of trimethylpentane, 2-aminopropane, acetonitrile and ethanol. Compounds in the eluent were oxidised with $KMnO_4$ in a post-column reaction coil, the excess $KMnO_4$ removed in a second coil with H_2O_2 and the products measured by spectrofluorimetry. This work demonstrated not only the applicability of LC to phenothiazine plasma determinations but also the use of post-column reactions. The application of LC to the separation of phenothiazine and tricyclic antidepressants was reported in 1976 (Knox and Jurand).

Phenothiazines have ultraviolet absorption maxima, with high extinction coefficients ($\approx$ 30 000 M^{-1} cm^{-1}) in the region 250 to 260 nm and detectors using mercury discharge lamps and interference filters at 254 nm are eminently suitable. Until recently, fixed-wavelength detectors, with their higher energies, were more stable than corresponding variable-wavelength ones, but now sensitivities as low as 0.002 or 0.001 absorbance units full-scale deflection are possible with both. It can be calculated that 1 ng of chlorpromazine should give a response in the order of 10% of full scale. As practically all of an extracted sample can be injected, sensitivities of this order are sufficient for plasma analysis following single doses of chlorpromazine. This was demonstrated by Midha *et al.* in 1981. Using 2-ml samples they were able to quantify 1 ng ml^{-1} with a c.v. of 4%. Earlier, u.v. detection had been used to determine fluphenazine after ion-pair chromatography (Johansson *et al.*, 1976). At 1 ng ml^{-1} the precision was 7%. As phenothiazines are readily oxidised to semi-quinone ion radicals, electrochemical detection is an alternative approach—indeed, potentially, it is superior. Coulometric detection, using a custom-made glassy carbon cell, was described for perphenazine and fluphenazine (Tjaden *et al.*, 1976). Curry and Brown (1981) and Wallace *et al.* (1981b) used a commercially available amperometric detector to measure several phenothiazines. Wallace *et al.* (1981b) reported a sensitivity of 0.2 ng ml^{-1} (c.v. = 15.4%) for promethazine. Depending upon the compound, size of sample, chromatographic conditions etc., it would seem reasonable to expect a lower limit of detection in the order of 0.5 ng ml^{-1}. Radioimmunoassay has been applied to fractions of LC eluent to detect fluphenazine, its metabolites and related phenothiazines (Goldstein and Vunakis, 1981).

Not surprisingly, the development of LC assays of tricyclic antidepressants closely follows that for the phenothiazines. Alkyl-bonded phases, C_8 or C_{18}, eluted with acid-buffered eluents, are popular. Bannister *et al.* (1981) chromatographed eight compounds on a C_8 column eluted with acetonitrile-phosphate buffer, pH 3.3. U.V. detection at 205 nm was used. Using a C_{18} phase, Breutzmann and Bowers (1981) measured amitriptyline, nortriptyline, imipramine and desipramine to a sensitivity of ≈ 1 ng ml^{-1}, using a detector at 215 nm. Cyanopropyl-bonded columns, eluted with ammonium acetate-methanol mixtures, much as described for chlorpromazine, have been used (Lehrer and Cannon, 1982). Alkaline eluents with unmodified silica have been reported. Edelbrook *et al.* (1982) separated amitriptyline, nortriptyline, desmethylnortriptyline, 10-hydroxyamitriptyline, amitriptyline *N*-oxide, *cis*-10-nortriptyline and *trans*-10-hydroxynortriptyline on a silica column eluted with acetonitrile-methanol-1M-NH_4-OH (250 : 55 : 13, by vol.). Butylamine has been used instead of aqueous ammonia to separate amitriptyline, imipramine, nortriptyline and desipramine (Gupta *et al.*, 1982).

Silica, for either adsorption or ion-pair chromatography, and alkyl-bonded silica have been used for the liquid chromatography of tricyclic antidepressants (Scoggins, 1980). Cyanopropyl columns are popular for chromatographing phenothiazines (Midha *et al.*, 1981a; Curry and Brown, 1981; Wallace *et al.*, 1981a). Usually, eluents were buffered between pH 2.5 and pH 7.5 to reduce the risk of dissolving the silica or hydrolysing the surface coating. At these pH values the compounds are ionised (Table 6.1) and counter ions such as heptane sulphonic acid may be added to improve the chromatography (McCutcheon, 1979). Recently there has been a growing number of reports of the use of alkaline eluents. Wheals (1979) investigated the use of cation-exchange columns which were prepared by oxidising the SH-groups of mercapopropyl-modified silica to sulphonic acid. The chromatographic properties of 41 phenothiazines in various mixtures of methanol and ammonium-nitrate buffers were documented. Buffer concentrations as high as 1.0M with a pH of 10 were used successfully. Methanol-acetonitrile-ammonium carbonate (1 : 1 : 1, by vol.) has been used with surface-modified silica to separate fluphenazine and fluphenazine esters (Heyes and Salmon, 1978). In a later method to separate fluphenazine oxides, methanol-aqueous ammonia (9 : 1, by vol.) was used (Heyes *et al.*, 1980). Li Wan Po and Irwin (1978) eluted a 5-μm silica column with ethyl acetate-methanol-3% (w/v) ammonia (85 : 15 : 1, by vol.) to separate *cis*- and *trans*-isomers of fluphenthixol, clopenthixol, chlorprothixene, doxepin and dothiepin. Organic bases have been used, rather than ammonia, for example butylamine (Skinner *et al.*, 1981) and ethanolamine (Mehta, 1981).

Metabolites may be chromatographed (1) because these are to be quantified or (2) to demonstrate that they do not interfere with the determination of the parent compound. The separation of fluphenazine N- and S-oxides has been demonstrated (Heyes *et al.*, 1980). Preskorn *et al.* (1980) separated amitriptyline metabolites: nortriptyline, desmethylnortriptyline, 10-hydroxynortriptyline and 10,11-dihydroxynortriptyline. Thioridazine metabolites, which are difficult to separate on GC, have been separated by LC (Muusze and Huber, 1974; Skinner *et al.*, 1981). A typical separation is shown in Figure 6.6 (Watkins, unpublished).

6.2.6 Problems in analysis

Sample collection and storage can seriously affect the results. Loss of imipramine from plasma when blood was collected in Vacutainer Tubes has been shown to be due to the plasticiser, tris-(2-butoxyethyl)phosphate, in the rubber stoppers. The plasticiser displaced imipramine from protein binding sites and so increased the red-cell–plasma ratio (Borga *et al.*, 1977). The problem may be widespread (Shah *et al.*, 1982). A similar effect has been shown to occur when samples are collected in heparinised tubes; the red-cell–plasma ratios for amitriptyline, imipramine and maprotiline were significantly increased in heparinised blood compared with blood containing EDTA (Maguire *et al.*, 1980). However, heparin may be reducing the plasma concentrations by another mechanism. The recovery of chlorpromazine *added* to heparinised plasma was reduced compared with that obtained with water or oxalated plasma (Curry, 1974). Plasticisers may also cause problems by giving rise to spurious peaks on chromatographic traces. We traced a 'forest' of interfering peaks as being due to cap liners in screw-capped tubes used during the extraction of chlorpromazine. The peaks suddenly appeared after a new carton of tubes had been opened.

Metabolites are a potential source of trouble. Obviously it is important to test as many potential metabolites as possible to demonstrate that they will not interfere in the assay (Figures 6.3 and 6.4). The method of McCutcheon (1979) for the LC assay of thioridazine and mesoridazine could not be applied to biological samples, as these compounds were not resolved from their respective 5-sulphoxides (Watkins, unpublished). Decomposition of metabolites to parent compound is another problem. The elimination of water from amine oxides on GC columns is to be expected, but reduction to the tertiary amine may also occur (Curry and Evans, 1976). On column reduction of promethazine sulphoxide has been reported (Patel and Welling, 1981). The addition of sodium metabisulphite or ascorbic acid as 'preservatives' is not to be recommended as these agents will reduce N-oxide metabolites, giving an overestimate of the parent-amine concentration. Amine oxides are labile in alkali and this may be another source of error (Whelpton, 1978).

Another potential problem that we have encountered concerns the phenothiazine, thioridazine (Figure 6.5). 5-sulphoxides of 2-substituted phenothiazines are chiral but, naturally, the enantiomers do not separate during chromatography. However, thioridazine is chiral and so thioridazine 5-sulphoxide can exist in four isomeric forms. The diastereoisomers are separable by thin-layer and column chromatography (Watkins, unpublished). Without a full set of reference compounds it would be easy to confuse these isomers. An unknown metabolite reported by Muusze (1975) is probably a diastereoisomer of thioridazine 5-oxide.

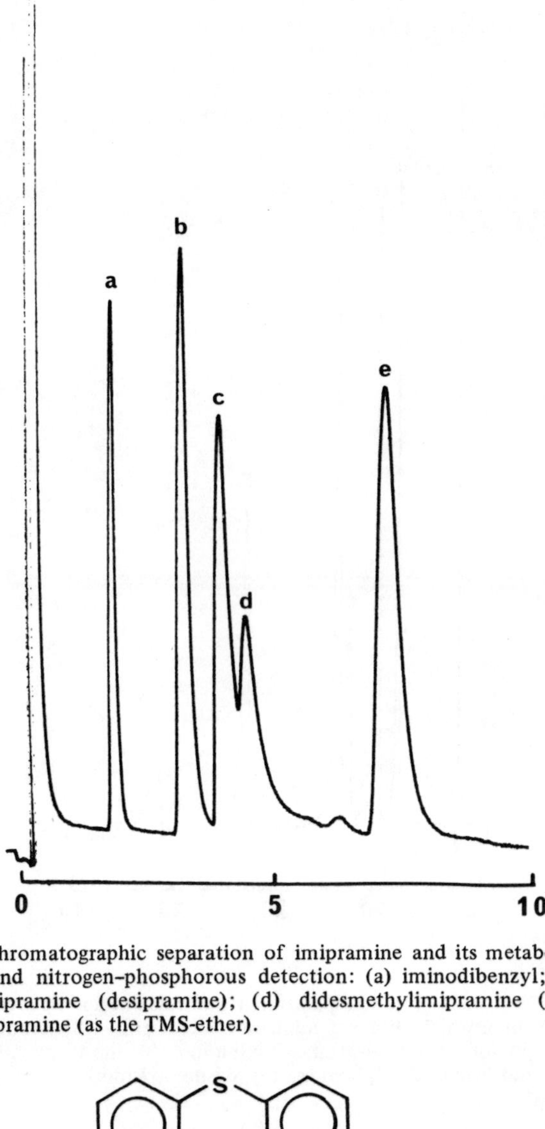

Figure 6.4 Gas-chromatographic separation of imipramine and its metabolites using a 3% OV-17 column and nitrogen-phosphorous detection: (a) iminodibenzyl; (b) imipramine; (c) desmethylimipramine (desipramine); (d) didesmethylimipramine (nordesipramine); (e) 2-hydroxyimipramine (as the TMS-ether).

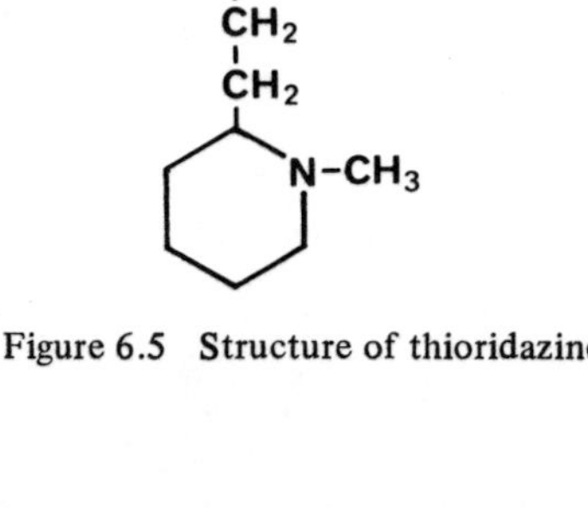

Figure 6.5 Structure of thioridazine.

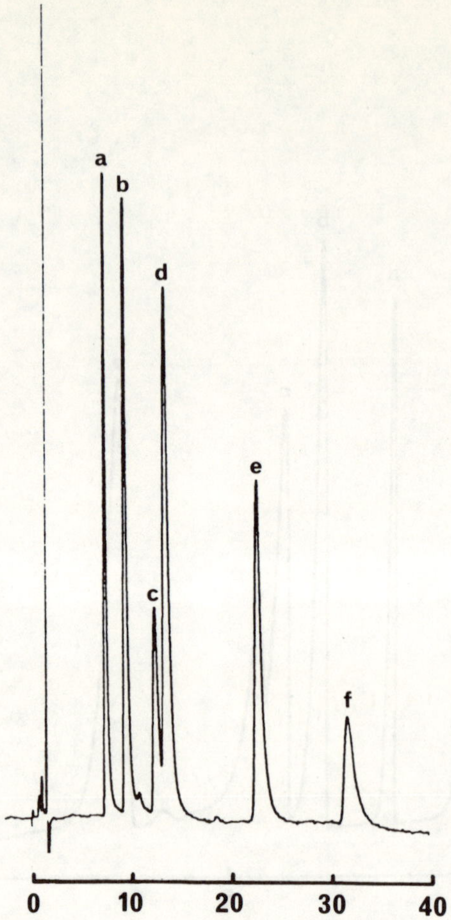

Figure 6.6 Liquid-chromatographic separation of thioridazine and its metabolites. Column: 250 × 4.6 mm Spherisorb 5. Eluent: methanol–acetonitrile–0.88 ammonium hydroxide (500 : 500 : 1.25, by vol.). (a) Thioridazine-2-sulphone, (b) thioridazine, (c) thioridazine-5-sulphoxide, (d) thioridazine-2-sulphoxide, (e) desmethylthioridazine, (f) desmethylthioridazine-2-sulphoxide.

Similarly the 2-sulphoxide and N-oxide are chiral and with all three positions oxidised there are sixteen possible isomers. The diastereoisomers of thioridazine N-oxide are separable (Table 6.2), but to date we have not separated isomers of the 2-sulphoxide.

Table 6.2 R_f Values of thioridazine 5- and N-oxides

Compound	R_f
thioridazine	0.62
thioridazine 5-oxide	0.44
thioridazine 5-oxide	0.39
thioridazine N-oxide	0.30
thioridazine N-oxide	0.24

System: SiO_2; $CHCl_3$-ethanol–ammonia, 80 : 10 : 1, by vol.

6.2.7 Choice of method

If the available apparatus is limited there may not be a choice. On the other hand, if there is, it will be influenced by previous experience, particular compound or compounds to be assayed, reasons for doing the assay, number of samples, etc.

GC–NPD appears to be applicable to practically all the compounds and is suitable for the less-experienced analyst. The sensitivity should be adequate for the majority of the compounds under most conditions, although assaying samples below about 1 to 2 ng ml^{-1} may need some perseverance.

GC–ECD methods are not to be recommended unless nitrogen detection is unsuitable. Preparing electron-capturing derivatives can be fraught with difficulties, as extraneous peaks are prone to arise from coextractants, solvent impurities, decomposition of the reagent, etc. If the compound is naturally electron-capturing then the selectivity of the ECD can be very useful.

The problems of low volatility, high polarity and thermal instability of metabolites make LC an attractive alternative to GC. Modern LC is a newer and rapidly expanding analytical technique. Versatility is a major advantage. The instrumentation is more 'modular' than GC and the various components are easily plumbed together. Two or three detectors may be connected in series and as most are nondestructive the sample can be recovered if needs be. Ultraviolet detectors are stable and have good linearity—the limitations of using 254 nm may be overcome by using variable-wavelength detectors (modern ones now offer 0.001 absorption units, full-scale deflection) or Zn or Cd lamps for detection at 214 or 229 nm respectively. Electrochemical detectors are less stable and less versatile than ultraviolet and in many ways are LC's equivalent of electron-capture detectors but are potentially more sensitive for phenothiazines. Commercial coulometric detectors look promising.

Small sample volumes, high sensitivities and high throughput make radioimmunoassay very appealing, although selectivity is likely to be a problem. Separation techniques to improve the selectivity reduce the number of samples that can be assayed in a given time. Radioimmunoassay is often described as inexpensive, but this appears to neglect the cost of developing the antisera. If several compounds and their metabolites are to be assayed then a chromatographic approach is probably preferable. Antisera that cross-react with most members of a group are useful for initial screening of unknown samples to determine the chemical class (e.g., is it a phenothiazine or a tricyclic antidepressant?) prior to a more selective technique.

GC–MF is thought of as a specialist technique and the high capital cost limits its use. With the introduction of newer systems based on quadrapole 'ion-filters', the cost in real terms has declined sharply. GC–MF is the most specific method available and when a number of compounds are to be determined is competitive with radioimmunoassay.

ACKNOWLEDGEMENTS

I thank Miss Geraldine Watkins for providing Figure 6.6 and the data of Table 6.2, and the MRC for financial support under grant No. G 979/342/N.

REFERENCES

Alfredsson, G., Wode-Helgodt, B., and Sedvall, G. (1976). A mass fragmentographic method for the determination of chlorpromazine and two of its active metabolites in human plasma and CSF. *Psychopharmacology* **48**, 123–31.

Bannister, S. J., Van der Wal, S., Dolan, J. W., and Snyder, L. R. (1981). Liquid chromatographic analysis for common tricyclic antidepressant drugs and their metabolites in serum or plasma with the Technicon 'FAST-LC' system. *Clin. Chem.* **27**, 849–55.

Beckett, A. H., Essien, E. E., and Smyth, W. F. (1974). A polarographic method for the determination of the N-oxide, N-oxide-sulphoxide and sulphoxide metabolites of chlorpromazine. *J. Pharm. Pharmac.* **26**, 399–407.

Bickel, M. H., and Weder, H. J. (1969). Buccal absorption and other properties of pharmacokinetic importance of imipramine and its metabolites. *Ibid.* **21**, 160–8.

Biggs, J. T., Holland, W. H., Chang, S., Hipps, P. P., and Sherman, W. R. (1976). Electron beam ionization mass fragmentographic analysis of antidepressants in human plasma. *J. Pharm. Sci.* **65**, 261–8.

Borga, O., Palmer, L., Linnarsson, A., and Holmstedt, B. (1971). Quantitative determination of nortriptyline and desmethylnortriptyline in human plasma by combined gas-chromatography–mass-spectrometry. *Analyt. Lett.* **4**, 837–49.

Borga, O., Piafsky, K. M., and Nilsen, O. G. (1977). Plasma protein binding of basic drugs. 1: Selective displacement from alpha$_1$-acid glycoprotein by tris(2-butoxyethyl)phosphate. *Clin. Pharmacol. Ther.* **22**, 539–44.

Braithwaite, R. A., and Widdop, B. (1971). A specific gas-chromatographic method for the measurement of 'steady-state' plasma levels of amitriptyline and nortriptyline in patients. *Clin. Chim. Acta.* **35**, 461–72.

Breutzmann, D. A., and Bowers, L. D. (1981). Reversed-phase liquid chromatography and gas chromatography/mass fragmentography compared for determination of tricyclic antidepressant drugs. *Clin. Chem.* **27**, 1907–11.

Breyer, U., and Schmalzing, G. (1977). A thin-layer chromatographic method for the measurement of trifluoperazine and its metabolites in rat tissues. *Drug Metab. Dispos.* **5**, 97–115.

Brunswick, D. J., Needelman, B., and Mendels, J. (1978). Radioimmunoassay of imipramine and desipramine. *Life Sci.* **22**, 137–46.

Brunswick, D. J., Needelman, B., and Mendels, J. (1979). Specific radioimmunoassay of amitriptyline and nortriptyline. *Br. J. Clin. Pharmacol.* **7**, 343–8.

Chatten, L. G., and Harris, L. E. (1962). Relationship between pK_b (H_2O) of organic compounds and $E\frac{1}{2}$ values in several non aqueous solvents. *Analyt. Chem.* **34**, 1495–1501.

Cornis, G., Godbillon, J., and Metayer, (1976). Determination of clomipramine in plasma or urine by the double-radioisotope derivative technique. *Clin. Chem.* **22**, 817–23.

Crammer, J. L., and Rolfe, B. (1970). Metabolism of ^{14}C-imipramine. 3: Conversions by rat tissues. *Psychopharmacologia* **12**, 263–77.

Crammer, J. L., Woods, H., and Roffe, B. (1968). Metabolism of ^{14}C-imipramine. 1: Excretion in the rat and in man. *ibid.* **12**, 263–77.

Crammer, J. L., Scott, B., and Rolfe, B. (1969). Metabolism of ^{14}C-imipramine, 2: Urinary metabolites in man. *Ibid.* **15**, 207–25.

Creese, I., and Snyder, S. H. (1977). A simple and sensitive radioreceptor assay for antischizophrenic drugs in blood. *Nature, Lond.* **270**, 180–2.

Curry, S. H. (1968). Determination of nanogram quantities of chlorpromazine and some of its metabolites in plasma using gas–liquid chromatography with an electron-capture detector. *Analyt. Chem.* **40**, 1251–5.

Curry, S. H. (1974). In Forrest, I., Carr, C. J., and Usdin, E. (eds), *Phenothiazines and Structurally Related Drugs*, Raven, New York.

Curry, S. H., and Brown, E. A. (1981). HPLC assay of phenothiazine, thioxanthene and butyrophenone neuroleptics and antihistamines in plasma. 3: Quantitative aspects and clinical data. *IRCS Med. Sci.* **9**, 170–1.

Curry, S. H., and Evans, S. (1976). A note on the assay of chlorpromazine N-oxide and its sulphoxide in plasma and urine. *J. Pharm. Pharmac.* **28**, 467–8.

Curry, S. H., and Mould, G. P. (1969). Gas chromatographic identification of thioridazine in plasma. *Ibid.* **21**, 674–7.

Curry, S. H., Whelpton, R., de Schepper, P. J., Vranckx, S., and Schiff, A. A. (1979). Kinetics of fluphenazine after fluphenazine dihydrochloride, enanthate and decanoate administration to man. *Brit. J. Clin. Pharmac.* **7**, 325–31.

Dekirmenjian, H., Jarvaid, J. I., Duslak, B., and Davis, J. M. (1978). Determination of antipsychotic drugs by gas–liquid chromatography with a nitrogen detector using a simple acetylation technique. *J. Chromatogr.* **160**, 291–6.

Driscoll, J. L., Martin, H. F., and Gudzinowicz, B. J. (1964). A gas chromatographic method for the quantitative analysis of some urinary metabolites of chlorpromazine. *J. Gas Chromatogr.* **2**, 109.

Edelbroek, P. M., de Haas, E. J. M., and de Wolff, F. A. (1982). Liquid-chromatographic determination of amitriptyline and its metabolites in serum, with adsorption onto glass minimized. *Clin. Chem.* **28**, 2143–8.

Efron, D. H., Harris, S. R., Manian, A. A., and Gaudette, L. E. (1971). Radioassay of chlorpromazine and its metabolites in plasma. *Psychopharmacologia* **19**, 207–10.

Faber, D. B., Mulder, C., and Man In't Veld, W. A. (1974). A thin-layer method for the determination of amitriptyline and nortriptyline in plasma. *J. Chromatogr.* **100**, 55–61.

Fishman, V., and Goldenberg, H. (1960). Metabolism of chlorpromazine organic-extractable fraction from human urine. *Proc. Soc. Exp. Biol. Med.* **104**, 99–103.

Fishman, V., and Goldenberg, H. (1963). Metabolism of CPZ. 4: Identification of 7-OHCPZ and its sulphoxide and demethyl derivatives. *Ibid.* **112**, 501–6.

Fishman, V., and Goldenberg, H. (1965). Side-chain degradation and ring hydroxylation of phenothiazine tranquillizers. *J. Pharm. Exp. Therap.* **150**, 122–8.

Fishman, V., Heaton, A., and Goldenberg, H. (1962). Metabolism of CPZ. 3: Isolation and identification of chlorpromazine-*N*-oxide. *Proc. Soc. Exp. Biol. Med.* **109**, 548–52.

Franklin, M., Wiles, D. H., and Harvey, D. J. (1978). Sensitive gas chromatographic determination for fluphenazine in human plasma. *Clin. Chem.* **24**, 41–4.

Gaertner, H. J., and Breyer, U. (1972). In vivo piperazine ring degradation in neuroleptic and antihistaminic drugs. *Arzhein-Forsch* **22**, 1084–5.

Gifford, L. A., Turner, P., and Pare, C. M. B. (1975). Sensitive method for the routine determination of tricyclic antidepressants in plasma using a specific nitrogen detector. *J. Chromatogr.* **105**, 107–13.

Goldstein, S. A., and Vunakis, H. V. (1981). Determination of fluphenazine, related phenothiazine drugs and metabolites by combined high-performance liquid chromatography and radioimmunoassay. *J. Pharm. Exp. Therap.* **217**, 36–43.

Gram, L. F., and Overφ, K. F. (1972). Drug interactions: inhibitory effect of neuroleptics on metabolism of tricyclic antidepressants in man. *Br. Med. J.* **i**, 463–5.

Green, A. L. (1967). Ionization constants and water solubilities of some phenothiazine tranquillizers and related compounds. *J. Pharm. Pharmac.* **19**, 10–16.

Gupta, R. N., and Molnar, G. (1980). Plasma levels and tricyclic antidepressant therapy. 1. A review of assay methods. *Biopharm. Drug. Disp.* **1**, 259–77.

Gupta, S. K., Robertson, S., Wellstead, C., and Skrinska, V. A. (1982). High pressure liquid chromatographic method for tricyclic antidepressants: Comparison with GC/MS. *Clin. Chem.* **28**, 1646.

Hammer, W. M., and Brodie, B. B. (1967). Application of isotope derivative technique to assay of secondary amines: Estimation of desipramine by acetylation with ^{3}H-acetic anhydride. *J. Pharmac. Exp. Ther.* **157**, 503–8.

Hammer, C. G., Holmstedt, B., and Ryhage, R. (1968). Mass fragmentography. Identification of chlorpromazine and its metabolites in human blood by a new method. *Analyt. Biochem.* **25**, 532–48.

Hansen, C. E., and Larsen, N. E. (1974). Perphenazine concentration in human whole blood. *Psychopharmac.* **37**, 31–6.

Hansen, L. B., and Larsen, N. E. (1977). Plasma concentrations of perphenazine and its sulphoxide metabolite during continuous oral treatment. *Ibid.* **53**, 127–30.

Harris, S. R., Gaudette, L. E., Efron, D. H., and Manian, A. A. (1970). A method for the measurement of plasma imipramine and desmethylimipramine concentrations. *Life Sci.* **9**, 781–8.

Hartvig, P., and Naslund, B. (1977). Simultaneous determination of plasma amitriptyline and nortriptyline as trichloroethyl carbamates by electron-capture gas chromatography. *J. Chromatogr.* **133**, 367–71.

Heyes, W. F., and Salmon, J. R. (1978). Some aspects of the high-performance liquid chromatography of fluphenazine and its esters. *Ibid.* **156**, 309–16.

Heyes, W. F., Salmon, J. R., and Marlow, W. (1980). High performance liquid chromatographic separation of the N- and S-oxides of fluphenazine and fluphenazine decanoate. *Ibid.* **194**, 416–20.

Jarvaid, J. I., Dekirmenjian, H., Liskevych, V., Lin, R. L., and Davis, J. M. (1981). Fluphenazine determination in human plasma by a sensitive gas chromatographic method using nitrogen detector. *J. Chromatogr. Sci.* **19**, 439–43.

Johansson, R., Borg, K. O., and Gabrielsson, M. (1976). Determination of fluphenazine in plasma by ion-pair partition chromatography. *Acta Pharma. Suecica* **13**, 193–200.

Jφrgenson, A. (1978). A sensitive and specific radioimmunoassay for *cis*(Z)-flupenthixol in human serum. *Life Sci.* **23**, 1533–42.

Kaul, P. N., Conway, M. W., Clark, M., and Huffine, J. (1970). Chlorpromazine metabolism. 1: Quantitative fluorometric method for 11 chlorpromazine metabolites. *J. Pharm. Sci.* **59**, 1745–9.

Kaul, P. N., Whitfield, L. R., and Clark, M. L. (1978). Quantitative determination of amitriptyline in blood. *Ibid.* **67**, 60–2.

Kawashima, K., Dixon, R., and Spector, S. (1975). Development of radioimmunoassay for chlorpromazine. *Eur. J. Pharmac.* **32**, 195–202.

Knox, J. H., and Jurand, J. (1975). Separation of tricyclic psychosedative drugs by high-speed ion-pair partition and liquid–solid adsorption chromatography. *J. Chromatogr.* **103**, 311–26.

Kresse, M., Schley, J., and Miller-Oblinghausen, B. (1980). Reliable routine method for determination of perazine in serum by thin-layer chromatography with an internal standard. *Ibid.* **183**, 475–82.

Larsen, N. E., and Marinelli, K. (1978). Determination of zimeldine and its demethylated metabolite in human plasma by gas-chromatography. *Ibid.* **156**, 335–9.

Larsen, N. E., and Naestoft, J. (1973). Determination of perphenazine and fluphenazine in whole blood by gas-chromatography. *Med. Lab. Tech.* **30**, 129–32.

Lehr, R. E., and Kaul, P. N. (1975). Chlorpromazine metabolism. 4: Quaternization as a key to determination of picomoles of chlorpromazine and other tertiary amine drugs. *J. Pharm. Sci.* **64**, 950–3.

Lehrer, M., and Cannon, P. (1982). Rapid quantification of tricyclic antidepressant drugs by HPLC. *Clin. Chem.* **28**, 1646.

Li Wan Po, A., and Irwin, W. J. (1979). A high performance liquid chromatographic assay of *cis-* and *trans-*isomers of tricyclic neuroleptic drugs. *J. Pharm. Pharmac.* **31**, 512–16.

McCutcheon, J. R. (1979). Reverse-phase HPLC determination of thioridazine and mesoridazine in whole blood. *J. Analyt. Toxicol.* **3**, 105–7.

Maguire, K. P., Burrows, G. D., Norman, J. R., and Scoggins, B. A. (1980). Blood/plasma distribution ratios of psychotropic drugs. *Clin. Chem.* **26**, 1624–5.

Mehta, A. C. (1981). High-performance liquid chromatographic determination of chlorpromazine and thioridazine hydrochlorides in pharmaceutical formulations. *Analyst* **106**, 1119–22.

Midha, K. K., Cooper, J. K., and Hubbard, J. W. (1980). Radioimmunoassay for fluphenazine in human plasma. *Commun. Psychopharmac.* **4**, 107–14.

Midha, K. K., Cooper, J. K., McGilveray, I. J., Butterfield, A. G., and Hubbard, J. W. (1981a). High-performance liquid chromatographic assay for nanogram determination of chlorpromazine and its comparison with a radioimmunoassay. *J. Pharm. Sci.* **70**, 1043–6.

Midha, K. K., Hubbard, J. W., Cooper, J. K., Hawes, E. M., Fournier, S., and Yeung, P. (1981b). Radioimmunoassay for trifluoperazine in human plasma. *Br. J. Clin. Pharmac.* **12**, 189–93.

Midha, K. K., MacKonka, C., Cooper, J. K., Hubbard, J. W., and Yeung, P. K. F. (1981c) Radioimmunoassay for perphenazine in human plasma. *Ibid.* **1**, 85–8.

Midha, K. K., Roscoe, R. M. H., Hall, K., Hawes, E. M., Cooper, J. K., McKay, G., and Shetty, H. V. (1982). A gas-chromatographic mass spectrometric assay for plasma trifluoperazine concentrations following single doses. *Biomed. Mass Spectr.* **9**, 186–90.

Muusze, R. G. (1975). Analysis of thioridazine and some of its metabolites in blood by liquid chromatography. PhD thesis, Amsterdam.

Muusze, R. G., and Huber, J. F. K. (1974). Determination of the psychotropic drug thioridazine and its metabolites in blood by means of high pressure liquid chromatography in combination with fluorometric reaction detection. *J. Chrom. Sci.* **12**, 779–87.

Nagy, A., and Treiber, L. (1973). Quantitative determination of imipramine and desipramine in human blood plasma by direct densitometry of thin-layer chromatograms. *J. Pharm. Pharmacol.* **25**, 599–603.

Ng, C. H., and Crammer, J. L. (1977). Measurement of thioridazine in blood and urine. *Br. J. Clin. Pharmacol.* **4**, 173–83.

Nyberg, G., and Martensson, E. (1977). Quantitative analysis of tricyclic antidepressants in serum from psychiatric patients. *J. Chromatogr.* **143**, 491–7.

Overø, K. F. (1972). Increased specificity of the ^{3}H-acetic anhydride coupling method for plasma analysis of drugs containing secondary amino groups. *Acta Pharmacol. Toxicol.* **31**, 433–40.

Patel, R. B., and Welling, R. G. (1981). On column reduction of promethazine metabolite during gas-chromatography. *Clin. Chem.* **27**, 1780–1.

Preskorn, S. H., Leonard, K., and Hignite, C. (1980). Liquid chromatography of amitriptyline and related tricyclic compounds. *J. Chromatogr.* **197**, 246–50.

Riess, W. (1974). The double radio-isotope derivative technique for the assay of drugs in biological material. 1: The measurement of maprotiline. *Analyt. Chim. Acta* **68**, 363–76.

Risk, C. A., and Hall, R. C. (1977). Evaluation of the Hall electrolytic conductivity detector for the analysis of narcotic alkaloid and phenothiazine drugs extracted from urine. *J. Chrom. Sci.* **15**, 156–9.

Robinson, J. D., and Risby, D. (1977). Radioimmunoassay for flupenthixol in plasma. *Clin. Chem.* **23**, 2085–88.

Rosseel, M. T., Bogaert, M. G., and Claeys, M. (1978). Quantitative GLC determination of *cis-* and *trans-*isomers of doxepin and desmethyldoxepin. *J. Pharm. Sci.* **65**, 802–5.

Scoggins, B. A., Maguire, K. P., Noirman, T. R., and Burrows, G. D. (1980). Measurements of tricyclic antidepressants. *Clin. Chem.* **26**, 5–17.

Shah, V. P., Knapp, G., Skelly, J. P., and Cabana, B. E. (1982). Interference with measurements of certain drugs by a plasticiser in vacutainer tubes. *Ibid.* **28**, 2327–8.

Skinner, T., Gochnauer, R., and Linnoila, M. (1981). Liquid chromatographic method to measure thioridazine and its active metabolites in plasma. *Acta. Pharmacol. Toxicol.* **48**, 223–6.

Spector, S., Spector, N. L., and Almeida, M. P. (1975). Radioimmunoassay for desmethylimipramine. *Psychopharmac. Comm.* **1**, 421–9.

Spirtes, M. A. (1974). Two types of metabolically produced trifluoperazine N-oxides. In Forest, I. S., Carr, C. J., Denber, H. C. B., and Usdin, E. (eds). *Phenothiazines and Structurally Related Drugs.* Raven, New York.

Tjaden, U. R., Lankelma, J., Poppe, H., and Muusze, R. G. (1976). Anodic coulometric detection with a glassy carbon electrode in combination with reversed-phase high-performance liquid chromatography. *J. Chromatogr.* **125**, 275–86.

Volin, P. (1981). Therapeutic monitoring of tricyclic antidepressant drugs in plasma or serum by GC. *Clin. Chem.* **27**, 1785–7.

Wallace, J. E., Shimck, E. L., Harris, S. C., and Stavchansky, S. (1981a). Determination of promethazine in serum by liquid chromatography. *Ibid.* **27**, 253–5.

Wallace, J. E., Schimck, E. L., Stavchansky, S., and Harris, S. C. (1981b). Determination of promethazine and other phenothiazine compounds by liquid chromatography with electrochemical detection. *Analyt. Chem.* **53**, 960–2.

Wheals, B. B. (1979). Simple preparation of a bonded cation-exchange packing material and its application of the separation of phenothiazines by high-performance liquid chromatography. *J. Chromatogr.* **177**, 263–70.

Whelpton, R. (1978). Lipophilicity as a factor in the biochemical pharmacology of tranquillizing drugs. PhD thesis, London.

Whelpton, R., and Curry, S. H. (1975). Gas-chromatography separation of chlorpromazine, diazepam and *N*-desmethydiazepam. *J. Pharm. Pharmac.* **27**, 970–1.

Whelpton, R., and Curry, S. H. (1976a). Chromatographic properties of imines formed from delinethylchlorpromazine and various aldehydes and ketones. *J. Chromatgr.* **121**, 88–92.

Whelpton, R., and Curry, S. H. (1976b). Methods for the study of fluphenazine kinetics in man. *J. Pharm. Pharmac.* **28**, 869–73.

Whelpton, R., Curry, S. H., and Watkins, G. M. (1982). Analysis of plasma trifluoperazine by gas chromatography and selected ion monitoring. *J. Chromatogr.* **228**, 321–6.

Wiles, D. J., and Franklin, M. (1978). Radioimmunoassay for fluphenazine in human plasma. *Brit. J. Clin. Pharmac.* **5**, 265–8.

Zehnder, K., Kalberer, F., Kreis, W., and Rutschmann, J. (1962). The metabolism of thioridazine and one of its pyrrolidine analogues in the rat. *Biochemical Pharmacol.* **11**, 535–50.

Zingales, I. (1967). Systematic identification of psychotropic drugs by thin-layer chromatography, 1. *J. Chromatogr.* **31**, 405–19.

7
Analysis of local anaesthetics

G. T. TUCKER and M. S. LENNARD

7.1 THE MAJOR AGENTS

Modern regional anaesthesia is practised with a relatively small armamentarium of agents. These can be divided into esters of the procaine type and amides of the lignocaine type; their chemical structures are shown in Table 7.1. Of the compounds listed, bupivacaine and lignocaine are currently the most widely used in anaesthetic practice. The former is especially popular for providing epidural analgesia during labour and vaginal delivery, owing to its relatively long duration of action and an ability to produce a marked differential blockade favouring sensory rather than motor loss. Etidocaine is a new, long-acting analogue but a tendency to produce a differential motor block largely confines its use to surgical anaesthesia. Prilocaine has fallen out of favour for epidural anaesthesia because of methaemoglobinaemia associated with high doses, although a relatively low propensity for central-nervous-system toxicity commends it for peripheral nerve blocks and intravenous regional anaesthesia. Like lignocaine it is widely used in dentistry.

Of the ester compounds, procaine is now largely relegated to use as an infiltration agent; amethocaine, in common with cocaine and benzocaine, is restricted to topical application, although some centres still use it as a spinal anaesthetic; while chloroprocaine has lately been resurrected in the USA for obstetric applications following reports of fetal morbidity associated with paracervical injection of more toxic agents such as mepivacaine.

Apart from its value as a local anaesthetic, lignocaine is extensively used as an intravenous cardiac anti-dysrhythmic agent. Cocaine is also set apart from the other local anaesthetics owing to the forensic implications of its abuse potential. Procaine has been used in high dose by i.v. infusion as an analgesic and together with other drugs, such as penicillin, to produce slow-release i.m. preparations.

Table 7.1 Chemical structures of clinically important local-anaesthetic agents

	Aromatic ring	Linkage group	Carbon chain	Amino group
Esters				
cocaine	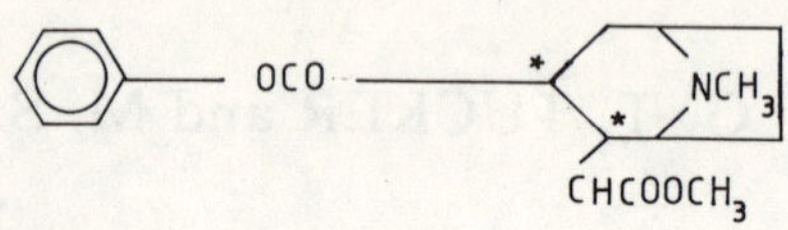			
benzocaine	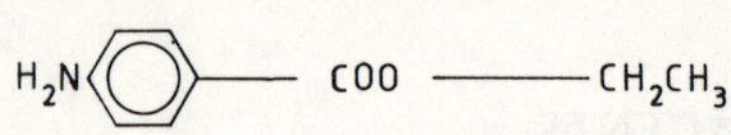			
procaine (Novocaine)	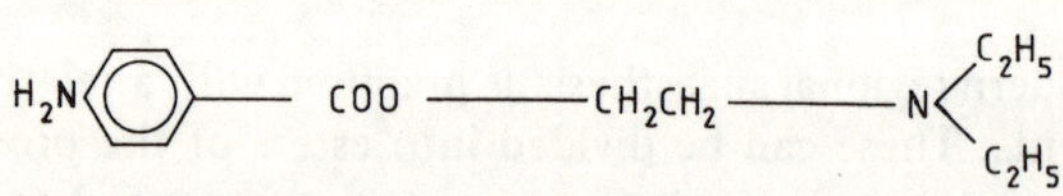			
2-chloroprocaine (Nesacaine)	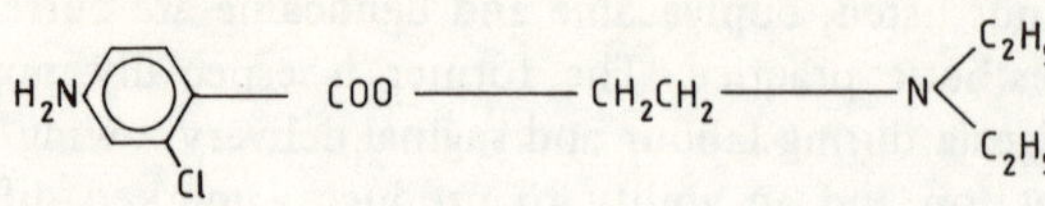			
amethocaine (Tetracaine, Pontocaine, Decicaine)	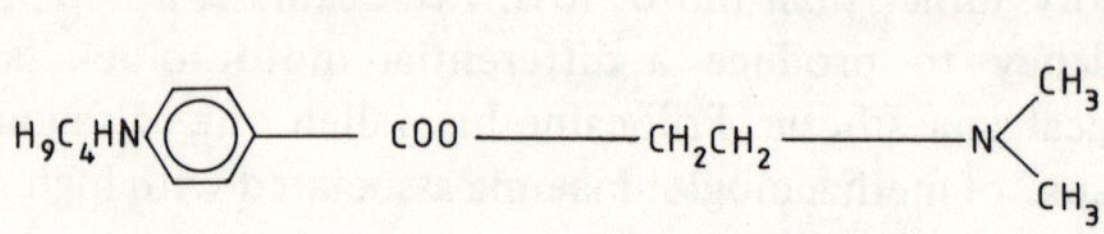			
Amides				
cinchocaine (Dibucaine, Nupercaine)				
prilocaine (Citanest)	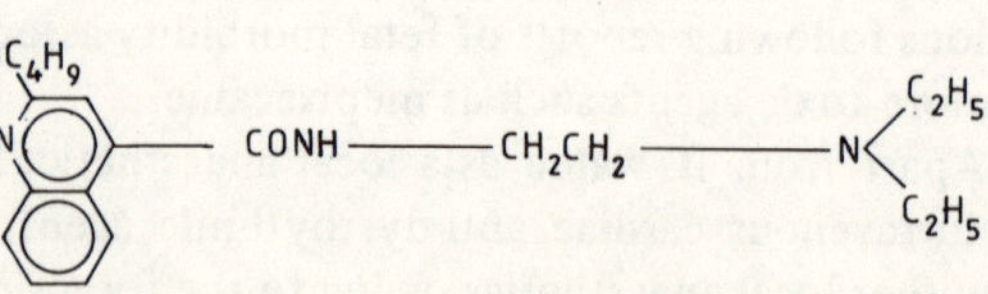			

lignocaine (Lidocaine, Xylocaine)

mepivacaine (Carbocaine)

bupivacaine (Marcaine)

etidocaine (Duranest)

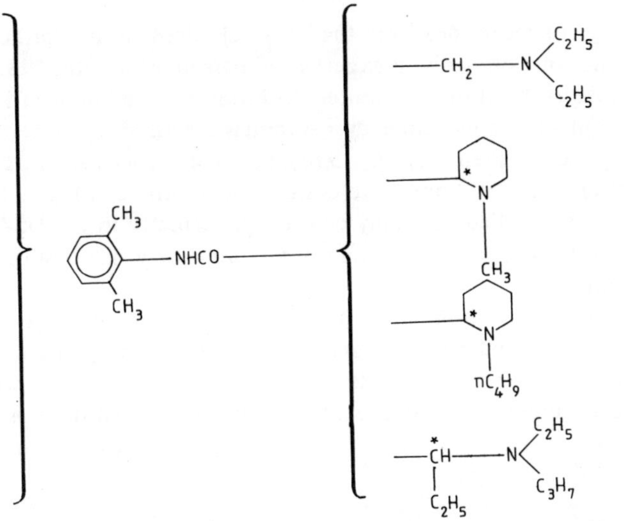

*Indicates an asymmetric carbon atom and, therefore, the existence of stereoisomers.

For detailed information on the pharmacology and toxicology of local anaesthetics the reader is referred to a number of recent reviews (e.g. Cousins and Bridenbaugh, 1980; Covino and Vassallo, 1976; De Jong, 1977; Mather and Cousins, 1979; Tucker and Mather, 1979, Tucker, 1983a,b).

7.2 ADVERSE REACTIONS

Measurement of the concentrations of local anaesthetics in biological fluids is of value in assessing their safety since their presence in the circulation can be associated with unwanted effects, mediated principally through the central nervous and cardiovascular systems.

In an anaesthetic context, adverse reactions are usually due to rapid inadvertent intravenous injection of normal extravascular doses intended for neural blockade, administration into highly vascular areas, or the extravascular injection of an excessive dose. The incidence of serious local-anaesthetic-induced reactions is unknown but probably very low. For example, a review of the world literature on epidural anaesthesia in 1969 revealed a 0.2% frequency of toxicity in more than sixty thousand cases (Dawkins, 1969). Nevertheless, the safety margins of local anaesthetics in terms of systemic toxicity are generally lower than those normally considered clinically desirable. It is important that they be injected carefully by trained and informed clinicians, a point which is emphasised by a number of recent deaths in the UK of children given bupivacaine for intravenous regional anaesthesia by inexperienced personnel (Heath, 1982).

Adverse reactions attributed to intravenous administration of lignocaine for the control of ventricular dysrhythmias occurred at a rate of 6.5% in a series of 750 patients (Pfeifer *et al.*, 1976). In 12 of the 47 patients exhibiting an adverse reaction, the reactions were considered life-threatening and 8 of these patients subsequently died. In many centres, particularly in the USA, plasma lignocaine concentrations are now monitored routinely in post-myocardial infarction patients.

A resurgence in the illicit use of cocaine in the 1970s has emphasised the need for sensitive and specific assays for the parent drug and its metabolites in biological fluids. Such methods have become increasingly important for epidemiological studies of cocaine abuse and in the clinical diagnosis of cocaine intoxication.

7.3 ANALYTICAL TECHNIQUES

For screening and forensic purposes qualitative and semi-quantitative thin-layer chromatographic methods still provide the fastest and most inexpensive approach to the analysis of local anaesthetics. A vast number of reports on the TLC determination of cocaine exist in the literature (Wallace *et al.*, 1975) and systems for most of the other local anaesthetics can be found in standard texts (e.g. Clarke, 1969). This review will concentrate on quantitative methods, principally those based upon gas–liquid chromatography (GLC), high-pressure liquid chromatography (HPLC) and immunoassay. Earlier colorimetric techniques based upon ion-pair extraction with acidic dyes (methyl orange, bromocresol purple) suffered from lack of specificity and sensitivity (Woods *et al.*, 1951, Sung and Truant, 1954; Bromage and Robson, 1961; Braid and Scott, 1965).

7.4 SAMPLE COLLECTION AND STABILITY

The amide-type local anaesthetics are stable at all pH values (Goto and Itano, 1979) and can be stored in blood at 4 °C for at least 1 to 2 months (Reynolds and Beckett, 1968; Gal *et al.*, 1981; Alkalay *et al.*, 1981). Their metabolites may be less stable, however. Thus, monoethylglycinexylidide (MEGX) and glycinexylidide (GX), the *N*-dealkylation products of lignocaine, hydrolyse slowly (Goto and Itano, 1979) and show significant loss after 1 month in neutral or alkaline solution at 4° to −20 °C. 4-hydroxyxylidine (4OHX), the primary urinary metabolite of lignocaine in man, is highly unstable after deconjugation (Adjepon-Yamoah and Prescott, 1974; De Gelder *et al.*, 1981).

Unlike the amides, the ester-type local anaesthetics undergo chemical hydrolysis at neutral and alkaline pH and are also substrates for plasma pseudocholinesterase and red-cell esterases (Foldes *et al.*, 1965; Stewart *et al.*, 1977; Calvo *et al.*, 1980). *In vitro* half-lives in plasma for normal adults are less than one minute for chloroprocaine and procaine and a little longer for amethocaine. Accordingly, it is necessary to stabilise the esters by collecting blood into cooled tubes containing a cholinesterase inhibitor. Various inhibitors have been investigated including sodium arsenite, sodium fluoride, physostigmine and ecothiophate iodide (Green *et al.*, 1974; Smith *et al.*, 1978; O'Brien *et al.*, 1979; Kuhnert *et al.*, 1981a). Only the last-mentioned, in a concentration of 2 mg ml^{-1} blood, gives optimal protection for both procaine and chloroprocaine and even then up to 25% of the latter may be lost before mixing becomes effective (O'Brien *et al.*, 1979).

Data on the stability of cocaine are somewhat confusing. This compound is hydrolysed nonenzymatically to benzoylecgonine at neutral and alkaline pH and by pseudocholinesterase to ecgonine methyl ester (Stewart *et al.*, 1977; Stewart *et al.*, 1979). Jatlow and Bailey (1975) found a maximum loss of 30% cocaine in blood frozen at −15 °C, although plasma extracts were stable in a desiccator at −15 °C for 72 h. In contrast, Dvorchik *et al.* (1977) showed cocaine to be stable in blood for at least 6 weeks when collected on ice and rapidly frozen to −15 °C with liquid nitrogen, while plasma extracts were unstable at −15 °C. Addition of sodium fluoride was shown by Javaid *et al.* (1978) to be necessary to stabilise cocaine in blood and Barnett *et al.* (1981) claim this to be effective for up to one year. Recently, Liu *et al.* (1982) found that storage of blood at neutral pH and 16 °C was associated with a 7% and 30% loss of cocaine after 1 and 36 days, respectively. All of this loss was accounted for by hydrolysis to benzoylecgonine with no evidence of any conversion to enzymatic products. The consensus of these findings suggests that it is prudent to collect blood samples containing cocaine on ice and in tubes containing a cholinesterase inhibitor. Both blood and urine samples should be analysed immediately; if this is not possible then they should be stored frozen at an acidic pH.

Certain types of blood collection tube must be avoided when measuring plasma concentrations of the amide-type local anaesthetics. Thus, leaching of the plasticiser from the stoppers of some Vacutainer tubes is associated with displacement of these agents from binding sites on plasma α_1-acid glycoprotein, leading to their redistribution into erythrocytes and spuriously low plasma or serum concentrations (Stargel *et al.*, 1979). Such artifacts may be important in the therapeutic monitoring of lignocaine and could result in inappropriate adjustment of dosage.

7.5 GLC METHODS

Historically, methods for the amide-type agents have preceded those for the esters. This largely reflects the greater demands on sensitivity for the analysis of the latter owing to their rapid metabolism and disappearance from the circulation.

7.5.1 Amides

7.5.1.1 Parent drugs

Salient features of the main methods, listed in chronological order for each amide, are summarised in Table 7.2. The basic analytical approach is very simple and overall there are no substantial differences in the techniques for the various analogues. The development of methods for each agent has followed closely on their introduction into clinical practice and one is immediately struck by the remarkable number of 'me-too' assays that have been reported.

The first methods appeared in the mid-1960s and were generally based upon the addition of an internal standard and alkali to the sample, extraction into a medium-polarity organic solvent, back-extraction into acid, re-extraction into organic solvent after alkalinisation and concentration by evaporation prior to injection. The column coatings used included SE-30, XF-1112 and Carbowax 20M/KOH; detection was by flame-ionisation detector (FID) and precise results could be obtained down to concentrations of about 50 to 200 ng ml^{-1} using 1 to 2 ml samples.

The 1970s saw several refinements to the basic method. By dissolving final residues in carbon disulphide it was possible to attenuate the solvent response of the FID (Tucker, 1970; Rowland *et al.*, 1971). Time-consuming evaporation steps were avoided by minimising the volume of the back-extract and by effecting the final solvent extraction into a microlitre volume (Benowitz and Rowland, 1973; Mather and Tucker, 1974). This also reduced losses during evaporation resulting from the volatility of the amines (Tucker, 1970). OV-series columns with higher temperature limits were introduced; the alkali-flame ionisation detector (AFID, nitrogen-selective detector) became reliable and allowed shorter retention times without interference from the solvent front and helped to push routine sensitivity down to the 10 to 20 ng ml^{-1} level. Sensitive methods for metabolites were reported (see below) and the first assays using the mass spectrometer as detector were described (Strong and Atkinson, 1972).

Recent interest in the therapeutic monitoring of plasma lignocaine has stimulated demands for rapid assays. Single alkaline extraction into benzene or, preferably, toluene and direct injection without further concentration into an AFID system was found to be perfectly adequate for measuring lignocaine concentrations in the 'therapeutic range' of 2 to 5 μg ml^{-1} (Hucker and Stauffer, 1976; Kruczek, 1981; Gal *et al.*, 1981). Alkali-coated columns have also made a comeback (Irgens *et al.*, 1976; Nation *et al.*, 1976; Hawkins *et al.*, 1982) owing to the relatively poor chromatographic characteristics (on-column decomposition?) of MEGX and GX and interference from slowly eluting cholesterol on OV-packings. They also help to eliminate the need for a back-extraction step. The latest innovation in methodology has been to use a combination of a support-coated open tubular column (SCOT column) with a nitrogen-selective detector and a solid injection technique (Burm *et al.*, 1982). This ensures high resolution with sharp peaks and extends reliable sensitivity down to 1 to 2 ng ml^{-1}.

Although most of the reported methods are claimed to be specific, only a few have documented freedom from interference by other commonly co-administered drugs such as pethidine, benzodiazepines or anti-dysrhythmic agents in addition to lignocaine (Tucker, 1970; Cameron, 1974; Holt *et al.*, 1979a; Karch and Chmielewski, 1981; Gal *et al.*, 1981; Hawkins *et al.*, 1982, Kacprowicz, 1982; Burm *et al.*, 1982).

Several techniques for measuring lignocaine in animal tissues have been described involving wet oxidation with perchloric acid and hydrogen peroxide (Keenaghan and Boyes, 1972), a complex deproteinisation and solvent wash procedure (Ahmad and Medzihradsky, 1971), solubilisation with sodium hydroxide (Benowitz and Rowland, 1973) and freezing in liquid nitrogen followed by perchloric acid treatment (Naito *et al.*, 1977). Holt *et al.* (1979b) reported an elegant method for lignocaine in samples of myocardium using Subtilisin, a proteolytic enzyme, to digest the tissue.

7.5.1.2 Metabolites

Identification of the biotransformation products of the amide-type local anaesthetics in human urine indicates three major sites of metabolic attack, namely aromatic hydroxylation, *N*-dealkylation and amide hydrolysis. Boyes (1975) and Tucker (1975) have reviewed limited data available on the pharmacological activity and toxicity of the various products. MEGX, GX and the 4-hydroxy product formed from lignocaine, as well as pipecolylxylidide (PPX) from mepivacaine and bupivacaine, and the mono-dealkylated derivatives of etidocaine, have all been measured in human plasma (Table 7.2). Of these, there is only evidence that MEGX contributes to the systemic effects of the parent drug in a small minority of patients.

MEGX can be measured in urine and plasma without derivatisation if an alkali-coated support is used (Beckett *et al.*, 1965; Nation *et al.*, 1976; Hawkins *et al.*, 1982). Alternatively, a SCOT column will allow direct determination of both MEGX and GX in urine (De Gelder *et al.*, 1981). However, neither approach is ideal for low plasma concentrations of these metabolites when adsorption (and, possibly, decomposition) becomes a problem with both alkali-coated and nonpolar phases (DiFazio and Brown, 1971; Strong and Atkinson, 1972). Therefore, various methods incorporating derivatisation of the amines have been developed. These include a time-consuming procedure involving temperature-programming and N-selective detection after acetylation of the metabolites (Adjepon-Yamoah and Prescott, 1974) and sensitive assays based upon electron-capture detection of MEGX as its pentafluorobenzoyl derivative (Halkin *et al.*, 1975), conversion of the de-ethylated metabolites to *N*-propyl derivatives by treatment with propionaldehyde and sodium cyanoborohydride followed by mass fragmentography (Hignite *et al.*, 1978) and determination of the amines as trifluoroacetyl derivatives using a SCOT column and N-selective detection (Rosseel and Bogaert, 1978).

Table 7.2 GLC methods for amide-type local anaesthetics and their metabolites (see the Keys in the Appendix to this chapter)

Author(s)	Compounds assayed	Internal standard	Primary extracting solvent	Evaporation step	Stationary phase	Detector	Sample (ml)	Sensitivity (μg ml^{-1})	c.v. % (μg ml^{-1})	
LIGNOCAINE										
Svinhufved *et al.*, 1965	L	–	CT	no	XF-1112	FID	p, s, b, u, t (0.5 to 4)	0.5	7 (> 2)	
Beckett *et al.*, 1965	L, MEGX	Cy	DE	yes	PEG 20M/KOH	FID	b (2) u (5)	1*R*	3 (2.4)	
Beckett *et al.*, 1966	L	Cy	CT	yes	PEG 20M/KOH	FID	b (2)	–	–	
Keenaghan, 1968	L	Pr	MC	yes	XF-1112	FID	b (2)	<0.5	7 (2.5)	
Reynolds and Beckett 1968	L	Md	DE	yes	SE-30	FID	b (2)	0.04	6.5 (0.1)	
Thomas *et al.*, 1968	L	Ca	DE	yes	UCW-98	FID	p (1)	–	–	
Spechtmayer and Steinbach, 1969	L	P	Bz	yes	SE-30	FID	b (1)	1	<10	
Lurie and Weiss, 1970	L	M or Pr	DE	yes	SE-30	FID	b (2)	–	5 (1.6)	Solid injection.
Rowland *et al.*, 1971	L	methyl DEGA methoxy DEGA	DE	yes	OV-17	FID	p, b (0.5 to 2)	0.2	5 to 7 (0.2 to 2)	
Edhorn, 1971	L	Tr	DE	yes	XF-1112	FID	b (1)	<0.5	–	
Di Fazio and Brown, 1971	L, MEGX, GX	M	Ch	yes	UCW/98 or Carbowax 20M/KOH	FID	p (2)	–	–	
Strong and Atkinson, 1972	L, MEGX	Tr	Bz	yes	SE-30/OV-17	MS (EI)	p (1)	0.3 to 0.5*R*	3 to 7 (0.3 to 0.5)	
Keenaghan and Boyes, 1972	X 4OHX	*o*-T –	MC	yes	OV-17 XF-1112	FID	u	–	0.2	Acid hydrolysis. Derivatisation with chloroacetic anhydride (X), heptafluorbutyryl imidazole (4OHX).
Thomas and Meffin, 1972	L, MEGX 3OHL, 4OHL	DM diMGX	DE MC	yes	OV-225 OV-17	FID	u (1)	–	–	Acetylated derivatives of 3OHL, 4OHL.
Benowitz and Rowland, 1973	L	DEA, DEABA	DE	no	OV-17	FID	p, b (0.5 to 1.5) t	0.01 (b)	~2 (0.2)	
Adjepon-Yamoah and Prescott, 1974	L, MEGX, GX 4OHX	APT NBAP	MC	yes	cyclohexane dimethanol succinate Carbowax 20M	AFID FID	p, u (2) u (1)	0.05 to 0.1 3	3 to 8 (0.1 to 40) 6 (10 to 100)	Metabolites acetylated after hydrolysis.
Ishikawa, 1974	L	Pr	DE	yes	XF-1105	FID	b, csf (0.5)	0.5	0.7 to 4 (3 to 10)	
Cameron, 1974	L	Cy	DE	yes	OV-17	AFID	p (2)	0.05	4 (1)	
Halkin *et al.*, 1975	MEGX	MEAA	PAc	no	OV-17	ECD	p, b (0.05 to 1)	0.01	0.8 (0.03)	Pentafluoro benzoyl derivative.
Strong *et al.*, 1975	X	TMA	Ch	yes	SE-30/OV-17	MS (EI)	u (0.5 to 1)	–	–	Acid hydrolysis

	4OHX L, MEGX, GX	2-N Tr	EAc Bz				p (1), u	0.1 to 0.5	-	of conjugates 4OHX as trimethyl silyl derivative.
Blankenbaker *et al.*, 1975	X, 4OHX	-	Ch	yes	UCW-98	FID	p, u (1)	-	-	Conjugates hydrolysed with glucuronidase.
Hucker and Stauffer, 1976	L	EMGX	Bz	no	OV-17	AFID	p, b (1)	0.1	7 (0.1 to 5)	
Nation *et al.*, 1976	L, MEGX	Bh	DE	yes	UCON-75/KOH	FID	p (1)	0.05*R*	3 to 5 (0.1 to 0.25)	
Irgens *et al.*, 1976	L, MEGX	Py	Bz	yes	PEG/KOH	AFID	p (2.5)	0.1 to 0.25	6 to 18 (0.1 to 0.25)	
Naito *et al.*, 1977	L	M	Ch	yes	OV-17	FID	t (0.3)	0.5	1	
Caille *et al.*, 1977	L	AP	MC	yes	OV-17	FID	p (2)	0.1*R*	-	
Vigouroux *et al.*, 1978	L	EMGX	MC	yes	OV-17	FID	p, s (0.5)	0.05	-	
Rosseel and Bogaert, 1978	L, MEGX, GX	Tm	MC	yes	OV-17 (SCOT)	AFID	p (2)	0.025 to 0.05	4 to 7 (0.5)	Metabolite as trifluoroacetates.
Kline and Martin, 1978	L	M	CS	no	OV-17	FID	p (1)	0.5	6 (2)	Deproteinisation with with trichlor-acetic acid.
Hignite *et al.*, 1977	L, MEGX, GX	M	DE	yes	OV-1	MS (EI)	p (0.5) u (1)	0.05	4 to 10	Propyl derivatives of metabolites.
Zylber-Katz *et al.*, 1977	L	Cy	Hx	no	OV-17	FID	p (1)	0.1	2 to 5 (1 to 2.5)	
Mihaly *et al.*, 1978	X	Cm	DE	yes	OV-17	FID	u (2)	0.1*R*	-	Acid hydrolysis.
Holt *et al.*, 1979a	L	Ei	Ch	no	OV-101	FID	p (0.2)	0.2	5 to 6 (2 to 9) 10 (0.2)	Also measured mexiletine.
Holt *et al.*, 1979b	L	Mi	DE	no	OV-101	FID	t (0.05 to 0.1g)	1 ($\mu g\ g^{-1}$)	6 to 13 (4–18 $\mu g\ g^{-1}$)	Tissue digested with proteolytic enzyme.
Park *et al.*, 1980	L	M	DE	yes	OV-1 or OV-17	AFID	p (1)	0.025	<2 (0.05 to 0.5)	
De Boer *et al.*, 1980	L	MHx	Pe	yes	Carbowax 20M (SCOT)	AFID	b (0.1)	≈0.05	-	Solid injection.
Karch and Chmielewski, 1981	L	M	CS	no	OV-17	FID	p (1)	0.04	3–10 (0.04–4)	Deproteinisation with trichloro-acetic acid. Temperature programming.
Kruczek, 1981	L	M	Bz	no	OV-17	AFID	s (1)	0.1	9 (3)	
Desch *et al.*, 1981	L	M	MC	yes	SE-30 or OV-17	FID	p (0.3)	0.1	11 (0.1 to 20)	
Gal *et al.*, 1981	L	CMPT	Tol	no	OV-1	AFID	p (0.1)	0.5*R*	6 to 7	
Breuer, 1982	L	M	MC	yes	OV-17	FID	p (0.9)	0.1 to 0.5	2 (5 to 10)	

Table 7.2 (continued)

Author(s)	Compounds assayed	Internal standard	Primary extracting solvent	Evaporation step	Stationary phase	Detector	Sample (ml)	Sensitivity ($\mu g\ ml^{-1}$)	c.v. % ($\mu g\ ml^{-1}$)	
Hawkins *et al.*, 1982	L, MEGX	Tm	EAc	no	Carbowax 20M/KOH	AFID	p, s (0.25)	0.3*R*	3 to 10 (3 to 10)	
Kacprowicz, 1982	L	E	Ch	no	Carbowax 20M/KOH	FID	p (0.2)	0.02	2 to 5	
De Gelder *et al.*, 1982	L, MEGX, GX, 3OHL, 3OHMEGX, 4OHX	B Pz B	MC MC/EAc DE	yes	Carbowax 20M (SCOT)	AFID	u (5)	–	–	Hydrolysis of urine. Solid injection.
Abernathy *et al.*, 1982	L	M	Hx/1PA	no	OV-101	AFID	p (0.25 to 2)	0.0025	1 to 6.5 (0.005 to 0.5)	
PRILOCAINE										
Svinhufved *et al.*, 1965	Pr	–	CT	no	XF-1112	FID	p, s, b, u, t (0.5 to 4)	0.5	7 (>2)	
Keenaghan, 1968	Pr	L	MC	yes	XF-1112	FID	b (2)	<0.5	7 (2.5)	
Ishikawa, 1974	Pr	L	DE	yes	XF-1105	FID	b, csf (0.5)	0.5	0.7 to 4 (3 to 10)	
Pratt *et al.*, 1967	M	5α-A	DE	yes	SE-30	FID	b (2)	0.05	10 (1 to 5)	
Reynolds and Beckett, 1968	M	Md	DE	yes	SE-30	FID	b (2)	0.04	4 (0.1)	
Maes *et al.*, 1969	M	CCy	Ch	yes	OV-1	FID	b (5), u (10)	0.5	1 to 4 (0.5 to 5)	
Asling *et al.*, 1969	M	Cp	DE	yes	OV-17	FID	b (0.2 to 1)	0.04	–	
Lurie and Weiss, 1970	M	L or Pr	DE	yes	SE-30	FID	b (2)	–	8 (2.5)	
Thomas and Meffin, 1972	M, PPX, 3OHM, 4OHM	B diMGX	DE MC	yes	OV-225 OV-17	FID	u (1)	–	–	
Ishikawa, 1974	M	Pr	DE	yes	XF-1105	FID	b, csf (0.5)	0.5	0.7 to 4 (3 to 10)	
Park *et al.*, 1980	M	B or E	DE	yes	OV-1 or OV17	AFID	p (1)	0.025	<2 (0.05 to 0.5)	
Reynolds and Beckett, 1968	B	Md	DE	yes	SE-30	FID	b (2)	0.04	5 (0.1)	
Thomas *et al.*, 1969	B	Dy	DE	yes	UCW-98	FID	p (1)	1*R*	15 (1)	
Tucker, 1970	B	Cy	DE	yes	OV-17	FID	p, b (1)	0.02	4 (0.1)	
Wilkinson and Lund, 1970	B	Cy	DE	yes	OV-17	FID	p (1) csf (0.05 to 0.1)	0.05*R*	–	
Berlin *et al.*, 1973	B	PXCP	MC	no	OV-17	FID	b (0.2)	0.015	3 to 17 (0.015 to 0.2)	
Goehl *et al.*, 1973	B, PPX, 40HB, 40HPPX, PA	– – –	DE EC ion-exchange column	yes	OV-17	FID	u (1)	–	–	4OH metabolites as trimethylsilyl derivatives. PA as acetyl derivative.

Bouche and Minetti, 1974	PPX			yes	OV-17	ECD	p	0.025R	3 to 5 to (0.025 to 1.5)	Heptafluoro-butyryl derivative.
Caldwell *et al.*, 1977	B	PXCP	DE	yes	OV-1	MS (EI)	b (0.02 to 1)	0.001R	6 to 13 (0.001 to 0.01)	
Zylber-Katz *et al.*, 1978	B	Cy	Hx	no	OV-17	FID	p (1)	0.1	2 to 5 (1 to 2.5)	
Lesko *et al.*, 1980	B, PPX	L	DE	yes	OV-17	AFID	s (0.1)	0.1	8 to 10 (0.1)	
Verheesen *et al.*, 1980	B	-	charcoal/ MC	yes	SE-30	FID	s (1)	0.05	5 (0.05)	
Park *et al.*, 1980	B	E	DE	yes	OV-1 or OV-17	AFID	p (1)	0.025	<2 (0.05 to 0.5)	
Kuhnert *et al.*, 1981b	B, PPX	W-12174	DE	yes	OV-17	MS (EI)	p, u (0.2 to 1)	<0.004	2 to 11 (0.015–0.5)	
Desch *et al.*, 1981	B	M	MC	yes	SE-30 or OV-17	FID	p (0.3)	0.1	11 (0.1 to 20)	
Burm *et al.*, 1982	B	PXCP	Pe	yes	Carbowax/20M/KOH (SCOT)	AFID	p (1)	0.001	6 (>0.003) 15 (0.001)	Solid injection.
ETIDOCAINE										
Bridenbaugh *et al.*, 1974	E	W-12141	DE	no	OV-17	FID	p (1)	0.1*R*	2 (0.1)	
Cameron, 1974	E	Dp	DE	yes	OV-17	AFID	p (2)	0.05	4 (1)	
Thomas *et al.*, 1976	E + 7 metabolites	Dy/p.T/1-N	DE	yes	OV-1	FID	u (1–5)	-	-	
Morgan *et al.*, 1977	E, PABX, EABX, ABX	B	DE	yes	OV-1/OV-17	FID	p, b, u	0.01*R* 0.01*R*	-	
Vigouroux *et al.*, 1978	E	EMGX	MC	yes	OV-17	FID	p, s (0.5)	0.05	-	
Park *et al.*, 1980	E	B	DE	yes	OV-1 or OV-17	AFID	p (1)	0.025	<2 (0.05 to 0.5)	
Desch *et al.*, 1981	E	M	MC	yes	SE-30 or OV-17	FID	p (0.3)	0.1	11 (0.1 to 20)	
CINCHOCAINE										
Alkalay *et al.*, 1981	Ci	deut	Hp+ iPA	yes	OV-1/OV-17	MS (EI or CI)	s (0.5 to 2)	0.001	8 (0.002)	

Pipecolylxylidide (PPX), the N-dealkylation product common to mepivacaine and bupivacaine, has been assayed without derivatisation in urine and blood using an FID (Reynolds, 1971; Thomas and Meffin, 1972; Goehl *et al.*, 1973), in serum using an AFID (Lesko *et al.*, 1980) and at concentrations down to 5 ng ml^{-1} in both plasma and urine by mass fragmentography (Kuhnert *et al.*, 1981b). Bouche and Minetti (1974) prepared a heptafluorobutyryl derivative and used an electron-capture detector. Treatment of the extracted residue with methanol was necessary to remove the acyl group from the amide nitrogen, leaving the monoacyl product substituted on the amine nitrogen. The three *N*-dealkylation products of etidocaine have been measured without derivatisation in urine and the two mono-*N*-dealkylated products in plasma (Thomas *et al.*, 1976, Morgan *et al.*, 1977).

Identification of the ring-hydroxy metabolites of the amide-type local anaesthetics and estimation of their urinary recoveries in man has been done following acid or enzymatic hydrolysis of their conjugates and extraction at pH 9 to 10. The products were chromatographed as such (Vine *et al.*, 1978; Dennhardt and Konder, 1980; De Geldeı *et al.*, 1981) or as acyl (Keenaghan and Boyes, 1972, Thomas and Meffin, 1972) or silyl derivatives (Goehl *et al.*, 1973). Several groups have also developed urine assays for the amide hydrolysis products xylidine and 4-hydroxy-2,6,-xylidine (Keenaghan and Boyes, 1972; Adjepon-Yamoah and Prescott, 1974; Strong *et al.*, 1975; Mihaly *et al.*, 1978; De Gelder *et al.*, 1981).

7.5.1.3 A recommended method

For the laboratory with access to a gas chromatograph fitted with an N-selective detector, we would recommend the procedures shown in Figures 7.1 and 7.2 for the rapid assay of lignocaine and MEGX. By appropriate selection of the internal standard and adjustment of the oven temperature the other amides can also be determined.

We routinely use these methods for the analysis of human plasma (concentration range: 0.1 to 5 μg ml^{-1}) and of rat-liver perfusate (concentration range: 10 to 100 ng ml^{-1}) and liver tissue samples.

7.5.2 Esters

7.5.2.1 Parent drugs

Green *et al.* (1974) described a method for measuring plasma procaine concentrations after intramuscular injection of procaine penicillin G for the treatment of gonorrhoea. The dosage of procaine in this context can be as high as 2 g and plasma drug concentrations of 4 to 11 μg ml^{-1} were observed, probably accounting for the frequency (0.9%) of neurological reactions in these patients. Deter-

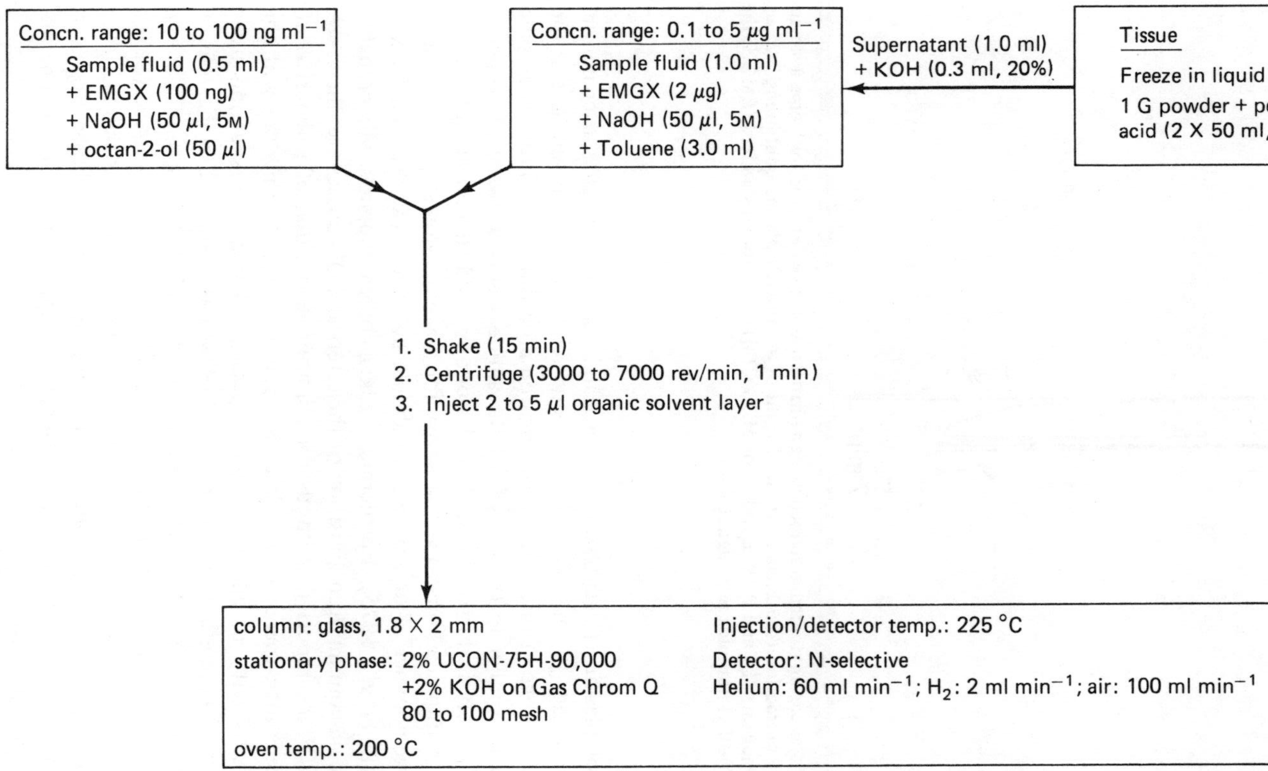

Figure 7.1 Simple GLC assays for lignocaine and its mono-*N*-de-ethylated metabolite MEGX. Note: by replacing toluene with octanol, a polar yet water-immiscible solvent, the solvent–aqueous volume ratio can be greatly decreased, allowing a corresponding enhancement in sensitivity. Octanol is also preferable to halogenated solvents when using N-selective detectors.

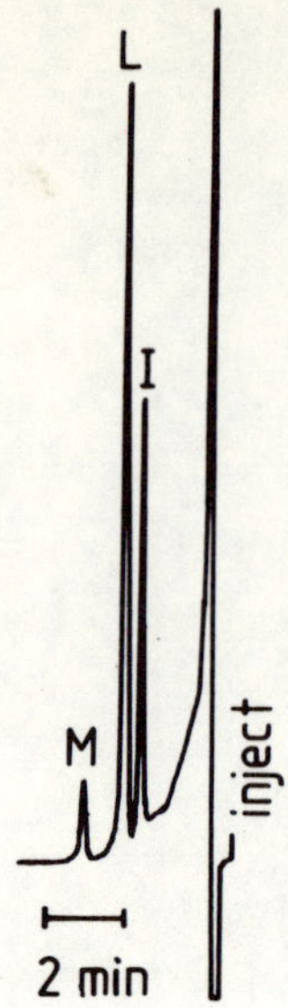

Figure 7.2 Gas chromatogram obtained using a nitrogen-selective detector following a single-step toluene extraction (see Figure 7.1) of 1.0 ml of a patient's plasma containing 2.25 μg ml^{-1} of lignocaine (L) and 0.19 μg ml^{-1} of MEGX (M). I = internal standard (EMGX, the *N*-methyl, *N*-ethyl homologue of lignocaine).

mination of plasma concentrations of procaine and its analogues after normal anaesthetic dosage is much more difficult and requires methods sensitive at the low ng mg^{-1} range (Table 7.3). The extraction procedures and chromatographic conditions are similar to those used for the amide agents. However, in order to minimise hydrolysis during the analytical work-up, mild alkaline conditions (pH 8.5 to 9.5; sodium carbonate) are necessary for the extraction steps and evaporation of large volumes of organic solvent should be avoided (Mather and Tucker, 1974; Tobin *et al.*, 1975). Furthermore, alkali-coated supports will probably cause some on-column decomposition of the esters and OV-phases are, therefore, preferred. Of the reported methods for chloroprocaine, that of Kuhnert *et al.* (1981a) using mass-spectroscopic detection appears to be the only one with the necessary sensitivity to allow a rigorous pharmacokinetic investigation using normal doses. The method of Smith *et al.* (1978) has been used to characterise the kinetics of procaine after high-dose i.v. infusions (1 to 1.5 mg min^{-1} kg^{-1}), when plasma clearances of 0.04 to 0.08 l min^{-1} kg^{-1} were observed (Seifen *et al.*, 1979). Park *et al.* (1980) have described a method which is claimed to be general for amide-type agents and amethocaine in biological fluids. However, specific details of the sensitivity, precision and applicability of the amethocaine assay were not given.

Quantitative GLC was first applied to the analysis of cocaine by Fish and Wilson (1969a), who showed that only about 1% of a dose is excreted unchanged in the urine in man (Fish and Wilson, 1969b). Subsequently, other urine methods have been reported using flame-ionisation detection (Wallace *et al.*, 1976; Von Minden and d'Amato, 1977; Kogan *et al.*, 1977; Valentour *et al.*, 1978) and electron-impact mass fragmentography (Jindal *et al.*, 1978; Jindal and Vestergaard, 1978; Ambre *et al.*, 1982) (Table 7.3).

Plasma concentrations of cocaine after normal doses are too low for serial determinations using an FID (Medzihradsky and Dahlstrom, 1975). Thus, peak concentrations after a typical intranasal application for surgery are about 40 to 500 ng ml^{-1} (Van Dyke *et al.*, 1976; Dvorchik *et al.*, 1977; Chinn *et al.*, 1980). Hence, other than in overdose cases (Valentour *et al.*, 1978), N-selective detectors have generally been used (Jatlow and Bailey, 1975; Dvorchik *et al.*, 1977; Kogan *et al.*, 1977; McCurdy, 1980) or else more sophisticated methods employing mass fragmentography in either the electron-impact (Barnett *et al.*, 1981) or the chemical-ionisation mode (Chinn *et al.*, 1980) with a deuterated internal standard. Javaid *et al.* (1978) have described a unique method in which cocaine is reduced with lithium aluminium anhydride to 2-hydroxytropine after mild alkaline extraction and then O-acylated with pentafluoropropionic anhydride and detected by electron capture. This technique was used to follow plasma and red-blood-cell concentrations and urinary excretion of cocaine after a 16-mg i.v. dose.

Many of the above methods for cocaine employ alkaline extraction at pHs between 8 and 10 with variable contact-times up to 20 min. This may lead to underestimation of cocaine, since Fletcher and Hancock (1981) have shown that significant hydrolysis to benzoylecgonine occurs after 1 h at pH values of 8 or more. Wallace *et al.* (1976) also advocate minimal contact of cocaine with acids, other than sulphuric, to avoid loss of the drug by hydrolysis.

7.5.2.2 Metabolites

The hydrolysis products of procaine and its analogues are considered to be pharmacologically inactive (Brodie *et al.*, 1948), although the *para*-amino benzoic acids may be responsible for the occasional allergic reaction to these drugs. 2-chloro-4-aminobenzoic acid (CABA), derived from chloroprocaine, has been measured in plasma following extraction at pH 2, conversion to its silyl derivatives and N-selective detection (Kuhnert *et al.*, 1980). Krogh and Jellum (1981) used GC–MS to determine CABA in urine as its methylated derivative. They also found that most of the CABA was further metabolised and excreted as the N-acetyl product. The latter may be the CABA conjugate observed in urine by Kuhnert *et al.* (1982) (Krogh and Jellum, 1982).

Small amounts of the N-oxide of amethocaine have been measured in animal urine using an FID following conversion to methyl *p*-(*N*-methyl-*N*-butylamino)-benzoate with trimethylanilinium hydroxide (Fukuda and Momose, 1975;

TABLE 7.3 GLC methods for ester-type local anaesthetics and their metabolites (see the Keys to the Appendix at the end of this chapter)

Author(s)	Compounds assayed	Internal standard	Primary extracting solvent	Evaporation step	Stationary phase	Detector	Sample (ml)	Sensitivity ($\mu g\ ml^{-1}$)	c.v. % ($\mu g\ ml^{-1}$)	
PROCAINE										
Green *et al.*, 1974	P	–	DE	yes	OV-101	FID	p (2)	2*R*	4 to 9 (5 to 20)	
Smith *et al.*, 1978	P	Pa	Tol	yes	OV-210	FID	p (1)	0.1	5 (1)	
CHLOROPROCAINE										
O'Brien *et al.*, 1979	CP	P	MC	yes	SE-30	FID	p (2)	0.1*R*	–	
Kuhnert *et al.*, 1980	CP, CABA	P PABA	MC	no yes	OV-17	AFID	p (1)	0.003 0.3	–	CABA as silyl derivative.
Kuhnert *et al.*, 1981a	CP	P	DE	yes	OV-1/OV-17	MS (EI)	p (0.3 to 1)	0.0015	4 to 8 (0.006 to 0.1)	
Krogh and Jellum, 1981	CABA, *N*-acetyl CABA	PAS	DE	yes	OV-17	MS (EI)	u (5)	–	–	As methyl derivatives.
AMETHOCAINE										
Park *et al.*, 1980	A	?	DE	yes	OV-1 or OV-17	AFID	p (1)	0.025	<2 (0.05 to 0.5)	
					OV-17				?	
COCAINE										
Fish and Wilson, 1969	C	Bh	DE	yes	OV-17	FID	u (5)	0.5*R*	3 (3 to 13)	
Medzihradsky and Dahlstrom, 1975	C	–	Bz/iPA	yes	OV-1	FID	p (1)	0.05 to 0.12	5 to 8 (0.25 to 4)	
Jatlow and Bailey, 1975	C	pr BE	Hp/iAA	yes	OV-17	AFID	p (2)	0.005 to 0.01	5 (0.05)	
Wallace *et al.*, 1976	C, BE	b-A	Ch/EA	yes	OV-17	FID	u (5)	0.2	5 to 6	Methylation of BE to C.
Dvorchik *et al.*, 1977	C	EM	Bz/iPA	yes	SP-2100-DB	AFID	p, b (1)	0.02	–	
Von Minden and d'Amato, 1977	C, BE	pBE	Ch/EA	yes	SP-2250 DA or SE-30	FID	u (5)	0.2	4 to 5	Propylation of BE with 1-iodopropane/organic base.
Kogan *et al.*, 1977	C	CPE	Hp/iAA	yes	SE-30 (u) OV-22 (p)	FID (u) AFID (p)	u p (0.5)	0.01	0.9 to 2	BE as pentofluorobenzyl derivative.
	BE	Sc	Ch/EA		OV-225 (p)	ECD (p)		0.005		
Javaid, *et al.*, 1978	C	–	CH	no	OV-225	ECD	p (1) RBC (1) u (5)	0.01	–	Reduced with lithium aluminium anhydride and acylated.

Valentour *et al.*, 1978	C, BE	pr BE	Ch/EA	no	OV-7 or OV-17 or OV-101	FID	b, u, t (5)	-	-	Ethylation of BE.
Jindal and Vestergaard, 1978	C, BE	deut.	CH and CH/iPA	yes	OV-1	MS (EI)	u (3)	0.002 to 0.005	5	BE as ethyl ester.
Jindal *et al.*, 1978	C, NC	deut.	CH	yes	OV-1	MS (EI)	u (1)	0.002	<5 (0.01)	NC as trifluoroacetyl derivative.
Chinn *et al.*, 1978	C, NC BE	deut	Tol/Hp/iAA Ch/iPA	no yes	OV-1	MS (CI)	b, p, u (1) t (10G)	<0.005	<10	Esterification of BE.
McCurdy, 1980	C, BE	pr BE	MC/EA (JETUBE®)	yes	OV-1	AFID	b (2)	0.1	4 to 9 (0.1 to 1)	Ethyl ester of BE.
Barnett *et al.*, 1981	C	deut	CH	yes	OV-1	MS (EI)	p (0.5)	0.002	-	
Ambre *et al.*, 1982	C, EME	PCy	MC	yes	OV-101	MS (EI)	u (0.5–2)	0.1	6 (100)	

Momose and Fukuda, 1976). No data are available on this metabolite in man.

Main routes of breakdown of cocaine in man are ester hydrolysis and *N*-demethylation. The former involves nonenzymatic loss of the methyl group to give benzoylecgonine, enzymatic loss of the benzoyl group in plasma and liver yielding ecgonine methyl ester and further hydrolysis of both of these compounds to ecgonine. Norcocaine, the product of N-demethylation, undergoes an analogous series of hydrolysis steps (Stewart *et al.*, 1977, 1979). Of these metabolites, only norcocaine is believed to have significant pharmacological activity, but it is not a major product (Hawks *et al.*, 1974; Nayak *et al.*, 1976). Norcocaine nitroxide has been suggested as a potential hepatotoxic metabolite of cocaine (Rauckman *et al.*, 1982). Measurements of benzoylecgonine and ecgonine methyl ester are used to detect and monitor cocaine use since these compounds are excreted to a much greater extent in urine than is the unchanged drug.

Benzoylecgonine is an amino-carboxylic acid and is therefore amphoteric and hydrophilic in nature. Accordingly, salting-out techniques or the use of alcohol–organic-solvent mixtures are necessary for efficient extraction. Any procedure, such as back-extraction, designed to eliminate contamination by polar compounds, will markedly lower the recovery of this metabolite. Derivatisation is also needed before chromatography and this is usually done by esterification, accomplished by means of methylation (Wallace *et al.*, 1976), ethylation (Jindal and Vestergaard, 1978; Valentour *et al.*, 1978; McCurdy, 1980) or propylation (Von Minden and d'Amato, 1977) (Table 7.3). The methyl ester is, of course, cocaine. Therefore, in this case the benzoylecgonine concentration is obtained by a difference method. It should also be noted that traces of methanol, which may be present in reagents, have been reported to methylate benzoylecgonine (Chinn *et al.*, 1980). Valentour *et al.* (1978) have streamlined the esterification process by using phase-transfer catalysis with tetrahexylammonium chloride. An FID is adequate to determine urinary concentrations of benzoylecgonine (Wallace *et al.*, 1976; Von Minden and d'Amato, 1977; Kogan *et al.*, 1977) or blood and tissue concentrations in overdose cases (Valentour *et al.*, 1978). Plasma concentrations of the metabolite after normal doses of cocaine have been measured by mass fragmentography (Chinn *et al.*, 1980) and with an electron-capture detector after conversion of the compound to the pentafluorobenzyl ester (Kogan *et al.*, 1977).

Ambre *et al.* (1982) advocate the measurement of urinary ecgonine methyl ester, rather than benzoylecgonine, in the routine monitoring of cocaine use. It is a major urinary metabolite and can be chromatographed on common stationary phases without derivatisation. However, its rapid elution along with other volatile compounds often found in urine extracts creates difficulties if a mass spectrometer is not available as the detector.

Norcocaine has been measured in human urine, plasma and tissues without derivatisation using chemical ionisation mass fragmentography (Chinn *et al.*, 1980) and in urine by electron-impact mass fragmentography (Jindal and

Vestergaard, 1978). It was found to have unusual chromatographic properties in that sensitivity was poor using OV-17 as the stationary phase, but not with OV-1, and the solvent used for injection affected the response (Chinn *et al.*, 1980). It is well established that chloroform should be avoided as a solvent for primary and secondary amines owing to their reaction with contaminants to form carbamoyl chlorides and carbamates. Norcocaine has recently been shown to be susceptible to these reactions (Cone *et al.*, 1982).

7.6 HPLC METHODS

Methods based upon HPLC have been reported recently for lignocaine and cocaine but have yet to be extended to the other local anaesthetics.

The analysis of metabolites of the agents is easier than with GLC procedures since derivatisation is not necessary to improve their chromatographic properties. On the other hand, sensitivity is more restricted with HPLC as the parent drugs are mostly tertiary amines which cannot be converted easily to highly fluorescent derivatives. Thus, measurement is currently limited to the use of u.v. detectors. Nevertheless, HPLC methods are ideal for the routine monitoring of therapeutic plasma concentrations of lignocaine and its N-de-ethylated metabolites and of the urinary excretion of cocaine and its products.

7.6.1 Lignocaine and metabolites (Table 7.4)

Most of the available procedures measure MEGX and GX as well as lignocaine and use reversed-phase systems eluted isocratically with aqueous buffered (pH 3.2 to 6.0) acetonitrile. An attractive alternative, however, involves the addition of low concentrations of ionic modifiers, such as perchloric acid, to methanolic eluents and chromatography on normal-phase, microparticulate silica columns (Lagerstrom and Persson, 1978; Flanagan *et al.*, 1982). This approach is claimed to have advantages in terms of high efficiency, stability, reproducibility and long column life. Furthermore, a high methanol content in the eluent is preferred since this solvent is cheap and it has a relatively low inhalation toxicity and a low u.v. cut-off (Flanagan *et al.*, 1982).

With one exception, all of the methods incorporate a preliminary solvent-extraction step. Wisnicki *et al.* (1979) favour direct injection of plasma onto a guard column. However, a representative chromatogram shows small, poorly characterised peaks and the pre-column requires repacking after fifteen injections.

Some authors report retention-time data on other drugs, mostly showing no interference with lignocaine and its metabolites (Adams *et al.*, 1976; Masoud *et al.*, 1978; Nation *et al.*, 1979; Hill *et al.*, 1980). The methods which only

Table 7.4 HPLC methods for lignocaine and its metabolites (see the Keys in the Appendix at the end of this chapter)

Author(s)	Compounds assayed	Internal standard	Primary extracting solvent	Evaporation step	Column	Mobile phase	λ (nm)	Sample (ml)	Sensitivity (μg ml^{-1})	c.v. % (μg ml^{-1})	
Adams *et al.*, 1976	L	P	charcoal/ MC	yes	ODS Sil-X-1	AN–0.2M p'ate (10:90), pH 6.0	205	s (1)	0.1*R*	11 (1)	
Narang *et al.*, 1978	L, MEGX, GX	EMGX	Ch/Hx/iPA	yes	C_{18} μ-Bondapak	AN–0.01M p'ate (8:92), pH 4.0	210	s (0.5)	<0.05	<5	
Masoud *et al.*, 1978	L	B	EAc	yes	ODS Sil-X-1	AN–0.2M p'ate (10:90), pH 4.0	205	p (0.5)	2*R*	–	
Lagerstrom and Persson, (1978)	L	–	MC	no	Lichrosorb S1.100	EC–MA–0.1M perchlorate (95.7:4:0.3)	228	p (1)	–	–	
Wisnicki *et al.*, 1979	L, MEGX, GX	–	–	no	C_{18} μ-Bondapak	AN–0.05M p'ate (5:95)	205	p (0.02)	1*R*	–	Direct injection with guard column.
Nation *et al.*, 1979	L, MEGX, GX	EMGX	EAc	no	Alkyl, phenyl μ-Bondapak	AN–0.006% phosphoric acid (30:70)	200	p (0.5)	0.02	5 to 8 (0.5)	
Hill *et al.*, 1980	L, MEGX, GX	–	MC	no	RP–8	AN–0.1M p'ate (18:82), pH 3.2	195	p (2)	0.04	<7	
Flanagan *et al.*, 1982	L, MEGX, GX			no	Spherisorb 5 silica	MA + 0.02% perchloric acid	215	p	–	–	

measure unchanged lignocaine do not establish lack of interference from its N-de-ethylated products (Adams *et al.*, 1976, Masoud *et al.*, 1978).

We routinely use an adaptation of the method of Nation *et al.* (1979), details of which are given in Figures 7.3 and 7.4.

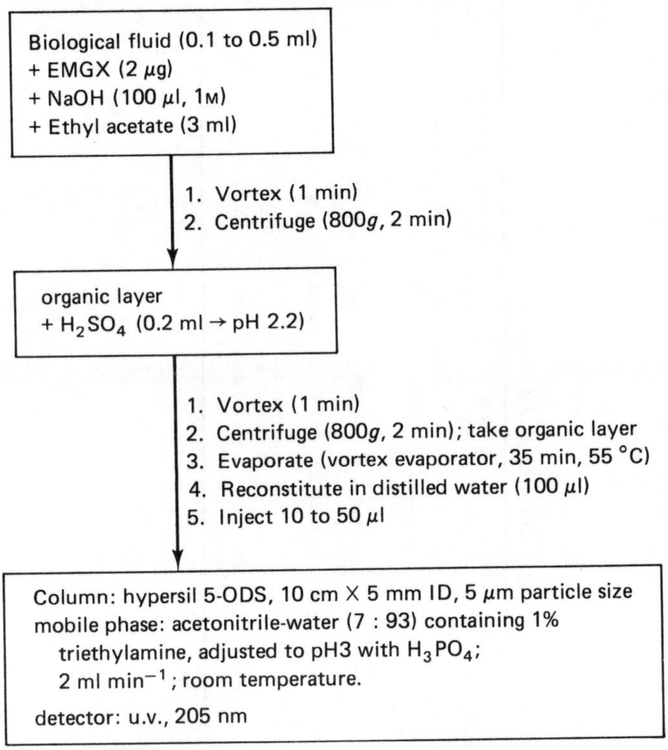

Figure 7.3 A simple HPLC assay for lignocaine and its *N*-de-ethylated metabolites. Note: improvement of chromatographic resolution by addition of triethylamine to the mobile phase results in faster analysis time. (After Nation *et al.* 1979).

7.6.2 Cocaine and metabolites (Table 7.5)

An early paper (Graffeo *et al.*, 1976) described a cumbersome technique using HPLC to purify benzoylecgonine from urine prior to its analysis by mass fragmentography. Subsequently, three methods using reversed-phase systems and u.v. detection have been reported. That of Jatlow *et al.* (1978) allows measurement of cocaine and benzoylecgonine in urine and that of Masoud and Krupski (1980) determines cocaine in plasma, providing that lignocaine, pethidine and droperidol are not present. Both of these techniques were validated with patient

Table 7.5 HPLC methods for cocaine and its metabolites (see the Keys in the Appendix at the end of this chapter)

Author(s)	Compounds assayed	Internal standard	Primary extracting solvent	Evaporation step	Column	Mobile phase	λ (nM)	Sample (ml)	Sensitivity ($\mu g\ ml^{-1}$)	c.v. % ($\mu g\ ml^{-1}$)	
Graffeo *et al.*, 1976	BE	deut.	direct injection	no	C_{18} μ-Bondapak	MA–water	254*	u (1)	0.001	–	*Fraction collected and detected with GC–MS (EI).
Jatlow *et al.*, 1978	C, BE	eBE	DE	yes	Partisil-10 ODS (40°)	AN–0.25M p'ate (17:83), pH 2.7	200 235	u (5)	0.5*R*	3 to 7 (2)	
Evans and Moriarty, 1980	C, BE, NC	L	Ch/iPA	yes	C_{18} μ-Bondapak	water AN–MA (8:1.1) + 1% acetic acid and 0.3M EDTA	235	p (0.5)	–	2 to 3	
Masoud and Krupski, 1980	C	A	DE	yes	ODS Sil-X-1	MA–0.05M p'ate (75:25), pH 6.6	232	p (1)	0.02*R*	5	

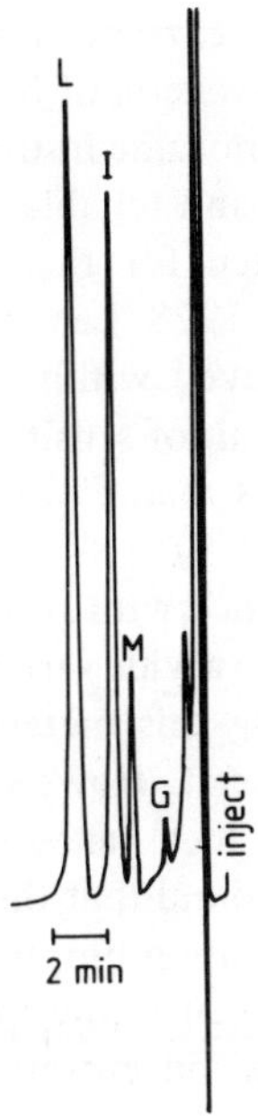

Figure 7.4 Chromatogram obtained after HPLC of lignocaine and its *N*-de-ethylated metabolites. (Method as described in Figure 7.3. In this case the sample (0.1 ml) was a suspension of human liver microsomes containing 4.22 μg ml^{-1} of lignocaine (L), 0.99 μg ml^{-1} of MEGX (M) and 0.51 μg ml^{-1} of GX (G). I = internal standard, EMGX, the *N*-methyl, *N*-ethyl homologue of lignocaine.)

samples. Evans and Moriarty (1980) described an assay for cocaine, norcocaine and benzoylecgonine in biological fluids but no data on its application to patient samples were given.

7.7 IMMUNOLOGICAL METHODS

Commercial kits are available for the measurement of lignocaine in serum by the enzyme multiplied immunoassay technique, EMIT (Syva Corp.), and of benzoylecgonine in urine by EMIT and by radioimmunoassay, RIA (Roche Diagnostics).

7.7.1 Lignocaine

The EMIT assay is based upon competitive binding between lignocaine in serum and lignocaine coupled to bacterial glucose-6-phosphate dehydrogenase for a lignocaine-specific antibody. The enzyme activity, monitored as a change in absorbance at 340 nm due to conversion of NAD^+ to NADH, correlates directly with the total concentration of lignocaine in the serum sample.

This method provides a rapid and reliable estimate of unchanged lignocaine concentration and is ideally suited for therapeutic monitoring (Cobb *et al.*, 1977; Pape *et al.*, 1978; Walberg, 1978, Lehane *et al.*, 1979; Miller *et al.*, 1981). Samples (8 to 50 μl) can be assayed within a few minutes either manually or with automatic equipment. The limit of sensitivity is routinely about 1 μm ml^{-1} with a coefficient of variation less than 5%, but this can be extended down to 50 ng ml^{-1} (Jain and Johnston, 1979).

There is an excellent concordance with results obtained using GLC methods and the EMIT assay is insensitive to a wide variety of other drugs. Cross-reactivity with MEGX is avoided by adding this metabolite to the lignocaine antibody preparation in order to desensitise it. However, the antibody still reacts significantly with other amide-type local anaesthetics, particularly mepivacaine (Pape *et al.*, 1978). Pape (1981) found that the effect of the latter was inversely related to its concentration and this prompted him to make the general point that special attention should be given to the specificity of the EMIT assay when it is used to measure very low drug concentrations such as those found in plasma ultrafiltrates or saliva samples.

7.7.2 Benzoylecgonine

The EMIT assay for benzoylecgonine in urine is one of the most widely used screening tests for cocaine use. However, it is only semi-quantitative at best and is subject to false positive results owing to antibody cross-reactivity (Wallace *et al.*, 1976; Ambre *et al.*, 1982). Therefore, it should be employed only as a preliminary to more specific chromatographic methods.

Kaul *et al.* (1976) developed an ^{125}I-RIA for cocaine and its metabolites using antibodies raised with an ecgonine–sheep-gamma-globulin conjugate. The assay was found to be sensitive to 5 to 10 ng of benzoylecgonine in human urine and reactivity decreased in the order: benzoylecgonine $>$ ecgonine $\gg$ cocaine $\gg$ norcocaine and ecgonine methyl ester, with insignificant cross-reactivity to a variety of other drugs. The Roche RIA for urinary benzoylecgonine also utilises an ^{125}I-labelled antigen. It is sensitive to 2 μg ml^{-1}, although a working limit of 100 μg ml^{-1} has been suggested. Results show a high concordance with GLC assay. Cross-reactivity occurs with cocaine itself (more reactive than benzoylecgonine) and other metabolites, although ecgonine methyl ester and ecgonine are essentially inactive. With the exception of thioridazine, other drugs and most tropane alkaloids do not cross-react (Mulé *et al.*, 1977; Budd, 1981).

7.8 OTHER METHODS

Lignocaine and its metabolites have been analysed in urine and plasma after organic solvent extraction followed by direct-insertion, chemical-ionisation mass spectrometry (Garland *et al.*, 1974). Deuterated lignocaine and metabolites served as internal standards and, using this technique, Nelson *et al.* (1977) were able to measure lignocaine, MEGX, GX, xylidine and the corresponding *para*-hydroxy products in human urine.

A rapid method based upon high-performance TLC with scanning at 220 nm was reported for the simultaneous measurement of lignocaine and other anti-dysrhythmic drugs in serum (Lee *et al.*, 1978).

APPENDIX: KEYS TO THE TABLES IN THIS CHAPTER

Compounds assayed

L = lignocaine
MEGX = monoethylglycinexylidide
GX = glycinexylidide
3OHL = 3′-hydroxy L
4OHL = 4′-hydroxy L
3OHMEGX = 3′-hydroxy MEGX
4OHX = 4′-hydroxy-2, 6-xylidine
X = 2, 6-xylidine
Pr = prilocaine
M = mepivacaine
PPX = pipecolylxylidide
3OHM = 3′-hydroxy M
4OHM = 4′-hydroxy M
B = bupivacaine
4OHB = 4′-hydroxy B
4OHPPX = 4′-hydroxy PPX
PA = pipecolic acid
E = etidocaine
PABX = 2-*N*-propylamino-2′-butyroxylidide
EABX = 2-*N*-ethylamino-2′-butyroxylidide
ABX = 2-amino-2′-butyroxylidide
P = procaine
CP = 2-chloroprocaine
CABA = 2-chloro-4-aminobenzoic acid
Ci = cinchocaine
C = cocaine

BE = benzoylecgonine
NC = norcocaine
EME = ecgonine methyl ester
A = amethocaine

Internal standards

Md = methadone
Ca = carbinoxamine
methyl DEGA = *m*-methyl-*N*-diethylglycylanilide
methoxy DEGA = *m*-methoxy-*N*-diethylglycylanilide
Tr = tripelennamine
DEA = 2-diethylaminoacetanilide
DEABA = 2-diethylamino-3′-bromoacetanilide
APT = aceto-*p*-toluidine
NBAP = *N*-butyryl-*p*-aminophenol
Cy = cyclizine
MEAA = 3′-methoxy-2-ethylaminoacetanilide
EMGX = *N*-ethyl, *N*-methyl analogue of L
Bh = benzhexol
Py = pyrrocaine
AP = aminopyrine
Tm = trimecaine
Ei = *n*-eicosane
Pz = pentazocine
MHx = methyl hexobarbitone
TMA = 2, 4, 6-trimethylaniline
2-N = 2-naphthol
Cm = chlormethiazole
o-T = *o*-toluidine
Dy = dicyclomine
Mi = mianserin
DM = dimethisoquin
diMGX = *N*-dimethyl analogue of L
5α-A = 5α-androstane
CCy = chlorcyclizine
Cp = chlorpheniramine
PXCP = 1-pentyl-2-(2, 6-xylylcarbamoyl)-piperidine
W-12174 = *N*-ethyl-*N*-*sec*-butylglycinexylidide
Dp = diphenhydramine
W-12141 = *N*-ethyl-*tert*-butylaminoacetyl-2′, 6′-xylidine
p-T = *p*-toluidine

1-N = 1-naphthylamine
Pa = procainamide
PABA = para-amino benzoic acid
PAS = para-amino salicyclic acid
deut. = deuterated compound
pr BE = propyl ester of BE
b-A = butyl anthraquinone
EM = ethyl morphine
CPE = chlorproethazine
Sc = scopolamine
PCy = phencyclidine
e BE = ethyl ester of BE
p BE = *n*-pentyl ester of BE
CMPT = 6′-chloro-α-methyl-1-pyrolidineaceto-*o*-toluidide

Solvents

CT = carbon tetrachloride
MC = methylene chloride
DE = diethyl ether
Ch = chloroform
PAc = pentyl acetate
Bz = benzene
CS = carbon disulphide
Hx = *n*-hexane
EAc = ethyl acetate
Pe = *n*-pentane
EC = ethylene chloride
Tol. = toluene
Hp = *n*-heptane
iPA = isopentyl alcohol
iAA = isoamylalcohol
EA = ethyl alcohol
iPrA = isopropylalcohol
CH = cyclohexane
AN = acetonitrile
ME = methyl alcohol

Detectors

FID = flame-ionisation detector
AFID = alkali flame-ionisation detector (N-selective detector)
ECD = electron-capture detector

MS (EI) = mass spectrometer (electron-impact)
MS (CI) = mass spectrometer (chemical-ionisation)

Samples

p = plasma
s = serum
b = blood
u = urine
t = tissue
c.s.f. = cerebrospinal fluid
RBC = red blood cells

Sensitivity

R signifies lowest concentration on the calibration range, assumed to be lower limit of assay in the absence of other information.
c.v. = coefficient of variation

REFERENCES

Abernathy, D. R., Greenblatt, D. J., and Ochs, H. R. (1982). Lidocaine determination in human plasma with application to single low-dose pharmacokinetic studies. *J. Chromatogr.* **232**, 180–5.

Adams, R. F., Vandenmark, F. L., and Schmidt, G. (1976). The simultaneous determination of lidocaine and procainamide in serum by use of high-pressure liquid chromatography. *Clin. Chim. Acta* **69**, 515–24.

Adjepon-Yamoah, K. K., and Prescott, L. F. (1974). Gas–liquid chromatographic estimation of lignocaine, ethylglycylxylidide, glycylxylidide and 4-hydroxy xylidine in plasma and urine. *J. Pharm. Pharmac.* **26**, 889–93.

Ahmad, K., and Medzihradsky, F. (1971). Distribution of lidocaine in blood and tissues after single doses and steady infusion. *Res. Comm. Chem. Path. Pharmac.* **2**, 813–28.

Alkalay, D., Carlsen, S., and Wagner, W. E. (1981). Quantitation of the local anesthetic dibucaine with gas chromatography/mass spectrometry. *Analyt. Lett.* **14**, 1745–56.

Ambre, J. J., Ruo, T.-I., Smith, G. L., Backes, D., and Smith, C. M. (1982). Ecgonine methyl ester, a major metabolite of cocaine. *J. Analyt. Toxicol.* **6**, 26–9.

Asling, J. H., Shnider, S. M., Wilkinson, G. R., and Way, E. L. (1969). Gas chromatographic determination of mepivacaine in capillary blood. *Anesthesiology* **31**, 458–61.

Barnett, G., Hawks, R., and Resnick, R. (1981). Cocaine pharmacokinetics in humans. *J. Ethnopharmac.* **3**, 353–66.

Beckett, A. H., Boyes, R. N., and Appleton, P. J. (1966). The metabolism and excretion of lignocaine in man. *J. Pharm. Pharmac.* **18** (suppl.), 76–81S.

Beckett, A. H., Boyes, R. N., and Parker, J. B. R. (1965). Determination of lignocaine in blood and urine in human subjects undergoing local analgesic procedures. *Anaesthesia* **20**, 294–8.

Benowitz, N., and Rowland, M. (1973). Determination of lidocaine in blood and tissues. *Anesthesiology* **39**, 639–41.

Berlin, A., Persson, B.-A., and Belfrage, P. (1973). Micromethod for the determination of bupivacaine in maternal and foetal blood during obstetric analgesia. *J. Pharm. Pharmac.* **25**, 466–9.

Blankenbaker, W. L., Di Fazio, C. A., and Berry, F. A. (1975). Lidocaine and its metabolites in the newborn. *Anesthesiology* **42**, 325–30.

Bouche, R., and Minetti, R. (1974). Quantitative micro-determination of 2,6-pipecolyl-xylidide by gas-liquid chromatography. *J. Chromatogr.* **90**, 191–4.

Boyes, R. N. (1975). A review of the metabolism of amide local anaesthetics. *Br. J. Anaesth.* **38**, suppl., 225–30.

Braid, D. P., and Scott, D. B. (1965). The systemic absorption of local analgesic drugs. *Ibid.* **37**, 394–404.

Breuer, H. (1982). Gas-liquid chromatographic determination of lidocaine in cat plasma using mepivacaine as internal standard. *J. Chromatogr.* **231**, 65–72.

Bridenbaugh, P. O., Tucker, G. T., Moore, D. C., Bridenbaugh, L. D., and Thompson, G. E. (1974). Preliminary clinical evaluation of etidocaine (Duranest): a new long-acting local anesthetic agent. *Acta Anaesth. Scand.* **18**, 165–71.

Brodie, B. B., Lief, P. A., and Poet, R. (1948). The fate of procaine in man following its intravenous administration and methods for the estimation of procaine and diethyl-aminoethanol. *J. Pharmac. Exper. Therap.* **94**, 366–95.

Bromage, P. R., and Robson, J. G. (1961). Concentrations of lignocaine in the blood after intravenous, intramuscular, epidural and endotracheal administration. *Anaesthesia* **16**, 461–78.

Budd, R. D. (1981). Cocaine radioimmunoassay–structure versus reactivity. *Clin. Toxicol.* **18**, 773–82.

Burm, A. G. L., Van Kleef, J. W., and De Boer, A. G. (1982). Gas chromatographic determination of bupivacaine in plasma using a support coated open tubular column and a nitrogen-selective detector. *Anesthesiology* **57**, 527–9.

Caille, G., LeLorier, J., Latour, Y., and Besner, J. G. (1977). GLC determination of lidocaine in human plasma. *J. Pharm. Sci.* **66**, 1383–5.

Caldwell, J., Moffatt, J. R., Smith, R. L., Lieberman, B. A., Beard, R. W., Snedden, W., and Wilson, B. W. (1977). Determination of bupivacaine in human fetal and neonatal blood samples by quantitative single ion monitoring. *Biomed. Mass Spectrom.* **4**, 322–5.

Calvo, R., Carlos, R., and Erill, S. (1980). Effects of disease and acetazolamide on procaine hydrolysis by red cell enzymes. *Clin. Pharmac. Ther.* **27**, 175–83.

Cameron, J. D. (1974). The gas chromatographic determination of plasma concentrations of some local anesthetics using a nitrogen detector. *Clin. Chim. Acta* **56**, 307–9.

Chinn, D. M., Crouch, D. J., Peat, M. A., Finkle, B. S., and Jennison, T. A. (1980). Gas chromatography–chemical ionization mass spectrometry of cocaine and its metabolites in biological fluids. *J. Analyt. Toxicol.* **4**, 37–42.

Clarke, E. G. C. (1969). *Isolation and Identification of Drugs.* Pharmaceutical Press, London.

Cobb, M. E., Buckley, N., Hu, M. W., Miller, J. G., Singh, P., and Schneider, R. S. (1977). Homogeneous enzyme immunoassay for lidocaine in serum. *Clin. Chem.* **23**, 1161.

Cone, E. J., Buchwald, W. F., and Darwin, W. D. (1982). Analytical controls in drug metabolism studies. 2: Artifact formation during chloroform extraction of drugs and metabolites with amine substituents. *Drug Metab. Disp.* **10**, 561–7.

Cousins, M. J., and Bridenbaugh, P. O. (eds) (1980). *Neural Blockade in Clinical Anesthesia and Management of Pain.* Lippincott, Philadelphia.

Covino, B. G., and Vassallo, H. G. (1976). *Local Anesthetics. Mechanisms of Action and Clinical Use.* Grune and Stratton, New York.

Dawkins, C. J. M. (1969). An analysis of the complications of extradural and caudal block. *Anaesthesia* **24**, 554–63.

De Boer, A. G., Breimer, D. D., Pronk, J., and Gubbens-Stibbe, J. M. (1980). Rectal bioavailability of lidocaine in rats: absence of significant first-pass elimination. *J. Pharm. Sci.* **69**, 804–7.

De Gelder, D. J., De Leede, L. G. J., and De Boer, A. G. (1981). Assay of lidocaine and 5 metabolites by capillary gas chromatography. *Proc. 41st Int. Congr. Pharmaceutical Sciences*, Vienna, abstr. No. 5.

De Jong, R. H. (1977). *Local Anesthetics*, 2nd ed. Charles C. Thomas, Springfield.

Dennhardt, R., and Konder, H. (1980). Metabolite von bupivacain beim menschen. *Regional Anaesth.* **3**, 25–6.

Desch, G., Cavadore, D., Jullien, Y., Mercier, L., Descomps, B., and De Rodez, M. (1981). *Analg. Anesth. Rean.* **2**, 158–68.

DiFazio, C. A., and Brown, R. E. (1971). The analysis of lidocaine and its postulated metabolites. *Anesthesiology* **34**, 86–8.

Dvorchik, B. H., Miller, S. H., and Graham, W. P. (1977). Gas chromatographic determination of cocaine in whole blood and plasma using a nitrogen-sensitive flame ionization detector. *J. Chromatogr.* **135**, 141–8.

Edhorn, G. A. (1971). Determination of lidocaine in whole blood by gas chromatography. *Canad. Anaesth. Soc. J.* **18**, 189–97.

Evans, M. A., and Moriarty, T. (1980). Analysis of cocaine and cocaine metabolites by high pressure liquid chromatography. *J. Analyt. Toxicol.* **4**, 19–22.

Fish, F., and Wilson, W. D. C. (1969a). Gas chromatographic determination of morphine and cocaine in urine. *J. Chromatogr.* **40**, 164–8.

Fish, F., and Wilson, W. D. C. (1969b). Excretion of cocaine and its metabolites in man. *J. Pharm. Pharmac.* **21**, 135–8S.

Flanagan, R. J., Storey, G. C. A., Bhamra, R. K., and Jane, I. (1982). High-performance liquid chromatographic analysis of basic drugs on silica columns using non-aqueous ionic eluents. *J. Chromatogr.* **247**, 15–37.

Fletcher, S. M., and Hancock, V. S. (1981). Potential errors in benzoylecgonine and cocaine analysis. *Ibid.* **206**, 193–5.

Foldes, F. F., Davidson, G. N., Duncalf, D., and Kuwabara, S. (1965). The intravenous toxicity of local anesthetic agents in man. *Clin. Pharmac. Ther.* **6**, 328–35.

Fukuda, J., and Momose, A. (1975). Determination of tetracaine N-oxide in urine by gas chromatography. *Yakugaku Zasshi* **95**, 480–83.

Gal, J., Freedman, M. D., Kumar, E., and Freed, C. R. (1981). A rapid and simple microassay for lidocaine in human blood plasma using gas–liquid chromatography with nitrogen detection. *Therap. Drug Monit.* **3**, 177–80.

Garland, W. A., Trager, W. F., and Nelson, S. D. (1974). Direct (non-chromatographic) quantification of drugs and their metabolites from human plasma utilizing chemical ionization mass spectrometry and stable isotope labeling: quinidine and lidocaine. *Biomed. Mass Spectrom.* **1**, 124–9.

Goehl, T. J., Davenport, J. B., and Stanley, M. J. (1973). Distribution, biotransformation and excretion of bupivacaine in the rat and the monkey. *Xenobiotica* **3**, 761–72.

Goto, S., and Itano, T. (1979). Hydrolysis of lidocaine and its metabolites. *Yakugaku Zasshi* **99**, 146–54.

Graffeo, A. P., Lin, D. C. K., and Foltz, R. L. (1976). Analysis of benzoylecgonine in urine by high-performance liquid chromatography and gas chromatography–mass spectrometry. *J. Chromatogr.* **126**, 717–22.

Green, R. L., Lewis, J. E., Kraus, S. J., and Frederickson, E. L. (1974). Elevated plasma procaine concentrations after administration of procaine penicillin G. *New Engl. J. Med.* **291**, 223–6.

Halkin, H., Meffin, P., Melmon, K. L., and Rowland, M. (1975). Influence of congestive heart failure on blood levels of lidocaine and its active monodeethylated metabolite. *Clin. Pharmac. Ther.* **17**, 669–76.

Hawkins, J. D., Bridges, R. R., and Jennison, T. A. (1982). A single-step assay for lidocaine and its major metabolite, monoethylglycinexylidide, in plasma by gas–liquid chromatography and nitrogen phosphorus detection. *Therap. Drug Monit.* **4**, 103–106.

Hawks, R. L., Kopin, I. J., Colburn, R. W., and Thoa, N. B. (1974). Norcocaine: a pharmacologically active metabolite of cocaine found in brain. *Life Sci.* **15**, 2189–95.

Heath, M. L. (1982). Deaths after intravenous regional anaesthesia. *Br. Med. J.* **2**, 913–4.

Hignite, C. E., Tschanz, C., Steiner, J., Huffman, D. H., and Azarnoff, D. L. (1978). Quantitation of lidocaine and its deethylated metabolites in plasma and urine by gas chromatography-mass fragmentography. *J. Chromatogr.* **161**, 243–9.

Hill, J., Roussin, A., LeLorier, J., and Caille, G. (1980). High-pressure liquid chromatographic determination of lidocaine and its active deethylated metabolites. *J. Pharm. Sci.* **69**, 1341–3.

Holt, D. W., Flanagan, R. J., Hayler, A. M., and Loizou, M. (1979a). Simple gas–liquid chromatographic method for the measurement of mexiletine and lignocaine in blood-plasma or serum. *J. Chromatogr.* **169**, 295–301.

Holt, D. W., Loizou, M., and Wyse, R. K. (1979b). Gas–liquid chromatographic measurement of lignocaine in small samples of canine myocardium after enzymatic digestion. *J. Clin. Pathol.* **32**, 225–8.

Hucker, H. B., and Stauffer, S. C. (1976). GLC analysis of lidocaine in plasma using a novel nitrogen-sensitive detector. *J. Pharm. Sci.* **65**, 926–7.

Irgens, T. R., Henderson, W. M., and Shelver, W. H. (1976). GLC analysis of lidocaine in blood using an alkaline flame-ionization detector. *Ibid.* **65**, 608–610.

Ishikawa, T. (1974). Determination of local anesthetics in the blood and cerebrospinal fluid by gas chromatography. *Jap. J. Anesthesiol.* **23**, 246–50.

Jain, S., and Johnston, A. (1979). The measurement of lignocaine at low concentrations in plasma, a comparison of gas liquid chromatography with enzyme immunoassay. *Br. J. Clin. Pharmac.* **8**, 598–9.

Jatlow, P. I., and Bailey, D. N. (1975). Gas-chromatographic analysis for cocaine in human plasma, with use of a nitrogen detector. *Clin. Chem.* **21**, 1918–21.

Jatlow, P. I., Van Dyke, C., Barash, P., and Byck, R. (1978). Measurement of benzoylecgonine and cocaine in urine, separation of various cocaine metabolites using reversed-phase high-performance liquid chromatography. *J. Chromatogr.* **152**, 115–21.

Javaid, J. I., Dekirmenjian, H., Davis, J. M., and Schuster, C. R. (1978). Determination of cocaine in human urine, plasma and red blood cells by gas–liquid chromatography. *Ibid.* **152**, 105–13.

Jindal, S. P., and Vestergaard, P. (1978). Quantitation of cocaine and its principal metabolite, benzoylecgonine, by GLC–mass spectrometry using stable isotope labeled analogs as internal standards. *J. Pharm Sci.* **67**, 811–4.

Jindal, S. P., Lutz, T., and Vestergaard, P. (1978). Mass spectrometric determination of cocaine and its biologically active metabolite, norcocaine, in human urine. *Biomed. Mass Spectrom.* **5**, 658–63.

Kacprowicz, A. T. (1982). Improved gas-chromatographic determination of lignocaine in plasma. *Clin. Chem.* **28**, 545–6.

Karch, F. E., and Chmielewski, K. F. (1981). GLC assay for lidocaine in human plasma. *J. Pharm. Sci.* **70**, 229–30.

Kaul, B., Millian, S. J., and Davidow, B. (1976). The development of a radioimmunoassay for detection of cocaine metabolites. *J. Pharmac. Exper. Ther.* **199**, 171–8.

Keenaghan, J. B. (1968). The determination of lidocaine and prilocaine in whole blood by gas chromatography. *Anesthesiology* **29**, 110–2.

Keenaghan, J. B., and Boyes, R. N. (1972). The tissue distribution, metabolism and excretion of lidocaine in rats, guinea pigs, dogs and man. *J. Pharmac. Exper. Ther.* **180**, 454–63.

Kline, B. J., and Martin, M. F. (1978). Simplified GLC assay for lidocaine in plasma. *J. Pharm. Sci.* **67**, 887–8.

Kogan, M. J., Verebey, K. G., DePace, A. C., Resnick, R. B., and Mulé, S. J. (1977). Quantitative determination of benzoylecgonine and cocaine in human biofluids by gas–liquid chromatography. *Analyt. Chem.* **49**, 1965–9.

Krogh, K., and Jellum, E. (1981). Urinary metabolites of chloroprocaine studied by combined gas chromatography-mass spectrometry. *Anesthesiology* **54**, 329–32.

Krogh, K., and Jellum, E. (1982). Urinary metabolites of chloroprocaine. *Ibid.* **56**, 483–4.

Kruczek, M. E. (1981). A rapid gas–liquid chromatographic determination of serum lidocaine using a nitrogen–phosphorus specific detector. *J. Pharmac. Methods.* **5**, 137–41.

Kuhnert, B. R., Kuhnert, P. M., and Reese, A. L. P. (1981a). Measurements of 2-chloro-2-chloroprocaine in obstetric patients and their neonates after epidural anesthesia. *Anesthesiology* **53**, 21–5.

Kuhnert, B. R., Kuhnert, P. M., and Reese, A. L. P. (1981a). Measurements of 2-chloroprocaine in plasma by selected ion monitoring. *J. Chromatogr.* **224**, 488–91.

Kuhnert, B. R., Kuhnert, P. M., and Reese, A. L. P. (1982). Urinary metabolites of chloroprocaine. *Anaesthesiology* **56**, 483.

Kuhnert, P. M., Kuhnert, B. R., Stitts, J. M., and Gross, T. L. (1981b). The use of a selected ion monitoring technique to study the disposition of bupivacaine in mother, fetus and neonate following epidural anesthesia for Cesarian section *ibid.* **55**, 611–17.

Lagerstrom, P.-O., and Persson, B.-A. (1978). Liquid chromatography in the monitoring of plasma levels of antiarrhythmic drugs. *J. Chromatogr.* **149**, 331–40.

Lee, K. Y., Nurok, D., Zlatkis, A., and Karmen, A. (1978). Simultaneous determination of antiarrhythmia drugs by high-performance thin-layer chromatography. *Ibid.* **158**, 403–10.

Lehane, D. P., Wissert, P. J., Menyharth, P., Levy, A. L., and Kukucka, A. (1979). Enzyme immunoassay for serum lidocaine in antiarrhythmic therapy. *Clin. Chem.* **25**, 614–16.

Lesko, L. J., Ericson, J., Ostheimer, G., and Marion, A. (1980). Simultaneous determination of bupivacaine and 2,6-pipecoloxylidide in serum by gas–liquid chromatography. *J. Chromatogr.* **182**, 226–31.

Liu, Y., Budd, R. D., and Griesemer, E. C. (1982). Study of the stability of cocaine and benzoylecgonine, its major metabolite, in blood samples. *Ibid.* **248**, 318–20.

Lurie, A. O., and Weiss, J. B. (1970). Blood concentration of mepivacaine and lidocaine in mother and baby after epidural anesthesia. *Amer. J. Obstet. Gynecol.* **106**, 850–6.

Maes, R., Kananen, G., and Sunshine, I. (1969). Determination of mepivacaine in blood and urine. *Anesthesiology* **30**, 657–9.

Masoud, A. N., and Krupski, D. M. (1980). High-performance liquid chromatographic analysis of cocaine in human plasma. *J. Analyt. Toxicol.* **4**, 305–10.

Masoud, A. N., Scratchley, G. A., Stohs, S. J., and Wingard, D. W. (1978). Simultaneous determination of lidocaine (lignocaine) and thiopental in plasma using high pressure-liquid chromatography. *J. Liq. Chromatog.* **1**, 607–16.

Mather, L. E., and Cousins, M. J. (1979). Local anaesthetics and their current clinical use. *Drugs* **18**, 185–205.

Mather, L. E., and Tucker, G. T. (1974). Meperidine and other basic drugs: General method for their determination in plasma. *J. Pharm. Sci.* **63**, 306–7.

McCurdy, H. H. (1980). Quantitation of cocaine and benzoylecgonine after Jetube extraction and derivatization. *J. Analyt. Toxicol.* **4**, 82–5.

Medzihradsky, F., and Dahlstrom, P. J. (1975). Concurrent determination of narcotic drugs in plasma by gas–liquid chromatography. *Pharmac. Res. Commun.* **7**, 55–69.

Mihaly, G. W., Moore, R. G., Thomas, J., Triggs, E. J., Thomas, D., and Shanks, C. A. (1978). The pharmacokinetics and metabolism of the anilide local anaesthetics in neonates. 1: Lignocaine. *Eur. J. Clin. Pharmac.* **13**, 143–52.

Miller, E., Walberg, C., and Haywood, L. J. (1981). Rapid assessment of lidocaine in cardiac patients by enzyme immunoassay. *Ther. Drug Monit.* **3**, 85–9.

Momose, A., and Fukuda, J. (1976). A new metabolite of tetracaine. *Chem. Pharm. Bull.* **24**, 1637–40.

Morgan, D. J., Cousins, M. J., McQuillan, D., and Thomas, J. (1977). Disposition and placental transfer of etidocaine in pregnancy. *Eur. J. Clin. Pharmac.* **12**, 359–365.

Mulé, S. J., Jukofsky, D., Kogan, M., De Pace, A., and Verebey, K. (1977). Evaluation of the radioimmunoassay for benzoylecgonine (a cocaine metabolite) in human urine. *Clin. Chem.* **23**, 796–801.

Naito, E., Matsuki, M., and Shimoji, K. (1977). A simple method for gas chromatographic determination of lidocaine in tissues. *Anesthesiology* **47**, 466–7.

Narang, P. K., Crouthamel, W. G., Carliner, N. H., and Fisher, M. L. (1978). Lidocaine and its active metabolites. *Clin. Pharmac. Ther.* **24**, 654–62.

Nation, R. L., Triggs, E. J., and Selig, M. (1976). Gas chromatographic method for the quantitative determination of lidocaine and its metabolite monoethylglycinexylidide in plasma. *J. Chromatogr.* **116**, 188–93.

Nation, R. L., Peng, G. W., and Chiou, W. L. (1979). High-performance liquid chromatographic method for the simultaneous determination of lidocaine and its N-dealkylated metabolites in plasma. *Ibid.* **162**, 466–73.

Nayak, P. K., Misra, A. Z., and Mulé, S. J. (1976). Physiological disposition and biotransformation of ^{3}H-cocaine in acutely and chronically treated rats. *J. Pharmac. Exper. Ther.* **196**, 556–69.

Nelson, S. D., Garland, W. A., Breck, G. D., and Trager, W. F. (1977). Quantification of lidocaine and several metabolites utilizing chemical-ionization mass spectrometry and stable isotope labeling. *J. Pharm. Sci.* **66**, 1180–90.

O'Brien, J. E., Abbey, V., Hinsvark, O., Perel, J., and Finster, M. (1979). Metabolism and measurement of chloroprocaine, an ester-type local anesthetic. *Ibid.* **68**, 75–8.

Pape, B. E. (1981). Antibody selectivity of a quantitative immunochemical assay for serum lidocaine. *Clin. Chem.* **27**, 2032–4.

Pape, B. E., Whiting, R., Parker, K. M., and Mitra, R. (1978). Enzyme immunoassay and gas–liquid chromatography compared for determination of lidocaine in serum. *Ibid.* **24**, 2020–2.

Park, G. B., Erdtmansky, P. E., Brown, R. R., Kullberg, M. P., and Edelson, J. (1980). Analysis of mepivacaine, bupivacaine, etidocaine, lidocaine and tetracaine. *J. Pharm. Sci.* **69**, 603–5.

Pfeifer, H. J., Greenblatt, D. J., and Koch-Weser, J. (1976). Clinical use and toxicity of intravenous lidocaine. A report from the Boston Collaborative Drug Surveillance Program. *Amer. Heart. J.* **92**, 168–73.

Pratt, E. L., Warrington, H. L., and Greco, J. (1967). The gas chromatographic determination of mepivacaine in blood with a note on other local anesthetics. *Anesthesiology* **28**, 432–7.

Rauckman, E. J., Rosen, G. M., and Cavagnaro, J. (1982). Norcocaine nitroxide. A potential hepatotoxic metabolite of cocaine. *Mol. Pharmac.* **21**, 458–63.

Reynolds, F. (1971). Metabolism and excretion of bupivacaine in man. A comparison with mepivacaine. *Br. J. Anaesth.* **43**, 33–37.

Reynolds, F., and Beckett, A. H. (1968). The determination of bupivacaine, lignocaine and mepivacaine in human blood. *J. Pharm. Pharmac.* **20**, 704–8.

Rosseel, M. T., and Bogaert, M. G. (1978). Determination of lidocaine and its desethylated metabolites in plasma by capillary column gas–liquid chromatography. *J. Chromatogr.* **154**, 99–102.

Rowland, M., Thomson, P. D., Guichard, A., and Melmon, K. L. (1971). Disposition kinetics of lidocaine in normal subjects. *Ann. New York Acad. Sci.* **179**, 383–98.

Seifen, A. B., Ferrari, A. A., Seifen, E. E., Thompson, D. S., and Chapman, J. (1979). Pharmacokinetics of intravenous procaine infusion in humans. *Anesth. Analg.* **58**, 382–6.

Smith, R. H., Brewster, M. A., MacDonald, J. A., and Thompson, D. S. (1978). Measurement of chloroprocaine and procaine in plasma by flame ionization gas–liquid chromatography. *Clin. Chem.* **24**, 1599–1602.

Spechtmeyer, H., and Steinbach, H. (1969). Gaschromatographische bestimmung einiger lokalanasthetica und ihrer alkylamino-metabolite in biologischem material. *Arzneim. Forsch* **19**, 1754–6.

Stargel, W. W., Roe, C. R., Routledge, P. A., and Shand, D. G. (1979). Importance of blood-collection tubes in plasma lidocaine determinations. *Clin. Chem.* **25**, 617–9.

Stewart, D. J., Inaba, T., Lucassen, M., and Kalow, W. (1979). Cocaine metabolism: Cocaine and norcocaine hydrolysis by liver and serum esterases. *Clin. Pharmac. Ther.* **25**, 464–8.

Stewart, D. J., Inaba, T., Tang, B. K., and Kalow, W. (1977). Hydrolysis of cocaine in human plasma by cholinesterase. *Life. Sci.* **20**, 1557–64.

Strong, J. M., and Atkinson, A. J. (1972). Simultaneous measurement of plasma concentrations of lidocaine and its desethylated metabolite by mass fragmentography. *Analyt. Chem.* **44**, 2287–90.

Strong, J. M., Mayfield, D. E., Atkinson, A. J., Burris, B. C., Raymon, F., and Webster, L. T. (1975). Pharmacological activity, metabolism and pharmacokinetics of glycinexylidide. *Clin. Pharmac. Ther.* **17**, 184–94.

Sung, C. Y., and Truant, A. P. (1954). The physiological disposition of lidocaine and its comparison in some respects with procaine. *J. Pharmac. Exper. Ther.* **112**, 432–43.

Svinhufved, G., Ortengren, B., and Jacobsson, S. E. (1965). The estimation of lidocaine and prilocaine in biological material by gas chromatography. *Scand. J. Clin. Lab. Invest.* **17**, 162–4.

Thomas, J., and Meffin, P. (1972). Aromatic hydroxylation of lidocaine and mepivacaine in rats and humans. *J. Med. Chem.* **15**, 1046–9.

Thomas, J., Climie, C. R., and Mather, L. E. (1968). Placental transfer of lignocaine following lumbar epidural administration. *Br. J. Anaesth.* **40**, 965–71.

Thomas, J., Climie, C. R., and Mather, L. E. (1969). The maternal plasma levels and placental transfer of bupivacaine following epidural analgesia. *Ibid.* **41**, 1035–40.

Thomas, J., Morgan, D., and Vine, J. (1976). Metabolism of etidocaine in man. *Xenobiotica* **6**, 39–48.

Tobin, T., Tai, C. Y., and Arnett, S. (1975). Recovery of procaine from biological fluids.

Res. Commun. Chem. Path. Pharmac. **11**, 187–94.
Tucker, G. T. (1970). Determination of bupivacaine (Marcaine) and other anilide-type local anesthetics in human blood and plasma by gas chromatography. *Anesthesiology*, **32**, 255–60.
Tucker, G. T. (1975). Biotransformation and toxicity of local anaesthetics. *Acta Anaesth. Belg.* **26** (suppl.), 123–40.
Tucker, G. T. (1983a). Chemistry and pharmacology of local anaesthetic drugs. In Henderson, J. J., and Nimmo, W. S. (eds), *Practical Regional Anaesthesia.* Blackwell, Oxford.
Tucker, G. T. (1983b). Pharmacokinetics of local anaesthetic drugs. *Ibid.*
Tucker, G. T., and Mather, L. E. (1979). Clinical pharmacokinetics of local anaesthetics. *Clin. Pharmacokin.* **4**, 241–78.
Valentour, J. C., Aggarwal, V., McGee, M. P., and Goza, S. W. (1978). Cocaine and benzoylecgonine determinations in postmortem samples by gas chromatography. *J. Analyt. Toxicol.* **2**, 134–7.
Van Dyke, C., Barash, P. G., Jatlow, P., and Byck, R. (1976). Cocaine: Plasma concentrations after intranasal application in man. *Science* **191**, 859–61.
Verheesen, P. E., Brombacher, P. J., Cremers, H. M. H. G., and De Boer, R. (1980). Determination of low levels of bupivacaine (Marcaine) in plasma during epidural analgesia. *J. Clin. Chem. Clin. Biochem.* **18**, 351–3.
Vigouroux, M., Montay, G., Benoit, N., Duckert, L., Roquet, F., and Reynier, M. (1978). Methode de dosage dans le sang de la lidocaine (Xylocaine) et de l'etidocaine (Duranest) par chromatographie en phase gazeuse. *Anesth. Analg. Rean.* **35**, 1045–50.
Vine, J., Morgan, D., and Thomas, J. (1978). The identification of eight hydroxylated metabolites of etidocaine by chemical ionization mass spectrometry. *Xenobiotica* **8**, 509–13.
Von Minden, D. L., and d'Amato, N. A. (1977). Simultaneous determination of cocaine and benzoylecgonine in urine by gas-liquid chromatography. *Analyt. Chem.* **49**. 1974–7.
Walberg, C. B. (1978). Lidocaine by enzyme immunoassay. *J. Analyt. Toxicol.* **2**, 121–3.
Wallace, J. E., Hamilton, H. E., Schwertner, H., King, D. E., McNay, J. L., and Blum, K. (1975). Thin-layer chromatographic determination of cocaine and benzoylecgonine in urine. *J. Chromatogr.* **114**, 433–41.
Wallace, J. E., Hamilton, H. E., King, D. E., Bason, D. J., Schwertner, H. A., and Harris, S. C. (1976). Gas–liquid chromatographic determination of cocaine and benzoylecgonine in urine. *Analyt. Chem.* **48**, 34–8.
Wilkinson, G. R., and Lund, P. C. (1970). Bupivacaine levels in plasma and cerebrospinal fluid following peridural administration. *Anesthesiology* **33**, 482–6.
Wisnicki, J. L., Tong, W. P., and Ludlum, D. B. (1979). Analysis of lidocaine and its dealkylated metabolites by high-pressure liquid chromatography. *Clin. Chim. Acta* **93**, 279–82.
Woods, L. A., Cochin, J., Fomefeld, E. J., McMahon, F. G., and Seevers, M. H. (1951). The estimation of amines in biological materials with critical data for cocaine and mescaline. *J. Pharmac. Exper. Ther.* **101**, 188–99.
Zylber-Katz, E., Granit, L., and Leby, M. (1978). Gas-liquid chromatographic determination of bupivacaine and lidocaine in plasma. *Clin. Chem.* **24**, 1573–5.

8

Indirect atomic absorption in toxicology

A. V. KOVATSIS

8.1 INTRODUCTION

In the past decade there has been considerable progress in atomic absorption spectroscopy (AAS), a method which may be divided into direct and indirect techniques. This division is due to the fact that at the outset the technique was applicable only in metallic analysis, AAS then being (as it still is) a very convenient method for the direct determination of metals.

With nonmetals, which have their resonance lines in the vacuum-ultraviolet region, difficulties arise from the strong absorption of light by the oxygen in the light path and from the flame gases. Goleb (1966) checked about 300 spectral lines in the 300 to 850 nm region and found that approximately one-third of these showed significant absorption of radiation from the source. The source was a hollow-cathode lamp with aluminium electrodes filled with the particular noble gas under study. The absorption tube had a copper cylindrical cathode and contained about 10^{-5} mol of the gas. The absorption under these conditions ranged up to 74%. Hence it is impossible for these elements to be determined directly by AAS. On the other hand, indirect AAS opened the route for a wide application in toxicological analysis. Thus, nonmetals or organic compounds or radicals which are able to form organometallic complexes or insoluble salts with metallic ions or to show chemical interferences in certain metallic determinations can be analysed by using the conversional absorption apparatus (Kovatsis, 1978a).

The indirect methods may be divided in three groups, according to the way by which the determination is achieved, as follows (Figure 8.1).

1. The first group of indirect methods involve techniques utilising chemical interference. The underlying principle here is that the amount of chemical

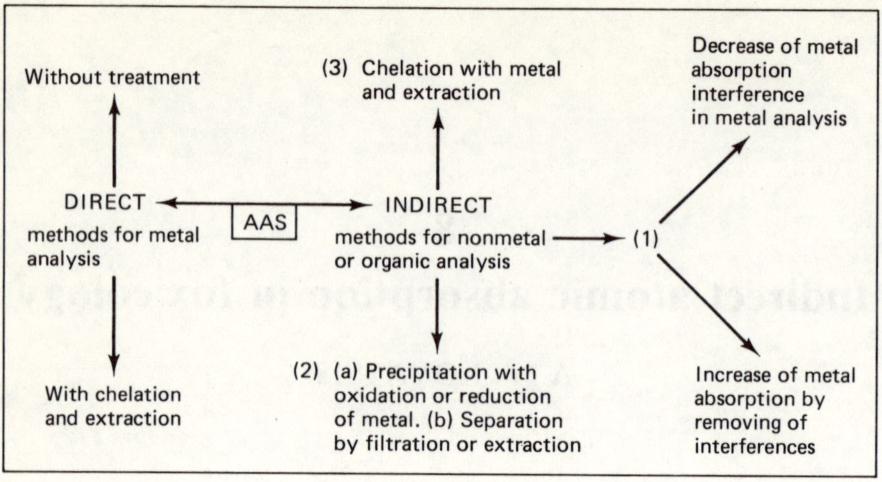

Figure 8.1 AAS methods.

interference is proportional to the concentration of the test substance. There are two modes for such determinations:

(a) Direct chemical interference in the flame. Sulphate or orthophosphate in aqueous solution causes a decrease in calcium absorption proportional to the anion concentration.

(b) Removal of chemical interference in the flame by the test substance. Glucose, for example, causes a linear increase in calcium absorption in the presence of fixed amount of sulphate. In the zirconium method, phosphate still interferes and alkali metals and ammonium ion enhance the absorption by suppressing ionisation.

2. The second group of indirect methods involve either precipitation of an equivalent amount of metal ion or the oxidation or reduction of it by an equivalent amount of the test substance.

In the first case either the precipitate can be dissolved and the amount of metal determined, or the amount of unreacted and unprecipitated metal in the filtrate can be analysed. A number of investigators have described determinations or orthophosphate based upon its reaction with molybdenum. Inorganic phosphate has also been determined by precipitating and then dissolving phosphomolybdate. Sheridan *et al.* (1966) determined some anionic surfactants by reaction with molybdenum, followed by the analysis of the excess molybdenum.

In the second case, it is possible to determine either the oxidised or reduced metal in the aqueous or organic layer, or, alternatively, the excess of unreacted metal. For example, Christian and Feldman (1968) were able to determine iodide by reacting with a slight excess of chromium (IV). Iodate ion, an oxidising agent, was determined by reacting with iron(II) and measuring the excess of iron(II) after removal of the iron(III) complex from N-HCl by extraction with ether. Iodine, as an oxidising agent, was determined by reducing selenium(IV) to the element and collecting the red selenium on Millipore filters (Newberry and Christian, 1965).

3. A third general type of determination is by extraction of an equivalent amount of metal. The test substance, dissolved either in water or in an organic solvent immiscible with water, forms a stable complex with a metal ion in the aqueous layer which can be extracted into the organic solvent; this is then aspirated into the flame. The amount of metal extracted is limited by the concentration of complex reagent. The chelate complex may be formed either by the test substance and the metal ion or by the test substance, the metal ion and another compound. In developing new techniques for the determination by indirect AAS a good knowledge of organometallic chemistry is of great advantage.

In this manner, Christian and Fieldman (1970) determined ADPC by extracting an equivalent amount of copper or cobalt into methyl isobutyl ketone (MIBK) or ethyl acetate (pH 6.5). Kumamaru *et al.* (1966a) determined phthalic acid by extracting copper in the present of neocuproine. An indirect method for the determination of nitrate based upon the same principle was proposed by Kumamaru *et al.* (1966). Pentachlorophenol was also determined by a procedure based on solvent extraction into nitrophenol of the ion pair formed between the tris-(1,10-phenanthroline)iron(II) cation and the anion of pentachlorophenol (Yamamoto *et al.* 1968).

The whole procedure involves three steps which can be summarised as follows:

1. formation of the complex;
2. isolation of the complex or the excess of metal added; and
3. clearing and aspiration into AAS.

The main step is the formation of the specific metal complex, which involves the study of all parameters which influence this formation, as well as the experimental detail condition under which this complex is formed. We should note here that in this stage there is a special difficulty which arises from the fact that in biological materials metal complexes may be formed by compounds other than those which are to be analysed. This difficulty cannot easily be avoided.

The solution of the above-mentioned problem comes from the second step, which involves isolating only the specific complex formed from the studied compound. Thus the main task is to find an organic solvent which would quantitatively extract, under specific conditions, only the complex of interest and at the same time be suitable for use in AAS.

Although these requirements involve a multiple experimental study, it is easy to discover a solvent which fulfils all the requirements. If this solvent extracts more than the interested complex then it is subjected to further treatment.

Up to the present, considerable work has been done on the applications of indirect AAS. Nevertheless, indirect AAS determination is a very promising technique and there are many possible procedures which are continuously published, while others will undoubtedly be reported in the near future. All these applications can be divided, according to the nature of the analysed compound, into two groups, namely inorganic and organic indirect AAS analysis, and we will now proceed on the basis of this division.

8.2 INORGANIC ANALYSIS

8.2.1 Iodine

Nomura and Karasawa (1981) proposed an indirect method for determination of iodine. When a solution (at pH 3.4–4.8) containing iodide and mercury(II) nitrate in a graphite tube is heated by increasing the temperature at a uniform rate, two mercury-absorption peaks appear because the decomposition temperature of mercury(II) iodide is higher than that of mercury(II) nitrate. Measurement of the second peak allows 1×10^{-6} to 1×10^{-5} M iodide to be determined with good reproducibility. Equimolar concentrations of cyanide, sulphide and thiosulphate interfered with this, but these anions could be destroyed with hydrogen peroxide. Cations that interfered were removed by extraction of 8-quinilinol complex.

8.2.2 Fluoride

The determination of fluoride by indirect AAS was proposed by Bond and O'Donnell (1968). Fluoride ion depresses the absorption of magnesium in the air–coal-gas flame, the change in absorbance of the magnesium resonance line at 285.2 nm being proportional to the fluoride concentration over the range 0.2 to 20 μg ml^{-1} (10^{-5} to 10^{-3} M). In the absence of interfering ions, principally sulphate and phosphate, the effect can be used to determine fluoride ion in this concentration range. An alternative, though somewhat less sensitive, technique is based on the enhancement of zirconium absorption by fluoride ion in the nitrous-oxide–acetylene flame; this allows determination to take place, with a high degree of freedom from the interference of fluoride ion, over the range 5 to 200 mg ml^{-1} (2.5×10^{-4} to 10^{-2} M). In the presence of phosphate, which interferes with the zirconium method, a similar enhancement of titanium absorption can be used for fluoride determination in the range 40 to 400 mg ml^{-1} (2×10^{-3} to 2×10^{-2} M).

These atomic absorption methods for fluoride determinations have been found to be considerably more rapid than more classical methods, and in many cases can be used directly without prior separation of fluoride. Their application has been demonstrated in the analysis of a wide range of inorganic fluorides.

8.2.3 Chloride

Westerlund-Helmerson (1966) developed a method for the rapid determination of chloride by indirect AAS. The method is based on the fact that after the addition of $AgNO_3$ the sample is dissolved in nitric acid. The AgCl precipitate is then dissolved in NH_4OH. Silver is determined in the ammonia solution by atomic absorption, and the corresponding content of chloride calculated.

Analytically the procedure is as follows. Boil 0.5 g of sample, 20 ml of 1% solution of $AgNO_3$, 20 ml of HNO_3, and about 60 ml of water in a 250-ml beaker. Allow the beaker to cool in darkness. Filter and rinse the filter paper ten times with 2% HNO_3. Wash the precipitate back into the same beaker with a little water, and boil with 20 ml of NH_4OH. Pour the solution through the used filter paper into a 200-ml volumetric flask and dilute to volume. Pipette a suitable proportion (e.g. 3·to 20 ml) of this solution into a 100-ml volumetric flask, add 5 ml of NH_4OH and dilute to volume. Measure the absorption and compare with silver standards of 1, 2, 5 and 10 p.p.m. silver. One p.p.m. silver corresponds to 0.329 p.p.m. chloride.

8.2.4 Halogen elements in organic compounds

The determination of halogen elements in organic compounds by indirect AAS was proposed by Kidani *et al.* (1973b). The recommended procedures are as follows. Nonsublimable compounds, such as *p*-chloroaniline and *p*-bromoacetanilide, were fused with metallic sodium of 10 to 20 times as much as their weight, and after an excess of metallic sodium had been decomposed with water the residues were filtered off and the filtrate was used for the measurement. Next, a proper amount of the sample solution (1 to 4 ml) was made acidic with nitric acid, after which 5 ml of 100 mg ml^{-1} silver nitrate solution was added, and the resultant solution warmed on a water-bath for 1 min. It was then kept standing for 30 min at a room temperature, the precipitates were filtered off, and the filtrate diluted to 100 ml with water; the excess amounts of silver were then determined by atomic absorption spectrophotometer.

The above procedure, however, is not applicable to the sublimable compounds such as 1-chlorophenazine. In this case the procedure is as follows. In a 50-ml capacity flask, the compound was dissolved in 2 ml of alcohol (*n*-butanol, iso-amyl alcohol etc.) with a reflux condenser and warmed. After an addition of metallic sodium, the resultant solution was boiled for 30 min and then kept standing for 10 min at a room temperature. After an addition of water, insoluble materials were filtered off and filtrate was used for the measurement. Standard solutions of Cl, Br and I for working curves were prepared according to similar procedures. In order to ascertain in the repeatability, the compounds with various halogen contents were analysed.

8.2.5 Fluorine in organic compounds

Kidani and Ito (1976a) also proposed an indirect method for determination of fluorine in organic compounds by AAS. This method is based on the decomposition of fluorine-containing compounds with sodium biphenyl, followed by atomic absorption spectrometry of iron in MIBK phase. The recommended procedure is as follows. The aqueous solution, separated after the decomposition with sodium biphenyl, was adjusted to a pH of 3.0 with 0.2N hydrochloric acid. To 5 ml of this solution was added first 1 ml of an excess of a ferric chloride solution which contains 10 mg ml^{-1} of Fe and then 1 ml of 2.5% ammonium thiocyanate solution. Excess iron was extracted with 2 ml of MIBK as ferric thiocyanate and the iron content extracted was measured by AAS. Fluorine is determined indirectly by this method and the calibration curve was linear in the range of 0.5 to 6.0 mg ml^{-1}. Metals which form more stable fluorine complexes than Fe(III) interfere, but the anions, other than CN^-, do not disturb the measurement.

8.2.6 Cyanides

There are two general indirect methods for the determination of cyanides by AAS.

One method involves the formation of an insoluble precipitate and the determination of either the metal incorporated in the precipitate or the excess metal ion in the supernatant solution. The second indirect method is based on the formation of a stoichiometric complex, the isolation of the complex by extraction, and the determination of the metal in the complex by atomic absorption measurement.

A method based on the first principle was proposed by Danchik and Boltz (1970) and includes the formation of the highly insoluble precipitate of silver cyanide. The silver cyanide is quantitatively precipitated and the excess of silver ion in the supernate is determined by AAS. This indirect method for cyanide has a higher sensitivity than either the spectrophotometric method or the indirect method based on the ferroin reagent.

The other method of the same authors, based on the second principle, includes the formation of the neutral dicyano-bis-(1, 10-phenanthroline) iron(II) complex which was extracted with chloroform. The ethanol solution is aspirated directly into the air–acetylene flame and the iron, equivalent to the definite amount of cyanide ion, is determined.

Another method based on the same first principle was proposed by Kovatsis and Tsougas (1979). The proposed method is based on the formation of a cyanonickel complex with $NiCl_2$, the elimination of the unreacted $NiCl_2$ by Na_2S and the determination of the nickelate complex by AAS.

The first step of the above-mentioned method involves the liberation of cyanide from the biological material and then bubbling it through a 0.1N-NaOH solution. This is conventionally accomplished by setting up three gas-washing bottles in series (Figure 8.2) with the appropriate materials and reagents in the respective bottles. Thus, 5 ml of 0.1N-NaOH solution are poured into a large

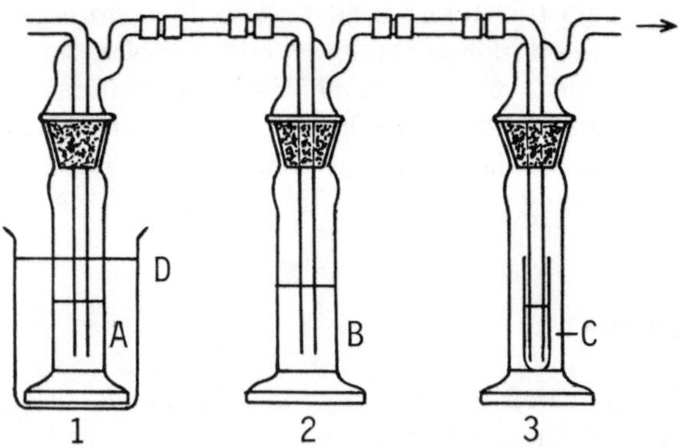

Figure 8.2 Diagram of the three gas-washing bottles in sequence: (1) specimen bottle, (2) scrubber bottle, (3) reaction bottle. (A) sample, (B) lead-acetate solution, (C) 0.1N-NaOH solution, (D) water-bath.

test-tube (approximately 12.5 by 15 cm), which is then inserted into the reaction bottle (3 in Figure 8.2). The inlet tubing is placed inside the test-tube containing the 0.1N-NaOH solution. 20 ml of buffered (Kovatsis and Tsougas, 1976) lead-acetate solution are placed in a reaction bottle (the scrubber bottle, 2 in Figure 8.2) with the glass tubing submerged in the lead-acetate solution to remove sulphides. To the specimen bottle (1 in Figure 8.2) is added 2 ml blood or 2 g homogenised tissue plus 15 ml water, an antifoam agent, and 2 ml of 50% H_2SO_4. The bottle containing the specimen is then placed in a bath at 90 °C. The water level in the bath is maintained at a higher level than the liquid in the specimen bottle. Suction (sufficient to produce 200 bubbles per minute) is then applied for 20 min. At the end of the aeration period the cyanide in the NaOH solution is ready to form the nickel complex by reacting with $NiCl_2$ (1% aqueous solution) at pH 7 to 8, the process being regulated by the acetic acid–sodium acetate.

The second step involves the elimination of the unreacted $NiCl_2$ by filtration after the formation of undiluted NiS salt by reaction with excess amounts of Na_2S. This excess may be up to double the theoretical amount which reacts with the added $NiCl_2$. The reaction is completed in 30 minutes.

The third step involves the determination of nickel in the nickelate complex by AAS, which is linear resulting from the liberated cyanide. Before each measurement the calibration curve is verified by utilising the standard solutions of potassium cyanide. The sensitivity of the proposed method is 1 μg ml^{-1} of sample.

8.2.7 Chlorate ion

Mitsui and Fujimura (1974a) proposed an indirect method for chlorate determination by AAS. The recommended procedure is as follows. To a sample solution was added 0.5 ml of 20% $FeSO_4$ solution, the resulting solution being heated on a water-bath for 10 min at 80 °C. After the solution had been cooled, the resulting chloride solution containing the Fe-complex salt was dissolved in 5 ml of 6N-HNO_3, and 2 ml of 5 mg ml^{-1} $AgNO_3$ solution was added to the solution. After the solution had been filtered, the AgCl precipitate was dissolved in 20 ml of 1.42N ammonia water. The solution was diluted to 1000 ml with water and was analysed by AAS.

8.2.8 Acid anhydrides

The indirect determination of acid anhydrides by atomic absorption spectrometry was proposed by Minami *et al.* (1980).

The recommended method is as follows. To 1 ml of ethanol solution of each sample (0.10 to 4.00 mg ml^{-1}) is added 4 ml of NH_2OH–HCl–NaOH solution (a mixture of 150 mg $NH_2OH \cdot HCl$ ml^{-1} solution and 85 mg NaOH ml^{-1} solution at a ratio of 2 : 1, by vol.). The mixture is allowed to stand for 10 min. To this solution is added 2 ml of 1.2N-HCl, 1 ml of 7 mg $FeCl_3 \cdot 6H_2O$ ml^{-1} solution and 5 ml of 5.5% NH_4OH solution. After standing for 10 min, the resulting solution is filtered. The iron in the filtrate is measured by AAS. There was no interference in the presence of 5- to 20-molar-fold of acetone, acetic acid, aniline, nitrobenzene, phenol, K^+, Mg^{2+}, or Ca^{2+} or in that of 1.5-molar-fold of ethyl acetate, but a marked interference was observed when 0.001- to 0.01-molar-fold of acetyl chloride, or Cu^{2+} or Al^{3+} was present.

8.2.9 Hydrogen sulphide

Hydrogen-sulphide determination by indirect AAS was proposed by Kovatsis and Tsougas (1976). In this method a known amount of buffered $Pb(CH_3COO)_2$ solution is added to the test sample and the excess reagent is measured by AAS. The proposed procedure is as follows. A sample of the ambient air to be examined for hydrogen sulphide is taken with a special vacu-sampler. This is brought back to the laboratory as quickly as possible (to prevent any possibility of hydrogen sulphide oxidation), where each vacu-sampler is injected with 50 ml of solution, buffered to pH 5.6 with $CH_3COOH \cdot CH_3COONa$, of $Pb(CH_3COO)_2$ containing up to 3000 p.p.m. of Pb.

After 30 min, with occasional shaking, the sampler is opened, the content filtered and the black precipitate of PbS washed with bi-distilled water. The filtrate is made up to a certain volume and then aspirated directly into the AAS flame for the determination of the excess of unreacted Pb. The difference between added and unreacted Pb represents the amount which was reacted with H_2S.

8.2.10 Hydrogen peroxide

Indirect determination of hydrogen peroxide by AAS was accomplished by Kidani and Ito (1980). The principle is as follows.

1. Cuprous–bathocuproine disulphonate chelate was prepared in advance by the reduction of cupric–bathocuproine disulphonate in the presence of reducing agents, L-ascorbic acid or Zn.

2. The Cu^+ chelates are oxidised to Cu^{2+} chelates in the presence of H_2O_2. The Cu^{2+} chelates are not so stable in water and they dissociate to Cu^{2+} ions and ligand. They remain in the aqueous phase, together with the unreacted Cu^+ chelates.

3. The Cu^{2+} dissociated in the aqueous phase is extracted with MIBK in the presence of acetylacetone. The stability constant of Cu^+ chelate in the aqueous phase is much larger than that of the copper acetylacetone in MIBK. The Cu^+-bathocuproine disulphonate chelate remaining unoxidised in the aqueous phase is removed by MIBK extraction.

4. The copper content in the MIBK extract is measured by flameless AAS.

The procedure which is based on the above-mentioned principle is as follows. To 3–5 ml of Cu^+-bathocuproine sulfonate was added 8 to 4 μg of H_2O_2. This was shaken and kept standing for 1.5 h. To this mixture was added 0.5 ml of 4% acetylacetone; after 5 min 5 to 10 ml of MIBK was added, after which followed a further 3 min shaking. The MIBK layer was analysed by flameless AAS.

8.2.11 Sulphur and sulphate

Roe *et al.* (1966) proposed an indirect method for estimation of sulphur in biological materials by AAS. The same method can be used for the determination of inorganic sulphate concentrations in urine. In the procedure, samples or urine, diet, faeces and biological tissues, oxidised by one of several techniques, were added to a solution containing an excess of barium chloride. The resulting precipitate of barium sulphate was dissolved in disodium ethylenediamine-tetra-acetic acid and the barium concentration of the resulting solution was analysed by AAS.

Determinations of inorganic sulphate concentration in urine samples were made directly in aliquots from which the sediment had been removed by centrifugation. Lanthanum chloride solution was added to all prepared samples, in order to eliminate phosphate interference in the AAS determination of barium.

8.2.12 Ammonia

Ammonia determination by indirect AAS was proposed by Mitsui and Fujimura (1974b). The method is based on the fact that the atomic absorption of silver is remarkably enhanced in the presence of ammonium ion, and the effect is proportional to the concentration of ammonium ion. The recommended procedure is as follows. Ammonium salts are dissolved in water to give concentrations of 17.6, 10.3 and 15.1 $\mu g\ ml^{-1}$, respectively. To 10 ml to each of the standards, 10 ml of aqueous solution containing 0.84 mg of NaOH and 12.8 μg of Ag is added, and the mixture is analysed by AAS.

8.3 ORGANIC ANALYSIS

The contribution of indirect AAS analysis of organic compounds is more extensive, since a great number of organic compounds are capable of forming organometallic complexes suitable for AAS analysis.

8.3.1 Carbon disulphide

Kneebone and Freiser (1975) proposed an indirect method for CS_2 determination in an industrial atmosphere, based on the formation of a complex with pyrrolidine and Cu^+ and the extraction of the formed chelate with isoamyl acetate. The detection limit of 7.0 μg CS_2 per sample can be lowered to one-fifth of this figure by reducing the volume of the extracting solvent. The procedure is as follows. To a 10.0 ml solution 10^{-2} M in pyrrolodine and 10^{-3} M in $CuSO_4$ was added CS_2 in the range 5–100 μg. The pH was adjusted to 2.0 to 2.5 with HCl. The solution was shaken with 10.0 ml of isoamyl acetate on a mechanical shaker for 5 minutes.

The phases were separated and the aqueous phase discarded. The absorbance of the copper chelate was measured in air–acetylene flame.

Kovatsis (1978b) proposed another method for indirect determination of CS_2 which may be used as an indicator for evaluation of dithiocarbamates as well as for CS_2 itself. The method is based on the formation of a unique and stable complex of zinc dibenzyl dithiocarbamate, $Zn(DBDC)_2$, from CS_2, $ZnCl_2$ and *NN′*-dibenzylamine. This complex is easily extracted with toluene in a 50% methanolic solution. The extraction is carried out at pH 9.1 and is quantitative. The procedure can be applied to a wide range of CS_2 concentrations, which quantitatively correspond to the dithiocarbamates decomposed in an acidic medium at a temperature of 95 to 100°C, since it is possible to dilute the final solution of the extracted complex. The procedure includes the digestion of dithiocarbamates, the formation of the complex and its extraction for AAS aspiration. The sensitivity of the proposed method is 0.2 μg/0.0044 abs. The detection limit is 0.165 $\mu g\,ml^{-1}$ for CS_2. Care should be taken to avoid rapid heating of the dithiocarbamate sample and to keep it at 95 to 100°C for 45 min. Below these temperatures the dithiocarbamates, together with CS_2, can also yield hydrogen sulphide. To increase the accuracy in that event, we proposed a second trap (Figure 8.2) with buffered lead-acetate solution (Kovatsis and Tsougas, 1976) to evaluate hydrogen sulphide and, indirectly, the dithiocarbamates which produce it. It is self-evident that the digestion of dithiocarbamates is carried out in the same apparatus that was previously mentioned as being used for cyanide determination (three gas-washing bottles in sequence).

8.3.2 Oxalic acid in urine

Menache (1974) proposed an indirect method to determine the oxalic acid in urine. Oxalates are precipitated from the urine with excess calcium ions at pH 5. The calcium in the precipitate is determined indirectly by AAS, subtracting the excess calcium measured in the supernate from the total calcium present, and added to a similar sample of the urine at pH 2. By multiplying this figure by the appropriate factor, the oxalic acid of the precipitate is deduced. There is no interference from phosphorus as coprecipitate if, before the pH is adjusted to pH 5, it is adjusted to pH 8. Urinary phosphorus also does not interfere in the AAS if, as in the usual determination of calcium with such instruments, the samples are diluted with lanthanum chloride.

The detailed procedure is as follows. Pipette two 5-ml samples of urine from a well-mixed 24-h collection into each of two test-tubes, marked 'test sample' and 'Control sample'. Adjust the pH of both to 2 with a few drops of hydrochloric acid 1 : 1 (v/v). Readjust the 'test sample' to pH 8 with a few drops of ammonium hydroxide (3 $mol\,l^{-1}$). Readjust the pH of the contents of the same tube to 5 with acetic acid (6 $mol\,l^{-1}$) drop by drop. Place the two tubes in boiling water, add to each 0.5 ml of calcium chloride (2 g of $CaCl_2 \cdot 6H_2O$ in 100 ml of water), mix, and continue heating for an additional 10 min. Cool the tubes in a refrigerator for at least an hour and centrifuge (3000 rev min^{-1}, 10 min). Oxalates are quantitatively precipitated at pH 5 (test sample) but not at pH 2 (control sample). Assay the supernate for calcium by AAS.

8.3.3 Halogen-containing compounds

Halogen-containing compounds can be determined by AAS according to the suggestions of Kidani *et al.* (1973a). The halogen-containing compounds were classified into three groups tentatively, that is, the compounds containing (1) ionic halogens, (2) nonionic halogens and (3) both ionic and nonionic single halogens. The recommended procedures are as follows. Samples containing ionic halogens, such as guanidine hydrochloride and propantheline bromide, were dissolved in water. It was found that desirable concentrations of the sample solution were 25 μg ml^{-1} for Cl-containing compounds, and 100 μg ml for both Br- and I-containing compounds for the measurements, respectively. Next, proper amounts of the sample solution (1 to 4 ml) were made acidic with nitric acid, this being followed by the addition of 5 ml of 100 μg ml^{-1} silver-nitrate solution, the whole then being warmed on a water-bath for 1 min. It was kept standing for 30 min at a room temperature, the precipitates were filtered off and the filtrate was diluted to 100 ml with water, after which excess amounts of silver were determined by AAS. Samples containing nonionic halogens, such as bromisovalum and iodoform, were fused with 10 to 20 times as much metallic sodium as was in the samples, and after the decomposition of unreacted metallic sodium with water the residues were filtered off and the filtrate used as a sample solution. The ensuing procedures were similar to those for ionic halogens.

8.3.4 Phosphorus in organic compounds

Phosphorus in organic compounds was determined by Kidani *et al.* (1974a). Their method is based on the fact that molybdophosphoric acid produced by the reaction of phosphoric acid with ammonium molybdate is extractable with organic solvents, and hence phosphorus can be determined indirectly by the measurement of the molybdenum extracted by AAS. Although nitrous oxide-air fuels have usually been employed for the determination of molybdenum, in this method an attempt was made to use an acetylene–air fuel instead of nitrous oxide–air. The recommended procedure was as follows. To 5 ml of a standard phosphorus solution (5 μg ml^{-1}), 5 ml of 60% perchloric acid was added and the mixture diluted to 40 ml with water. To this, 3 ml of 10% ammonium molybdate was added, the molybdophosphoric acid produced was extracted with MIBK, and the extract was washed twice with water. The MIBK was used for the measurement.

Using these conditions, an ionic sample such as histamine diphosphate was dissolved in water and treated by the usual procedure, while such nonionic samples as triphenylphosphine and pyridoxal phosphate were decomposed by boiling with concentrated sulphuric acid and concentrated nitric acid and then treated like the ionic sample.

8.3.5 Aliphatic amines

Minami *et al.* (1981a) proposed an indirect method for the determination of aliphatic amines by AAS, using the complex formation of amines and thiocyanate with cobalt followed by AAS. The recommended procedure is as follows: 0.5 ml of acetone solution of KSCN (32.6 mg ml^{-1}) and 0.5 ml of acetone solution of Co(II) [27.91 mg $Co(NO_3)_2 6H_2O$ ml^{-1}] are mixed in a 20-ml test-tube. The solvent is evaporated on a water-bath at 90 °C. To this test-tube is added 5 ml of benzene solution of each sample (0.01–0.13 mg ml). After being shaken for 1 min the benzene solution is dehydrated with anydrous sodium sulphate. To 1 ml of this solution is added 5 ml of methanol, and finally the cobalt content is measured by AAS. No interferences were observed in the presence of 2.2-molar- to 15.6-molar-fold of ethanol, diethylether, acetone, acetaldehyde, ethyl acetate, acetic acid, nitrobenzene, acetonitrile, or phenol and 1.4-molar-fold of diphenylamine.

8.3.6 Primary amines

The determination of primary amines by AAS was proposed by Mitsui and Fujimura (1974d). The recommended procedures are as follows. The complex-formation reagent solution is prepared by mixing 3.372 g of triethanolamine, 0.205 g of nitrosalicylaldehyde, 1 ml of 50% acetaldehyde solution, 5 ml of 4% cupric sulphate and water (final volume 50 ml). Each sample solution of amine is added to 1 ml of the complex-formation reagent solution and diluted to 10 ml with water. After standing 1 hour, the precipitate of copper–amine complex is filtered off. Then, *either* (1), by the filtrate method, 1 ml of the filtrate is diluted to 10 ml or 25 ml with water, and the copper content is measured by AAS; *or* (2), by the precipitate method, the precipitate (copper complex) is dissolved into 10 ml of 12.6 N nitric acid and diluted to a proper volume (100, 250, or 500 ml), then analysed by AAS. The coexistence of 20 to 30 times of secondary or tertiary amines does not interfere. Several metal ions such zinc, magnesium and calcium cause severe interferences and must be removed beforehand.

8.3.7 Aliphatic secondary amines

Mitsui and Fujimura (1974e) proposed an indirect method for the determination of aliphatic secondary amines by AAS. Diethylamine hydrochloride, ephedrine hydrochloride and methamphetamine hydrochloride are estimated by complexing the aliphatic secondary amines with copper, followed by solvent extraction of the copper complexes into MIBK and final determination of complexed copper by AAS. The recommended procedure is as follows. 1 ml of the sample solution, 1 ml of 0.5 N ammonia water, 1 ml of Cu^{2+} solution and 1 ml of carbon disulphide were mixed. The Cu^{2+} in the mixed solution was controlled to less than 0.25 in terms of aliphatic secondary-amine hydrochloride–Cu^{2+} (mol/mol) ratio. The mixed solution was shaken for 1 min with 25 ml of MIBK, and the whole allowed to stand for 10 min. The amount of copper in MIBK solution was determined by AAS.

8.3.8 Methamphetamine HCl in the presence of ephedrine HCl

Mitsui *et al.* (1975) proposed an indirect method for the determination of methamphetamine hydrochloride in the presence of ephedrine hydrochloride. Methamphetamine hydrochloride in a methaphetamine hydrochloride and ephedrine hydrochloride mixture was determined indirectly by AAS of bismuth. The recommended procedure is as follows. A sample is dissolved in water, to which 1 ml of 7% HCl and 1 ml of KI–$BiCl_3$ aqueous solution (7% KI solution saturated with $BiCl_3$) are added. The total volume of the solution is brought to 10 ml with water. The solution is allowed to stand for 30 min and filtered. To one ml of the filtrate is added 1 ml of conc. HCl; this is diluted to 25 ml with water, and bismuth then determined by AAS. The interference of metal ion and $Na_2S_2O_3$ on the determination of methamphetamine hydrochloride was eliminated by extraction of methamphetamine from the basic aqueous solution into chloroform.

8.3.9 Low-molecular-weight ketones and aldehydes

Minami *et al.* (1981b) proposed an indirect method for the determination of low-molecular-weight ketones and aldehydes by AAS. The recommended procedure is as follows. 1 ml of sample solution (0.01 to 2.01 mg ml^{-1}) is added to 2 ml of thiosemicarbazide solution (thiosemicarbazide 11 mg ml^{-1}) and 1 ml of copper acetate solution (copper acetate 15 mg ml^{-1}). The mixture is warmed on a water bath for 4 min at 70 °C and then cooled. It is then shaken with 5 ml of benzene for 5 min, and the two liquid layers are separated by centrifugation. The benzene layer is dehydrated and ethanol added (1 : 1). The copper in the solution is measured by AAS.

8.3.10 Anthranilic acid

Kidani *et al.* (1975a) proposed a method for indirect determination of anthranilic acid by AAS. The method is based on the extraction of its insoluble cobalt(II) chelate with MIBK in the presence of bathophenanthroline from phosphate buffer solution of pH 6.3 which was then subjected to AAS. The calibration curve obtained was shown to be linear in the range of 3 to 22 μg ml^{-1} and the recovery was 99.5%.

8.3.11 Phthalic acid

Kumamaru *et al.* (1966) proposed a method for indirect determination of phthalic acid by AAS. The procedure is as follows. Mix 1 ml copper(II) sulphate solution (1×10^{-2} M), 2 ml of 5% hydroxylamine sulphate solution, 5 ml of 0.25 M phosphate buffer solution and varying amounts of standard phthalic acid solution with water to 25 ml and shake for 2 min with 10.0 ml of an MIBK solution containing neocuproine (2×10^{-3} M). Measure the absorption using a copper hollow-cathode lamp as light source at the 324.7 nm copper line. Use an air–acetylene flame with an air flow-rate of about 70 l min^{-1}.

8.3.12 Polyhydric alcohols and acetaldehyde

Mitsui and Fujimura (1976) proposed a method for the determination of polyhydric alcohols and acetaldehyde in ethyl alcohol by indirect AAS. Periodic acid reacts with polyhydric alcohol in the sample to yield iodate which is then precipitated by silver nitrate. After being washed with diluted nitric acid and water to remove the excess silver nitrate, the precipitate is dissolved in ammonia-water for the determination of silver by AAS. Acetaldehyde in the sample (ethyl alcohol) reacts with Tollen's reagent to yield silver. The precipitate silver is filtered, washed with water, and then dissolved by addition of conc. nitric acid and water for the determination of silver by AAS. The limits of determinations are as follows: glycerol 0.16 mg, lactose 0.82 mg, saccharose 1.93, glucose 0.21, tartaric acid 1.22 mg, benzoine 1.07 mg, acetaldehyde 1.90×10^{-3} mg.

8.3.13 Amino acids

Kidani *et al.* (1976c) proposed an indirect method for the determination of amino acids by AAS. The proposed method is based on the fact that the amino acids react with salicylaldehyde to yield their Schiff's bases in alkaline solution, and the Schiff's bases–Cu(II) chelates formed by the addition of Cu(II)ion–are extractable with MIBK in the presence of bathophenathroline. Therefore amino acids can be determined indirectly by the estimation of copper in the organic phase by AAS. Two ml of 2.0×10^{-5} to 2.0×10^{-4} M amino acid solution, 2.0 ml of 1.0×10^{-2} M salicylaldehyde solution, 1.0 ml of 1.0×10^{-3} M cupric acetate solution and 5 ml of boric acid buffer solution of pH 10.0 were taken into a 30 ml centrifuge tube and mixed sufficiently. After the solution was allowed to stand for 5 min, 10.0 ml of chloroform was added. The mixture was shaken for 10 min and was centrifuged. After separation, 5.0 ml of upper aqueous phase was transferred into another 30 ml centrifuge tube and 10.0 ml of 1.0×10^{-4} M bathophenanthroline MIBK solution was added. Being shaken well for 5 min it was centrifuged and the copper in the organic phase was determined by AAS.

8.3.14 Folic acid

The determination of folic acid by AAS was proposed by Kidani *et al.* (1976b). 2-amino-4-hydroxypteridine-6-carboxylic acid, one of the oxidation products of folic acid with potassium permanganate, reacts with nickel ions to form a metal complex. The nickel complex is extracted with MIBK in the presence of bathophenanthroline. Therefore, quantitative determination of folic acid can be made indirectly by measuring nickel content in MIBK phase by AAS.

8.3.15 Barbituric acid and derivatives

Mitsui and Fujimura (1975) proposed an indirect method for the determination of barbituric acid by AAS. Barbituric acid derivatives react with copper–pyridine reagent to yield insoluble complexes in an alkaline medium. Barbiturates could therefore be indirectly determined by measuring the amount of copper in the filtrate or precipitate by atomic absorption spectrophotometry. The recommended procedures are as follows. The sample solution in 0.08 M sodium carbonate (containing 0.51 to 16.21 mg of barbiturates) is mixed with 1 to 3 ml of copper solution (3.37 mg of copper ion per ml) and 1 ml of pyridine, and then brought to 10 ml with water. The mixture is allowed to stand for 30 minutes and then filtered. *Method 1:* to 1 ml of the filtrate is added 10 ml of conc. nitric acid, mixed well, and then the mixture is diluted to 50 ml with water. The copper content of the resultant solution is measured by atomic absorption spectrophotometry. *Method 2:* the precipitates are washed with 100 ml of 5% pyridine, and dissolved by adding 20 ml of conc. nitric acid followed by diluting to 500 ml with water. The copper content of the resultant solution is assayed by atomic absorption spectrophotometry.

8.3.16 *p*-Aminobenzoic acid

Kidani *et al*. (1975b) proposed an indirect method for the determination of *p*-aminobenzoic acid (PABA) by AAS. Previously, the authors reported on the formation of 2 : 1 PABA–metal complexes with various metals. The complexes are not extractable with organic solvents, but copper–PABA complex is extracted wih MIBK in the presence of bathophenanthroline. Therefore PABA is determined indirectly by measuring copper in the MIBK extract by atomic absorption spectometry. To PABA–methanol solution was added cupric chloride–methanol solution, then the mixture was warmed on a water-bath until methanol was evaporated to dryness. After being cooled, the residue was washed with ethyl acetate twice in order to remove an excess of copper. The residue was then extracted with bathophenanthroline MIBK solution, and the copper in MIBK phase was measured by an atomic absorption spectrophotometer. The calibration curve obtained was linear in the range of 13.7 to 37.0 μg ml^{-1} and the recovery was 100.6%.

8.3.17 Flufenamic acid

Minamikawa *et al*. (1973) proposed an indirect method for the determination of flufenamic acid by AAS. In the presence of Cu and 2-(2-hydroxy-ethyl)pyridine, flufenamic acid formed a chelate compound, which could be extracted with propyl acetate. The amount of flufenamic acid was obtained indirectly by measuring Cu in this propyl-acetate solution by atomic absorption. When this method was applied to the perfusion of rat small intestine and to the analysis of preparations, good results were obtained without any interference. It was also found that flufenamic acid, Cu, and 2-(2-hydroxyethyl)pyridine combined in the ratio of 1 to 1 to form a chelate.

8.3.18 Isonicotinylhydrazine

Kidani *et al.* (1973d) proposed an indirect method for the determination of isonicotinylhydrazine by AAS. Isonicotinylhydrazine (INAH) reacts with cupric ion to produce INAH-Cu(II) chelate (2 : 1) at pH 4.5, which can be extracted with methyl isobutyl ketone (MIBK). Thus it is found that INAH can be quantitatively determined indirectly if the quantity of Cu(II) in the organic phase is measured by atomic absorption spectrophotometry.

Procedure for the determination was as follows: cupric chloride solution and aqueous INAH solution were mixed together with acetic acid–sodium acetate buffer solution which was adjusted to pH 4.5; this solution was extracted with MIBK for 15 minutes twice and then kept standing for 10 minutes. The organic phase was centrifuged at 3000 rev min^{-1} for 5 minutes, and the copper in the organic phase was measured by atomic absorption spectrophotometer.

8.3.19 Catechol

Kidani *et al.* (1974c) attempted to determine the catechol by AAS. According to their proposed method, catechol reacts with cupric ion to produce a yellowish, 2 : 1-ratio chelate at pH 10.0, which is extractable with chloroform in the presence of capriquat, tri-*n*-octylmethylammonium chloride. Therefore, catechol may be determined indirectly if the copper in the organic phase is measured by atomic absorption spectrophotometry.

The determination procedure is as follows. 1 ml of 1.0×10^{-3} M aqueous catechol solution and 1.0 ml of 5.0×10^{-3} M aqueous cupric chloride solution were added to 5.0 ml of Britton–Robinson buffer solution of pH 10.0 with mixing. After this had stood for 5 min, 10.0 ml of 1.0×10^{-3} M capriquat chloroform solution was added. The mixture was shaken well for 5 min, and was centrifuged at 3000 rev min^{-1} for a further 5 min. After separation, 5.0 ml of organic phase was transfered into a test-tube and was made up to 10.0 ml with methanol. The amount of copper was determined by atomic absorption spectrophotometry using a reagent blank as reference.

8.3.20 Chinoform

The determination of chinoform by AAS was proposed by Kidani *et al.* (1973c). Chinoform, being a derivative of oxine, forms metal chelate with various metal ion. It is known that chinoform reacts with zinc to produce a yellow chelate of 2 : 1 ratio and it is extractable with MIBK. Therefore, if zinc in the MIBK layer is measured by atomic absorption spectrophotmetry it follows that chinoform may be determined quantitatively. Chinoform zinc chelate can be extracted easily with chloroform, but MIBK is considered to be more suitable than chloroform as a solvent for atomic absorption spectrophotometry.

The procedure for the determination is as follows. 10 ml of 4.1×10^{-5} M chinoform MIBK solution was taken in a 100 ml separatory funnel, and then 10 ml of 2.0×10^{-4} M aqueous zinc sulphate solution and 10 ml of sodium borate–boric acid–sodium chloride buffer solution, adjusted to pH 7.9, were added. The mixture was shaken well for 10 minutes and kept standing for 10 minutes. First the lower aqueous layer was separated off and then the MIBK layer was transferred to a test-tube. After the MIBK layer was filtrated through filter paper, 2 ml of the filtrate was diluted to 10 ml with MIBK, and the absorbance then measured by atomic absorption spectrophotometry against a reagent blank.

8.3.21 Ethambutol

Kovatsis and Tsougas (1978) proposed an indirect method for the determination of ethambutol. The method is based on the fact that in the presence of cupric ions and sodium hydroxide, ethambutol forms a chelate compound which can be extracted with methyl ethyl ketone (2-butanone). The amount of ethambutol–copper complex was determine by measuring the copper by atomic absorption spectroscopy (AAS) in the methyl ethyl ketone extract. When this method was applied to pharmaceutical samples satisfactory results were obtained. The method is accurate for routine analyses and very simple to carry out.

8.3.22 Chlorpheniramine maleate

Kidani *et al.* (1974b) proposed an indirect method for the determination of chlorpheniramine maleate by AAS.

Chlorpheniramine maleate (MCP) itself does not form a metal complex because MCP has not any chelating functional groups. However, MCP will be extractable with chloroform at a pH 4.3, when it is reacted with Zincon to form a ternary complex. Zincon is known to produce a blue complex with copper in a 1 : 1 molar ratio. Therefore MCP is determined indirectly by measuring the absorbance of copper in the organic phase by atomic absorption spectrophotometry. A ternary complex of copper–Zincon MCP is extracted with MIBK for four times, while it is extracted with chloroform more easily, because MIBK is known to be superior to chloroform as a solvent for atomic absorption spectrophotometry.

The procedure for the determination is as follows. 1 ml of an aqueous solution of 1.3×10^{-3} M Zincon was taken into a 30 ml centrifuge tube, and to this were added 1 ml of an aqueous solution of 3.0×10^{-3} M cupric chloride and 7 ml of Britton-Robinson buffer solution, adjusted to pH 4.3. Then 1 ml of an aqueous solution of 5.0×10^{-4} M MCP was added and it was extracted with 10 ml chloroform. The mixture was shaken well for 5 minutes. After the upper aqueous layer had been separated off, 5.0 ml of the chloroform layer was transferred into test-tubes, and to this was added 5 ml of methanol. Finally, the copper content of the organic phase was measured by an atomic absorption spectrophotometer against a reagent blank.

8.3.23 Alkylbenzenesulphonate

Matsueda and Morimoto (1980) proposed an indirect method for the determination of alkylbenzenesulphonate (LAS). The method is based on the extraction with MIBK of the ion pairs formed between LAS and thiourea–copper(I) complex. Addition of thiourea to an aqueous medium containing copper(II) results in the formation of various thiourea–copper(I) complexes which are extractable as ion pairs with LAS into MIBK. Therefore, LAS can be determined indirectly by measurement of copper in the organic phase by atomic absorption spectrophotometry. LAS was preseparated from foreign anions by extraction with MIBK in the presence of sodium chloride. The effect of sodium chloride concentration on the extraction of LAS with MIBK, and the effects of the molar ratio of copper(II) to thiourea and the concentration of thiourea–copper(I) complex on the determination of LAS were examined. The recommended procedure is as follows. Place a water sample solution containing not more than 200 μg of LAS in a 120 ml graduated test-tube with 10 ml of the 30% (w/v) sodium chloride solution, and then adjust the volume to 100 ml with water. Add 10 ml of MIBK. Shake for 3 min and allow to stand for 5 min. Pipette a 5 ml aliquot of the MIBK layer into a 15 ml test-tube, containing 5 ml of the thiourea–copper(I)-complex solution (2×10^{-3} M-Cu; 8×10^{-3} M-thiourea), and shake for 3 min. Aspirate the MIBK layer directly to atomic absorption apparatus and measure the absorbance of copper. The linear relationship was observed between the absorbance and the concentration of LAS in the range of 0.01 to 20 μg ml^{-1}.

8.3.24 Biacetyl

Minami *et al.* (1979) proposed an indirect method for the determination of biacetyl by AAS. Biacetyl reacts with hydroxylamine hydrochloride-sodium acetate solution and nickel ion, and the water-insoluble complex which is Ni-dimethylglyoxime is formed. Biacetyl could therefore be determined directly by measuring the amount of nickel in precipitate by atomic absorption spectrophotometry (AAS). The recommended procedure is as follows: the sample solution containing 0.05 to 2.00 mg of biacetyl is mixed with 3 ml of hydroxylamine hydrochloride–sodium acetate solution ($NH_2OH \cdot HCl$ 80.68 mg ml^{-1}, CH_3COONa 40.21 mg ml^{-1}). The mixture is heated in a water bath at 75 °C for 10 min. After cooling, the mixture has added to it 2 ml of nickel solution (Ni^{2+} 6.30 mg ml^{-1}), and is then left to stand for 5 min. After filtration, the precipitate is washed with water, dissolved by adding 2 ml of conc. nitric acid, and diluted to 100 ml with water. The nickel content of the resultant is measured by AAS.

8.3.25 Phenols

Mitsui and Fujimura (1974c) proposed an indirect determination of phenols by AAS. The following compounds were investigated: phenol, *o*-cresol, *m*-cresol, *p*-cresol, *p*-ethylphenol, *o*-isopropylphenol, *o*-sec-butylphenol, 3, 4-xylenol, 3,5-xylenol, *o*-aminophenol, *o*-chlorophenol, *p*-chlorophenol, *p*-hydroxyphenylacetic acid, *o*-hydroxybenzoic acid, propyl-*p*-hydroxybenzoate, *p*-nitrophenol, 1-naphthol, 2-naphthol, and 1-nitroso-2-naphthol. To prepare the sample solutions, the phenol was dissolved in water, and the other phenols in methanol.

The recommended procedures are as follows: methanol was eliminated by evaporator when it was used as the solvent, and 3 ml of water was added (but in phenol, 1 ml of the phenol solution was added to 2 ml of water). To this solution were added 1 ml of 1.73 N acetic acid and 1 ml of 40.64 mg ml^{-1} of sodium cobaltinitrite, and the solution was heated in a water bath for 5 min at 100 °C. After the solution had been cooled, the cobalt complex containing phenols was extracted with 10 ml of MIBK. The extracted solution was centrifuged and was subjected to AAS.

8.3.26 Alkannin

Kovatsis *et al.* (1980a) proposed an indirect method for the determination of alkannin by AAS. The developed method is based on the formation of a Cu-alkannin complex. This complex was washed by ethyl acetate, to remove the unreacted Cu, and ingested by nitric acid. The resulting solution was diluted and filtered. The clear solution aspirated in AAS, which determined the Cu content of the complex on the basis of curves from a standard solution of Cu.

Parameters involved in this method were studied. The alkannin content was determined in the region of 1 to 10 mg. The method is accurate, quick and suitable for routine analysis for a variety of specimens.

8.3.27 Colchicine

Kovatsis *et al.* (1980b) proposed an indirect method for the determination of colchicine in biological samples. Our method is based on the formation of an isonicotinoyl hydrazone derivative of colchicine, which subsequently reacts with copper acetate and at pH 5 forms a copper complex. The formed complex is extracted with amyl alcohol and aspirated then into AAS.

The recommended procedure is as follows. In the first step the extraction of colchicine from biosamples is performed by chloroform, the volume of which must be ten times that of the sample volume. The solvent was centrifuged and evaporated in vacuum and at low temperature in the absence of light.

In the second step, the residue is dissolved in 2 ml of distilled water and then 1.7 ml of solution of anhydrous carbonate (20%) and 80 mg isonicotinohydrazide added. Warm for 10 minutes in a water bath of 100 °C and cool. Adjust the pH at 5 with acetic acid and add 10 ml of copper acetate (1 mg ml^{-1}). After 15 min the formed complex is extracted with amyl alcohol, which was subsequently aspirated into AAS.

8.3.28 1, 2-Diols

The determination of 1, 2-diol by indirect AAS was proposed by Tan *et al.* (1980). According to this work, 1, 2-diols were reacted with an excess of potassium periodate, the remaining periodate was precipitated with excess lead nitrate, and the lead periodate formed was separated from the medium by membrane filtration. The precipitate was then dissolved in 1M-HNO_3 and analysed for the lead content by AAS. The recommended procedure is as follows. To a 15-cm test-tube containing 1.00–2.30 ml of the diol sample in water was added 1.00 ml of 2.00×10^{-2} M-KIO_4; the contents of the tube were mixed well and left standing for 2 to 5 min. The concentration of the diol was 0.40 to 4.00 μmol ml^{-1}. One ml of 4×10^2 M-$Pb(NO_3)_2$ was added to the reaction mixture and the solution was mixed for approximately 30 s to precipitate the lead periodate. This solution must not be left standing for more than 2 min as lead periodate in aqueous solution adsorbs onto the test-tube. The contents of the test-tube were poured into a disposable filtration-unit and suction was applied. The test-tube was rinsed 3 times with approximately 6-ml portions of deionised and distilled water. The filtrate was then decanted through the suction vent under reduced pressure. The filtering and decanting processes were repeated twice with 20 ml of deionised and distilled water. Care must be taken to mix the filtrate each time before decanting to prevent localised concentration of any excess $Pb(NO_3)_2$ reagent. After the last decantation, 10.0 ml of 1M-HNO_3 was redistributed on to the membrane filter and allowed to remain standing for 30 s before suction was applied. This digestion step was repeated twice. The 30 ml of dissolved lead ion was poured out through the disconnected suction vent into a stoppered flask. The sample was then ready for AAS.

8.3.29 Pentachlorophenol

Pentachlorophenol was also determined by indirect AAS by a procedure based on the solvent extraction into nitrophenol of the ion-pair formed between the tris-(1,10 phenanthroline)iron(II) cation and the anion of pentachlorophenol and measuring the iron content in the extracted ion-pair (Yamamoto *et al*., 1967).

8.3.30 Alkaloids

Alkaloids such as strychnine, quinine, emetine, procaine, tetracaine and ephedrine were indirectly determined with good precision by AAS. The recommended procedures are as follows (Minami *et al*., 1981c). To 5 to 20 ml of each sample solution (1.5 to 100 μg ml in 0.1 N-HCl) is added 1 ml of Reinecke salt solution (ammonium tetrathiocyanodiammonochromate 6 mg ml^{-1}). After 5 to 10 ml of nitrobenzene is added, the mixture is shaken for about 2 min and then allowed to stand for 20 min. After the nitrobenzene layer is separated it is dehydrated and the chromium in the nitrobenzene solution measured by AAS.

REFERENCES

Bond, A. M., and O'Donnell, T. A. (1968). *Analyt. Chem.* **40**, 560–3.

Danchik, R. S., and Boltz, D. F. (1970). *Analyt. Chim. Acta* **49**, 567–9.

Christian, G., and Fieldman, F. (1968). *Ibid.* **40**, 173–9.

Christian, G., and Fieldman, F. (1970). In *Atomic Absorption Spectroscopy*. Wiley Interscience, p. 441.

Goleb, J. A. (1966). *Analyt. Chem.* **38**, 1059–61.

Kidani, Y., Takemura, H., and Koike, H. (1973a). *Bunseki Kagaku* **22**, 187–91.

Kidani, Y., Takemura, H., and Koike, H. (1973b). *Ibid.* **22**, 604–6.

Kidani, Y., Inagaki, K., Osugi, N., and Koike, H. (1973c). *Ibid.* **22**, 892–5.

Kidani, Y., Inagaki, K., Saotome, T., and Koike, H. (1973d). *Ibid.* **22**, 896–9.

Kidani, Y., Takemura, H., and Koike, H. (1974a). *Ibid.* **23**, 212–14.

Kidani, Y., Saotome, T., Kato, M., and Koike, H. (1974b). *Ibid.* **23**, 265–9.

Kidani, Y., Uno, S., Kato, Y., and Koike, H. (1974c). *Ibid.* **23**, 740–4.

Kidani, Y., Osugi, N., Inagaki, K., and Koike, H. (1975a). *Ibid.* **24**, 218–21.

Kidani, Y., Saotome, T., Inagaki, K., and Koike, H. (1975b). *Ibid.* **24**, 463–5.

Kidani, Y., and Ito, E. (1976a). *Ibid.* **25**, 57–60.

Kidani, Y., Nakamura, K., and Inagaki, K. (1976b). *Ibid.* **25**, 509–513.

Kidani, Y., Uno, S., and Inagaki, K. (1976c). *Ibid.* **25**, 514–18.

Kidani, Y., and Ito, E. (1980). In Kovatsis, A. (ed.), *Toxicological Aspects*. Technika, Thessaloniki, p. 55–70.

Kneebone, B. M., and Freiser, H. (1975). *Analyt. Chem.* **47**, 942–4.

Kovatsis, A. (1978a). In Heyndrickx, A. (ed.), *Human Toxicology*. European Press, Ghent, pp. 47–61.

Kovatsis, A. (1978b). *At. Absorpt. Newsl.* **17**, 104–6.

Kovatsis, A., and Tsougas, M. (1976). *Bull. Envir. Contam. Tox.* **15**, 412–20.

Kovatsis, A., and Tsougas, M. (1978). *Arzneim. Forsch.* **28(I)**, 248–50.

Kovatsis, A., and Tsougas, M. (1979). *Vet. Human Tox.* **21**, 190–3.

Kovatsis, A., Papageorgiou, V., and Christianopoulou, M. (1980a). In Kovatsis, A. (ed.) *Toxicological Aspects*. Technika, Thessaloniki, pp. 43–54.
Kovatsis, A., Christianopoulou, M., and Papageorgiou, V. (1980b). *Ibid*., pp. 220–30.
Kumamaru, T., Hayasashi, Y., Okamoto, N., Tao, E., and Yamamoto, Y. (1966). *Analyt. Chim. Acta* **35**, 524–5.
Matsueda, T., and Morimoto, M. (1980). *Bunseki Kagaku* **29**, 769–73.
Menache, R. (1974). *Clin. Chem.* **20**, 1444–5.
Minami, Y., Mitsui, T., and Fujimura, Y. (1979). *Bunseki Kagaku* **28**, 717–20.
Minami, Y., Mitsui, T., and Fujimura, Y. (1980). *Ibid.* **29**, 491–4.
Minami, Y., Mitsui, T., and Fujimura, Y. (1981a). *Ibid.* **30**, 475–7.
Minami, Y., Mitsui, T., and Fujimura, Y. (1981b). *Ibid.* **30**, 566–8.
Minami, Y., Mitsui, T., and Fujimura, Y. (1981c). *Ibid.* **30**, 811–3.
Minamikawa, T., Sakai, K., Hashitani, N., Fukushima, E., and Yamagishi, N. (1973). *Chem. Pharm. Bull.* **21**, 1632–40.
Mitsui, T., and Fujimura, Y. (1974a). *Bunseki Kagaku* **23**, 3–6.
Mitsui, T., and Fujimura, Y. (1974b). *Ibid.* **23**, 449–53.
Mitsui, T., and Fujimura, Y. (1974c). *Ibid.* **23**, 1303–8.
Mitsui, T., and Fujimura, Y. (1974d). *Ibid.* **23**, 1309–14.
Mitsui, T., and Fujimura, Y. (1974e). *Nippon Kagaku Kaishi* **10**, 1908–11.
Mitsui, T., Fujimura, Y., and Suzuki, T. (1975). *Bunseki Kagaku* **24**, 244–7.
Mitsui, T., and Fujimura, Y. (1975). *Ibid.* **24**, 575–8.
Mitsui, T., and Fujimura, Y. (1976). *Ibid.* **25**, 429–35.
Newberry, C. L., and Christian, G. D. (1965). *J. Assn Offic. Agr. Chemists* **48**, 332–7.
Nomura, T., and Karasawa, I. (1981). *Analyt. Chim. Acta* **126**, 241–5.
Roe, D. A., Miller, P. S., and Lutwak, L. (1966). *Analyt. Biochem.* **15**, 313–22.
Sheridan, J., Lau, E. P., and Senkowski, B. Z. (1966). *2nd Middle Atlantic Regional Meeting of the ACS*, New York, Fed. 6–7.
Tan, B., Melius, P., and Kilgore, M. (1980). *Analyt. Chem.* **52**, 602–4.
Westerlund-Helmerson, U. (1966). *At. Absorpt. Newsl.* **5**, 97.
Yamamoto, Y., Kumamaru, T., and Hayashi, Y. (1968). *Talanta* **14**, 611–5.

9

Capillary column gas chromatography and its application in toxicology*

B. S. THOMAS and E. BAILEY

9.1 INTRODUCTION

The prediction that capillary columns will totally replace conventional packed columns in toxicological investigations by gas chromatography (GC) is already more than half fulfilled (Van Boven and Sunshine, 1979). The importance of GC as an analytical tool has been re-emphasised by the now widespread use of capillary columns, particularly in multi-component analyses and trace-level determinations of selected compounds in complex biological and environmental samples. For example, in the Italian Seveso incident such a method was necessary to identify a highly toxic chloro-dioxin compound, TCDD, in tissue of dead animals from the contaminated area (Frigerio, 1978).

Probably the oldest adage in GC is that 'a chromatographic peak only represents what a substance is not.' Certainly at one time, this remark had an element of truth in it, especially when applied to separations from biological material (e.g. blood, urine) and when almost all analyses were performed with packed columns, which have a limited separating efficiency. Often the unsuspecting analyst could be misled by such 'favourable' factors as perfect peak symmetry and the same retention times as standard compounds. The use of mixed stationary-phase GC columns (and each individual analyst had their own special mixtures) would often separate peak contaminants which single phases would not resolve (Thomas, 1965). The use of GC combined with mass spectrometry (MS) would indicate the homogeneity or heterogeneity of such peaks, but such a combination was by no means universally available. Capillary columns of high separating efficiency were introduced twenty-five years ago by Desty *et al.* (1958) and Golay (1958) but it is not until comparatively recently that they have been universally adopted. It is now the considered opinion of the present authors that, except for prepara-

*For a glossary of terms and abbreviations used in this Chapter, see p. 256.

tive work, and for analysis of simple mixtures, capillary columns will replace packed columns for most GC applications.

A detailed account of the theory of GC is too well documented to warrant inclusion in this chapter, and it is presumed that the reader has a certain familiarity with the process. However, in order to obtain optimum performance with capillary columns the analyst must have an understanding of the basic principles, together with an acquaintance with some of the pitfalls, and how to avoid them during the analytical process (e.g. see Bremner, 1967; Jennings, 1978).

9.2 ADVANTAGES OF CAPILLARY COLUMNS

The obvious advantage in the use of capillary columns over conventional packed columns is their much greater separating efficiency. By this is meant the narrowness of the emergent peaks in relation to the start or injection point on the chromatogram (i.e. the recorder chart tracing). The efficiency of a particular column is expressed as the plate number, which is similar to that used for characterising the efficiency of the distillation column and is calculated from the following equation:

$$n = 16(t_r/w)^2$$

where n is the number of theoretical plates, t_r is the retention time of a particular substance and w is the width of the base of the peak. A more realistic assessment of plate measurement is to take into consideration the gas hold-up value, t_m, or retention time required for the injection air peak to pass through the column. This is termed the effective theoretical place value N. Some workers use the t_r of methane as an indicator of this value, which is subtracted from the t_r in the efficiency equation. It is considered more accurate to take w as the width of the peak at half-height × 2 with packed columns, but owing to the narrowness of the peak with a capillary column it is easier to revert to base measurement. The value of n is proportional to the column length and it is also affected by the nature of the test compound, column temperature and type of carrier gas. Because of their low density, hydrogen and helium are each particularly recommended for use with capillary columns. However, for gas chromatography and mass spectromety in combination (GC–MS), helium is essential.

A more detailed account of the parameters for measurement of column behaviour is given by Jennings (1978). A typical 2-m-long packed column may attain an n value of 3000 to 4000 theoretical plates whereas a capillary column with an average length of 25 m should have an efficiency of 50 000 to 150 000 theoretical plates.

Since the peaks in capillary chromatography are very sharp and symmetrical, small concentrations of solutes can be resolved and measured. This gives capillary columns an effective five- to tenfold increase in sensitivity over packed columns. The chromatograms illustrated in Figure 9.1a and b demonstrate the differences in both efficiency and sensitivity between a capillary column and a packed column. Another advantage to be gained by using a capillary column is that elution times are shorter, which gives rise to a much faster speed of analysis at a given temperature.

9.3 TYPES OF CAPILLARY COLUMN

The term capillary column is used to describe any narrow-bore GC column. By narrow bore is meant an internal diameter of less than 1 mm, whereas the internal diameter of a conventional packed column is usually 2 to 4 mm. The different types of capillary columns are illustrated in cross-section in Figure 9.2. They can be divided into two main types: micropacked and open tubular columns. Micropacked columns have internal diameters ranging from 0.5 to 1 mm and can be considered as miniaturised versions of ordinary packed columns. They have a high sample-loading capacity and can give relatively high separating efficiencies, but they are difficult to prepare. Also, they have a low specific permeability to the carrier gas, which limits the practical length of the column to a maximum of about 10 m. Their main application has been in the analyses of gases and low-boiling-point compounds.

Open tubular columns have an open diameter and therefore the carrier gas is less restricted, allowing very long lengths of columns to be used. There are two main types of open tubular columns:

1. wall-coated open tubular (WCOT);
2. support-coated open tubular (SCOT) and porous-layer open tubular (PLOT).

9.3.1 WCOT columns

This is now the most frequently used type of capillary column and has the highest plate efficiency. The columns contain no packing or support material and the stationary phase is either coated by adhesion or chemically bonded (cross-linked) as a thin film on the inner wall of the tubing. They are usually made from either glass or fused silica and they have an inside diameter of 0.1 to 0.5 mm. WCOT columns made from stainless steel or nickel have also been used, but they have never been successful in biological work because of problems caused by adsorption and catalytic decomposition. Although many analyses can be carried out successfully on short WCOT capillaries 10 m long or even less, generally columns of 20 to 25 m are used for most separations. However for analysis of very complex mixtures such as cigarette smoke, which contain many hundreds of volatile components, it may be necessary to use columns up to 100 m long (Grob, 1978).

The efficiency of the column is also dependent on its internal diameter. A wide-bore WCOT column (0.5 mm i.d.) is less efficient than a narrow-bore

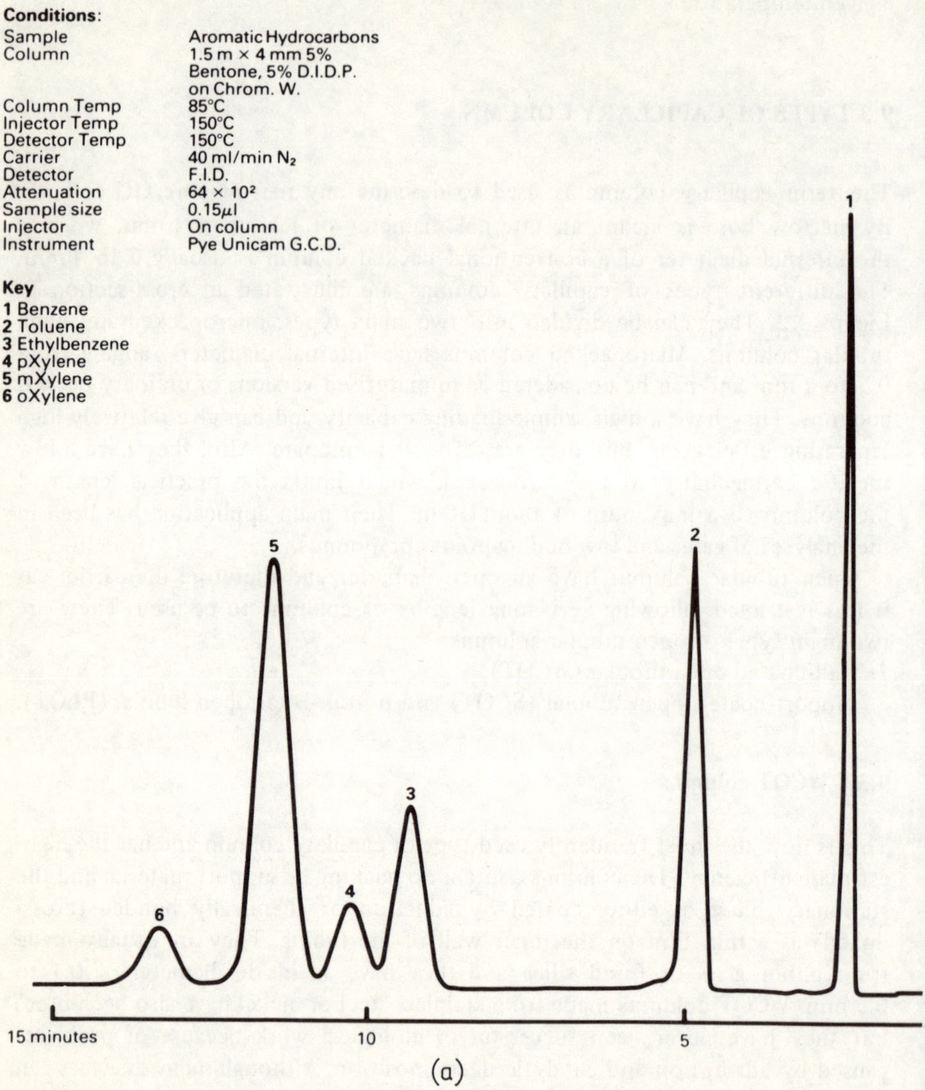

Figure 9.1 Comparison of packed (a) and capillary (b) column separations. Reproduced by kind permission of Pye Unicam.

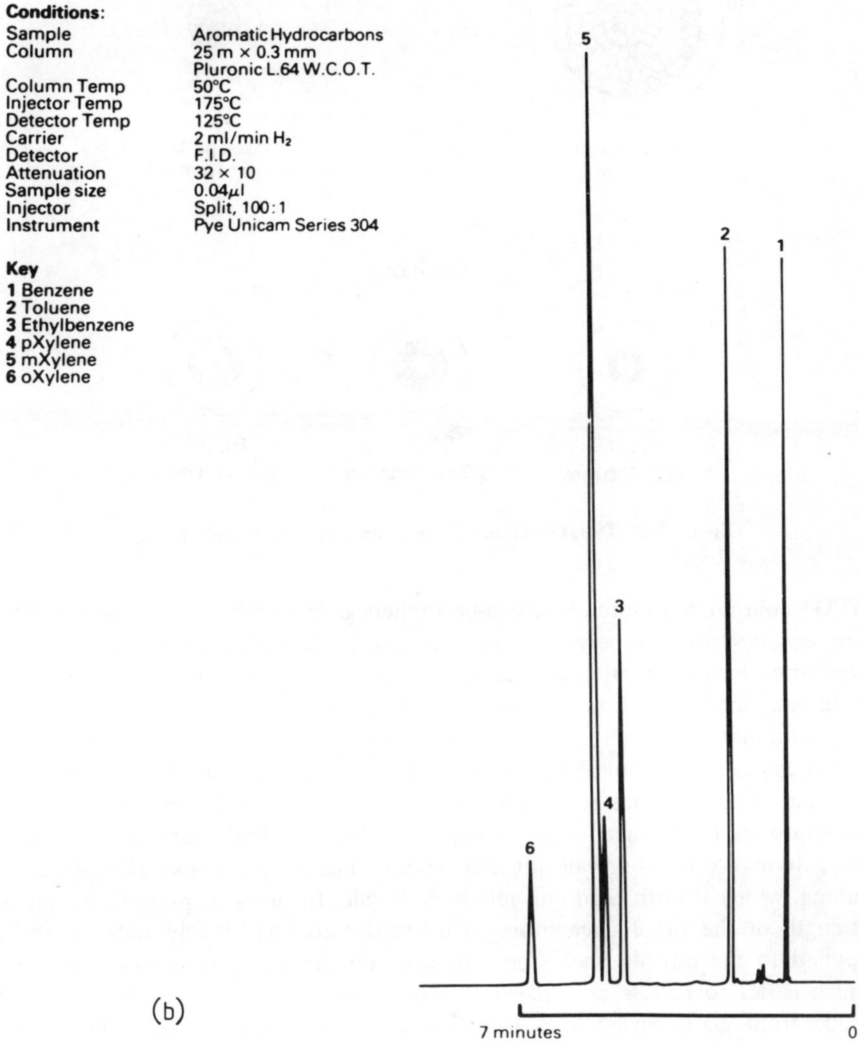

Figure 9.1 (continued)

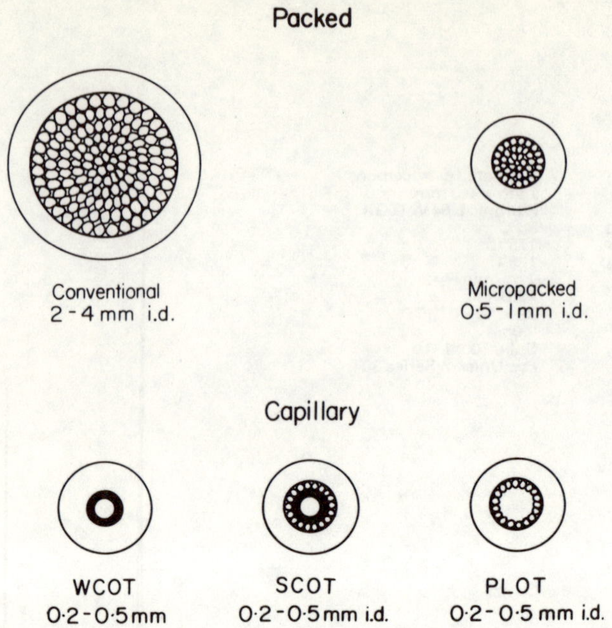

Figure 9.2 Types of capillary columns as shown in cross-section.

WCOT column, but more phase can be applied, giving it a higher sample capacity. The best compromise between efficiency and loading capacity is obtained with capillaries having an internal diameter ranging from 0.2 mm to 0.3 mm. The optimum carrier-gas flow-rate for this dimension of WCOT column is about 1 to 3 ml min^{-1}.

Fused-silica open tubular columns were first introduced in 1979 as a result of research in fibre-optics technology at the Hewlett-Packard Corporate Research Laboratories (Dandeneau and Zerenner, 1979). Capillaries drawn from fused silica have a very thin wall and are flexible and strong, unlike glass capillary tubing, which is both rigid and relatively fragile. In order to preserve the initial strength of the fused-silica tubing a protective coating of polyimide has to be applied to the outside wall. Capillary columns fabricated from fused silica are much easier to handle and install in the GC oven than are capillary columns made from glass. Fused silica is also a more inert material and although the columns still have to be deactivated before coating with stationary phase, less treatment of the wall surface is required to produce an inactive column.

Nonpolar polysiloxanes such as SE-30, OV-1 and SE-52 are the most extensively used phases with WCOT columns. They will spontaneously coat on the surface of glass and fused silica to give a stable, uniform film of phase, which is essential for producing columns of high separating efficiency. Capillary columns coated with these nonselective phases can invariably be operated at temperatures in excess of 300 °C without damage to the column. WCOT columns coated with polar phases are more difficult to prepare because of the poor wettability of the wall surface. Polar capillary columns are generally less efficient and do not have the same degree of thermal stability. In order to prepare polar WCOT columns, the wall surface has to be roughened either by etching or by deposition of particles of, e.g., NaCl or $BaCO_3$, or alternatively the surface must be chemically modified to improve its wettability.

9.3.2 SCOT columns

A capillary column of this type is typically made from glass and has an internal diameter of about 0.5 mm. It differs from a WCOT column in having a layer of solid support-particles, usually of a diatomacious earth, adhered to the inner wall, thereby increasing its surface area. This allows a thicker film of stationary phase to be applied and therefore the sample loading capacity is larger than with narrow-bore WCOT columns. The column is generally prepared in one step, the stationary-phase coating solution containing the support material as a suspension. SCOT columns will accept virtually any stationary phase, unlike WCOT columns which are more limited in this respect. Their plate efficiency, while lower than WCOT columns, is still considerably higher than those of packed columns. A separation of a standard mixture of derivatised amino acids on a 40-m glass SCOT column is shown in Figure 9.3.

9.3.3 PLOT columns

These have similar dimensions to SCOT columns but their inner wall is coated with a very porous layer of material, often aluminium oxide. PLOT columns are often used in gas–solid chromatography for, e.g., the analysis of low-molecular-weight hydrocarbons.

9.4 INSTALLATION OF CAPILLARY COLUMNS

Most modern gas chromatographs are designed for use with capillary columns. The capillary is usually suspended in the GC oven by a suitable bracket. The ends of glass capillaries have to be straightened and moulded into shape with a microflame or with a mechanical end-straightening device so that the ends approximately match the injector outlet and detector inlet. Fused-silica columns are inherently straight and therefore do not require this treatment. The most important factor when installing the columns is to ensure that there is no unswept dead volume in the system. Ideally the end of the column should be located inside the detector beyond the hydrogen inlet of the FID or the scavenger inlet of the ECD. If this is not possible, a make-up T-piece must be used and an

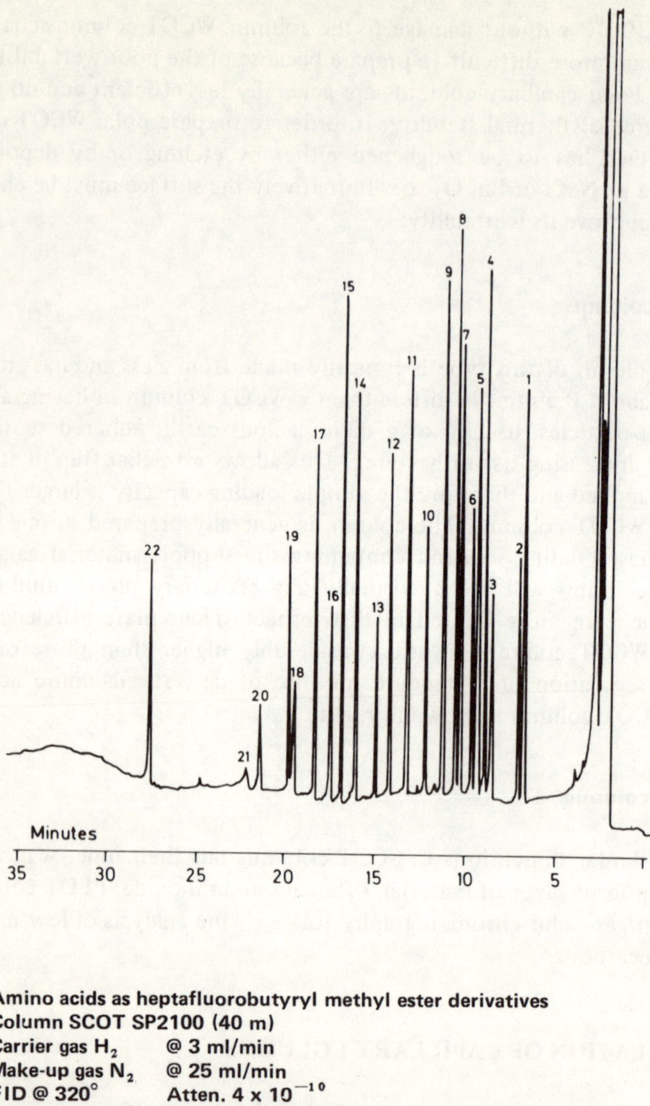

Amino acids as heptafluorobutyryl methyl ester derivatives
Column SCOT SP2100 (40 m)
Carrier gas H_2 @ 3 ml/min
Make-up gas N_2 @ 25 ml/min
FID @ 320° Atten. 4×10^{-10}
Injector @ 220°. Temp. Prog. 100° (2 min) → 8°/min
Amount – approx. 500 p mol of each

1) Alanine
2) Glycine
3) β-Alanine
4) Valine
5) Threonine
6) Serine
7) Leucine
8) iso-Leucine
9) Nor-Leucine
10) Proline
11) Homo-serine
12) OH-Proline
13) Methione
14) Asparagine
15) Phenylalanine
16) Ornithine
17) Glutamine
18) Lysine
19) Tyrosine
20) Arginine
21) Histidine
22) Cystine

Figure 9.3 Gas chromatogram (FID) of a standard mixture of amino acids. Reproduced by kind permission of the editor of the *Journal of High Resolution Chromatography and Chromatography Communications* (Thomas, 1980).

additional flow of carrier gas added to flush the effluent from the column quickly into the detector.

Wide-bore WCOT and SCOT columns are often the easiest types to use for those new to high-resolution GC. Since the carrier gas flows are higher than with narrow-bore WCOT columns, connections and injection techniques are less critical. An injector–detector connection system suitable for use with these columns, as used by one of the authors (B.S.T.) with a Pye gas chromatograph, is illustrated in Figure 9.4. Care must be taken to ensure correct coupling to the make-up T-

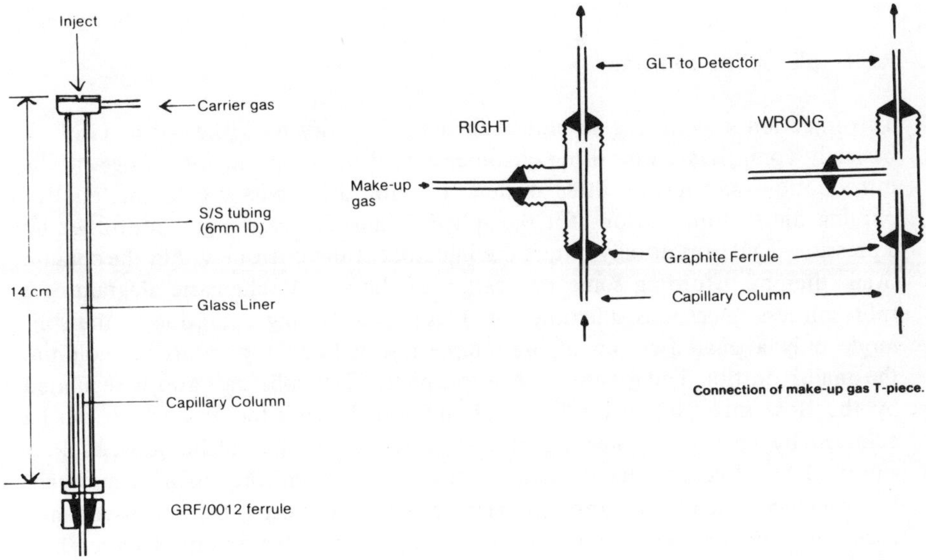

Figure 9.4 Method of connecting a wide-bore glass capillary column to the injector and to the FID. Reproduced by kind permission of the editor of the *Journal of High Resolution Chromatography and Chromatography Communications* (Thomas, 1980).

piece to avoid eddy currents which would reduce peak efficiency. Both the glass injection lines and the glass-lined, stainless-steel detector connection should be deactivated by treatment with a silanising agent before installation. An efficiency of 75 000 theoretical plates from a 40-m wide-bore WCOT column used for urinary steroid analysis has been obtained with this system (Thomas, 1980).

9.5 INJECTION SYSTEMS

In an ideal situation the analytical sample should vaporise completely into the carrier gas stream without decomposition, so that it enters the column as a homogeneous plug of vapour ready for its chromatographic journey. Special sampling techniques are required for narrow-bore capillary columns because of the low carrier-gas flows used and the need to introduce sample loads normally in the range 1 to 100 ng per component. Moreover, the sampling technique and the sampling parameters must be selected according to the type of sample (i.e. range of concentrations, thermal stability and volatilities of the components). There are essentially two basic methods of sample introduction: the split–splitless and solid-injection systems, where the sample is vaporised before it enters the column, and the nonvaporising systems, where the cold sample is introduced directly into the column.

9.5.1 Split–splitless injector

This injection system was developed in the late 1960s by Professor K. Grob. It basically comprises a vaporising chamber closed by a septum for syringe-needle introduction, and having three outlets, one for the capillary columns, one for purging the septum and one for the splitting line. The carrier gas, controlled by a pressure regulator, usually enters the injectors at the bottom within the column oven, thereby affording some preheating of the gas. A schematic diagram of a split–splitless injector is illustrated in Figure 9.5. During operation in the split mode only a small fraction of the sample injected actually enters the column, the major portion being vented to atmosphere. The splitting ratio is regulated by the flow through the capillary column and the splitting line, which can be adjusted by means of a needle valve. Typical split ratios can be between 1 : 5 and 1 : 1000. Because the flow rates through the vaporising chamber are high, the residence time of the sample in the injector is very short and as a consequence peak-band broadening does not occur to any appreciable extent. This method of injection is simple and easy to use, but it does suffer from two significant limitations. First, since a large proportion of the injection sample is discarded, the method is not suitable for trace analysis. Second, sample-component discrimination can occur with wide-range boiling-point mixtures, which can affect quantitation. This latter limitation can, however, often be overcome by the use of suitable internal standards added to the sample before the GC analysis.

When the injector is operated in the splitless mode the whole of the injected sample is allowed to enter the column. This is achieved by closing the split line during the injection and keeping the oven temperature 20 to 30 K below the boiling point of the solvent used. The less-volatile sample components with the solvent then condense on the first few turns of the capillary column. In order to avoid a tailing solvent peak, caused by residual vapour in the injector, the split line is opened after a suitable time (typically 30 to 60 s). The column temperature is then increased to start the chromatography analysis. The splitless mode of sample introduction is useful for dilute samples, and discrimination against high-boiling-point compounds is less likely to be observed than with the split injection.

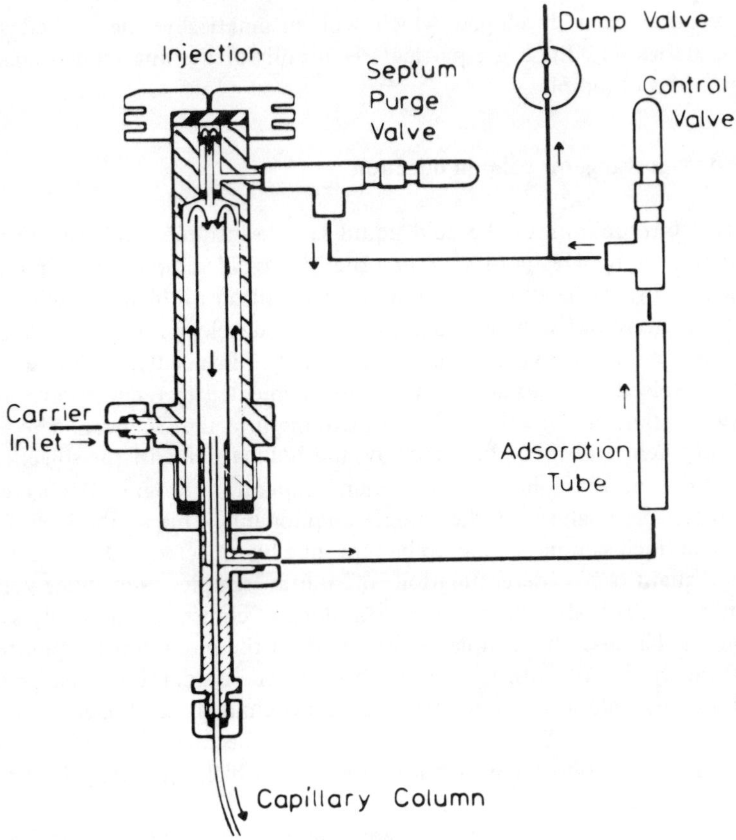

Figure 9.5 Schematic diagram of a split–splitless capillary column injector. By kind permission of SGE Ltd.

9.5.2 Solid injection

This method is suitable for high-boiling-point liquids and solids and has been successfully employed for biomedical applications such as steroids, fatty acids and drug estimations. By eliminating solvent from the column it overcomes some of the problems associated with liquid sampling. The best-known injector of this type was developed by Van den Berg and Cox (1972). It consists principally of a moving glass needle onto the tip of which the liquid sample is deposited from a microlitre syringe. The solvent is evaporated off the needle by a flow of carrier gas passing through and out of the top of the injector. The dried sample on the needle is lowered by a magnet into a vaporising inlet and the sample components then swept into the column by the carrier gas. Solid injectors have also been developed which will automatically inject dried samples into capillaries and these are particularly useful for the unattended analysis of large numbers of samples.

9.5.3 Nonvaporising, on-column injection

The direct introduction of the cold liquid sample into the capillary column was first advocated by Desty (1965) in order to avoid sample transfer onto the column and overcome discrimination and adsorption problems in the sampling insert. The nonvaporising, on-column injector developed by Grob and Grob (1978) uses a special microsyringe with a long thin needle, which allows the sample, dissolved in a suitable solvent, to be injected through a valve into the first few centimetres of the column protruding into the GC oven. The column is normally held at a temperature below the boiling point of the solvent during the injection and the column oven is then temperature-programmed as required to complete the analysis of the sample components. This method of sampling enables a defined sample volume to be reproducibly injected and is ideally suited for the quantitative determination of dilute samples and wide-volatility-range mixtures. It is also the injection technique of choice for thermally sensitive compounds, because the sample is subjected to the minimum temperature for the GC analysis. As with splitless sampling, on-column injection is usually limited to a sample size no greater than approximately 2 μl, otherwise a relatively large portion of the inlet end of the column becomes flooded by solution. This can result in solute-maldistribution effects, which ultimately lead to poor separating efficiencies and/or splitting of peaks.

A number of on-column injectors are commercially available. The one developed by SGE Ltd. is illustrated in Figure 9.6. This employs a seal, operated by pneumatic ram, which is opened as the syringe is inserted and then closed around the needle so that the system is pressurised, resulting in continual gas flow through the column during injection. The injector is cooled by the flow from a gas or air supply, which prevents evaporation of the sample from the syringe needle during the injection. It will accept both glass and fused-silica columns with inside diameters down to 0.2 mm and can be fitted to most GC instruments.

A new general-purpose sample-injection system based on the principle of cold injection by syringe into a small vaporising chamber, followed by temperature-programme vaporisation from the injection chamber, has been developed by Poy *et al.* (1981).

9.6 CHOICE OF STATIONARY PHASE

A glance through a modern catalogue of commercially available stationary phases is bewildering, but owing to the very high efficiencies of capillary columns

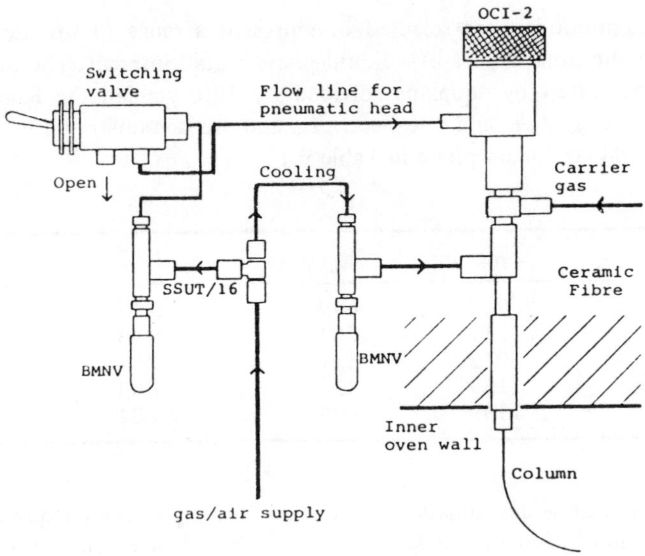

Figure 9.6 Schematic diagram of a septumless, nonvaporising on-column injector. By kind permission of SGE Ltd.

most separation problems can be solved using only one or two selected phases. However, choice of stationary phase can be scientifically exploited to resolve compounds according to their molecular size, weight and structure and the presence of functional groups (e.g. hydroxyl, carbonyl, amino etc.) by use of the Rohrschneider concept of plarity (Rohrschneider, 1966). It must be emphasised that no polarity index can take account of unknown substances that may be present in the analytical sample; this is particularly so with biological materials.

9.6.1 Rohrschneider index

If a solute were dissolved in a completely nonpolar solvent it would be affected only by nonpolar forces. Squalane (C30 H62), a highly branched nonpolar phase, was selected as the standard, and Kovats indices (Kovats, 1958) were used to describe solute retentions. Thus, a substance with a functional group X will exhibit its lowest polarity (i.e. lowest t_r or I) in squalane. If a phase contains polar forces (e.g. induction, charge transfer, molecular orientation or hydrogen bonding) these will interact with X, causing an increase in t_r. This difference in retention behaviour, which is a measure of the increased polarity of the second liquid phase over that of the first (i.e. squalane), is termed I and is expressed as follows:

$$I = I_{\text{polar phase}} - I_{\text{squalane}}.$$

Five test compounds were selected to represent a range of functional groups with which the polar forces of a liquid phase would interact. The increase in I over that exhibited by squalane, divided by 100, yielded the Rohrschneider constants of x, y, z, u and s respectively, and are demonstrated by the use of Carbowax 20M stationary phase in Table 9.1.

Table 9.1

Compound	I_{20M}	$I_{squalane}$	$I/100$	Constant
benzene	967	649	3.18	x
ethanol	917	384	5.33	y
butanone-2	912	531	3.81	z
nitromethane	1159	457	7.02	u
pyridine	1199	695	5.04	s

Thus the Rohrschneider constants x, y, z, u and s give both a qualitative and quantitative indication of the selectivity of a liquid phase (e.g. a high x-value indicating greater retentivity of double-bonded compounds, y-alcohols, z-carbonyl etc.).

Today it is common practice to refer to McReynolds constants (McReynolds, 1970) when describing the properties of a stationary phase. The McReynolds theory is identical to that of Rohrschneider but the number of reference compounds has been extended to 10, while from the original five only benzene and pyridine have been retained. In fact, neither will determine the best stationary phase for separation of compounds with similar separation characteristics, and it is often necessary to resort to trial and error. A test mixture specially composed for the testing of capillary columns, within the Rohrschneider context, has been suggested by Grob *et al.* (1978). This rigorously tests for presence of adsorption sites, including assessment of the acid–base characteristics of the column.

9.7 CHARACTERISATION OF SUBSTANCES BY GC (RETENTION INDICES)

The most common method of characterisation of unknown substances by GC is by their relative retention time, $t_{r,rel}$. By this is meant the time at which a peak is eluted in comparison with that of a standard compound of known structure and composition. This is not a satisfactory system, as standardised operating conditions cannot be accurately reproduced from one laboratory to another. Therefore other ways have been advocated for standardisation of gas-chromatography data of which the Kovats index (Kovats, 1958) is probably the best known. For capillary-column work, where temperature programming is often used, the methylene-unit (m.u.) system (Horning, 1968) is ideal for characterisation of high-molecular-weight compounds. This is based on the linear time interval between adjacent unbranched saturated hydrocarbons on a defined stationary phase. For example, if the interval between the retention times of, say, a C_{27} and a C_{28} hydrocarbon is divided into 100 units, then an unknown peak emerging somewhere between the two would be recognised as having an m.u. of 27 plus the number of linear units between the two known compounds divided by 100 and so on. Paraffin wax can be used as a suitable reference standard-hydrocarbon mixture for determining the m.u. values (Figure 9.7). It is of course necessary to spike the paraffin wax with at least one known

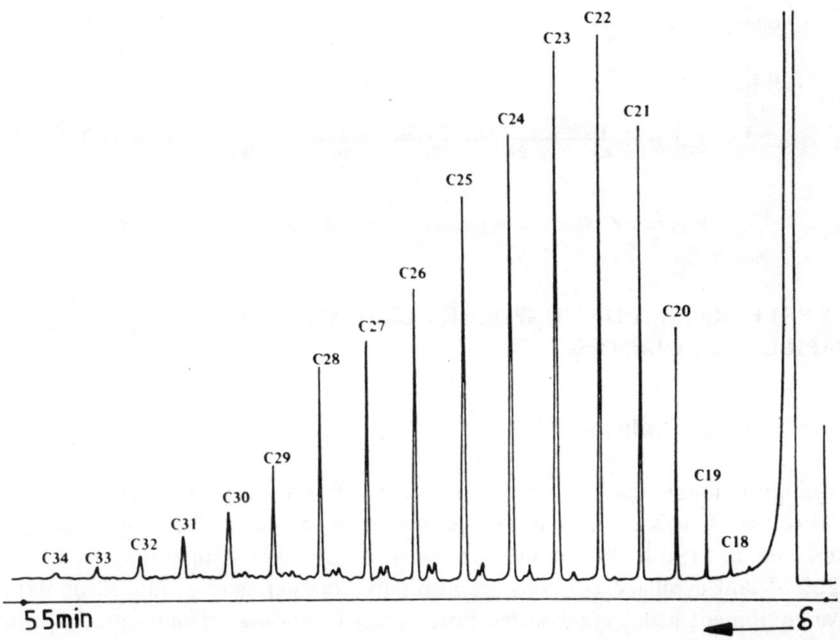

Figure 9.7 Gas chromatogram (FID) of paraffin wax. Conditions: 40-m SCOT SP2100 glass capillary programmed at 2 K min^{-1}, 190 to 300 °C. Reproduced by kind permission of the editor of the *Journal of High Resolution Chromatography and Chromatography Communications* (Thomas, 1980).

hydrocarbon for easy identification. A plot of the linear relationship of the m.u. value plotted against the relative retention time of the straight chain hydrocarbon peaks is shown in Figure 9.8. The advantage of this system is that it is reproducible from one laboratory to another.

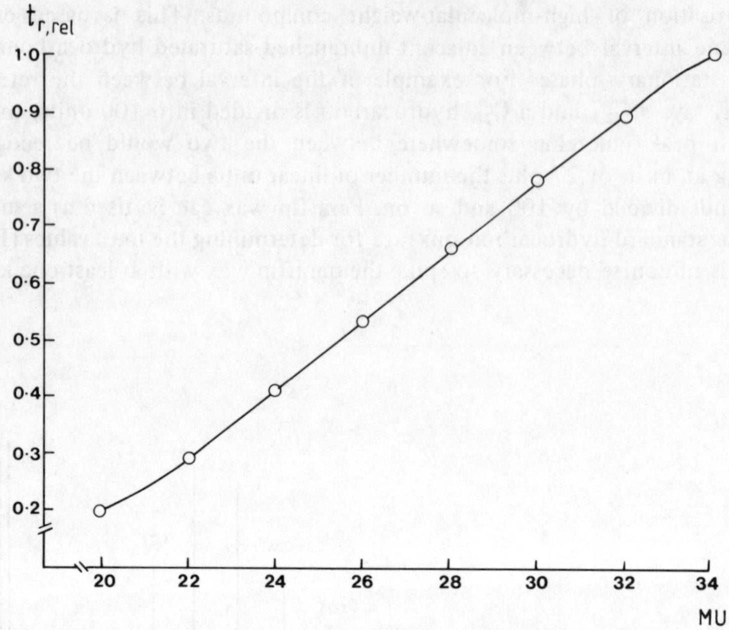

Figure 9.8 Graphic presentation of m.u. values from Figure 9.7.

9.8 PREPARATION OF NONPOLAR GLASS AND FUSED-SILICA CAPILLARY COLUMNS

9.8.1 Drawing of columns

Capillary columns made from soda or Pyrex glass are drawn at temperatures of 600 to 900 °C using relatively simple machinery based on the original design of Desty *et al.* (1960). Fused silica, however, requires a temperature of 2100 to 2200 °C and capillary columns are normally commercially produced on expensive equipment utilising advanced fibre-optics technology. The necessary protective polyimide coating, as previously mentioned, is applied to the outside directly the drawn column leaves the furnace.

9.8.2 Pre-coating treatment of columns

Activity in glass columns that can cause adsorption and peak tailing is due partly to the presence of metallic oxides acting as Lewis acid sites, and these must first be removed by leaching with acid as in the procedure described by Grob and Grob (1979). Fused-silica columns, which contain less than 1 p.p.m. metal oxides, do not require this treatment.

The activity associated with the presence of silanol groups and siloxane bridges is, however, common to both glass and fused silica, although much less so in the latter. High-temperature silylation using a mixture of hexamethyldisilazane and diphenyltetramethyldisilazane (Grob *et al.*, 1979), or octamethylcyclotetrasiloxane (Stark *et al.*, 1980), can be used to effect deactivation of the silanol groups.

Capillary columns deactivated by the above procedures can be coated with a nonpolar silicone gum phase (e.g. SE-30, OV-1, SE-52, SE-54) to give columns of high resolution, thermal stability and inertness. These phases can also be immobilised on the capillary surface by cross-linking *in situ* using dicumyl peroxide as a free-radical initiator. In the production of these so-called cross-linked columns, the peroxide is simply added to the coating solution, and the filled column is sealed and maintained at the requisite reaction temperature prior to conditioning. This cross-linking process increases both the thermal stability and durability of the column. It also renders the coated phase resistant to most solvents as well as allowing a much greater liquid-loading capacity.

9.8.3 Column coating and immobilisation

Column coating is generally performed by the static method originally introduced by Bouche and Verzele (1968). This method has the advantage of producing reliable columns with an accurately predetermined film thickness. A solution of stationary phase (0.02 to 4.0% in pentane) is selected to give a required film-thickness according to the following equation:

$$\text{film thickness } (\mu\text{m}) = \frac{\text{column i.d. (mm)} \times \text{stationary-phase conc. (\%)}}{0.4}$$

The peroxide is then added to the coating solution in an amount dependent on the type and concentration of the dissolved phase (Grob and Grob, 1982; Wright *et al.*, 1982).

The apparatus used by one author (E.B.) for the static coating is shown in Figure 9.9. The capillary column is filled from a reservoir using nitrogen pressure. A short length of solvent-resistant silicone-rubber tubing is fitted to the outlet end of the column, and when the solution emerges the tubing is closed with a clamp. The column, now sealed at one end, is placed in the thermostatically controlled cabinet or water bath (40 °C) and the solvent evacuated from the open end under reduced pressure, which for a 25-m column can take up to 12 h. Nitrogen is then passed through the open column at 50 °C for several minutes. It is then resealed at both ends and heated at 175 °C for 1 h. Finally the column is washed through with several column volumes of methylene chloride and conditioned overnight by slow programming to 300 to 320 °C using a carrier gas flow of 2 ml min^{-1}.

Recently, advances have been made in overcoming problems associated with

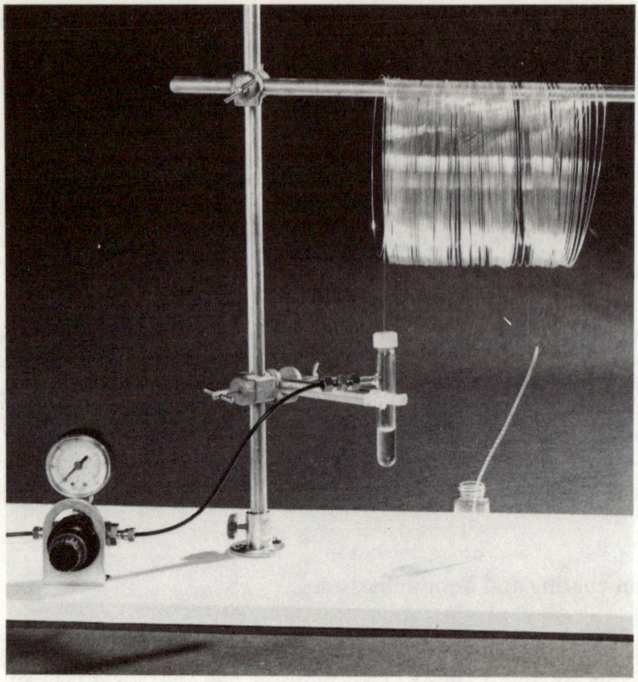

Figure 9.9 Apparatus for coating a capillary column. Shown are a pressure regulator, coating reservoir, column and supporting rod and container for collection of excess coating solution. The silicone-rubber tubing is closed with a Spencer-Wells clamp before the column is evacuated.

the preparation of capillaries coated with immobilised moderately polar and phases, and the reader is referred to the relevant papers presented at a recent meeting on capillary chromatography at Riva del Garde, Italy (Verzele *et al.*, 1983; Blomberg *et al.*, 1983; Richter *et al.*, 1983; Markides *et al.*, 1983).

9.9 CARE OF CAPILLARY COLUMNS

First priority in the care of capillary columns is inclusion of both O_2 and H_2O traps in the carrier-gas line prior to its entry into the gas chromatograph. Very convenient purification cartridges constructed in heavy Perspex, which may be changed without having to turn off the gas pressure, are available from commercial sources. These also contain indicators that change colour when the cartridge contents are exhausted.

A column must not be used for prolonged periods at or near its maximum operating temperature. It is far better to operate it 15 to 20 K below this and extend the analytical time instead. Above 350 °C the polyimide coating on fused silica columns undergoes oxidation, which renders the column too brittle for further use.

After extended use loss of column efficiency may occur, usually owing to a build-up of contaminants in the injector end. Droplet formation due to stationary phase condensation may also affect the column performance, but this problem is not encountered with immobilised-phase columns. Column efficiency can often be restored by removal of one or two coils from the inlet end of the column, but there are limits to the number of times this can be done. The problem can be avoided by connecting a length of uncoated deactivated glass or fused silica tubing from the injector to the column using a zero-dead-volume connector. This does not affect column performance and by timely renewal can increase the life of a column. Columns coated with immobilised phases can be rinsed with appropriate solvents to remove nonvolatile contaminants.

Samples containing involatile material are not always the hazard to capillary columns one might expect (Grob, 1978). However, most environmental and biological samples require an extraction and often one or more purification steps prior to GC analysis. A derivatisation of the extract may also be necessary.

9.10 DERIVATIVE FORMATION

The object of derivative formation in GC is to provide an altered structure that is more suitable than the original compound for qualitative or quantitative estimation. There are several reasons for using derivatives, but it must be emphasised that their use is not confined to capillary GC, being first introduced, at about the same time as GC itself, as methyl esters for fatty-acid analysis (Cropper and Heywood, 1953). In fact all derivatisation methods for use with packed columns can be used with capillary columns, and sometimes to advantage. For instance, haloalkylsilyl ethers (Eaborn *et al.*, 1969), which are highly sensitive to electron-capture detection (ECD) and have a prolonged retention time on packed columns, can be eluted in less than half the time on capillary columns.

The main reasons for using derivatives may be summarised as follows.

1. The compound may be nonvolatile; for example, bile acids are not amenable to direct separation by GC but the methyl esters (ME) and the methyl ester–trimethylsilyl ether (ME–TMSE) derivatives can be separated by GC.

2. The compound may be thermally unstable. For example, corticosteroids with a 17α, 21-dihydroxy-20-oxo side chain lose their side chain when gas-chromatographed and the compound eluted is a corresponding 17-oxosteroid. If these steroids are to be gas-chromatographed in their intact form then suitable derivatives which stabilise the labile side-chain must be used. The methyloxime–trimethylsilyl ether (MO–TMSE) derivatives can be used for this purpose.

3. Compounds containing polar functional groups are susceptible to irrevers-

ible adsorption because of their interaction with active sites on the column. If the column wall is suitably inactivated, and the film of stationary phase on the column wall is uniform, this adsorption phenomenon may often be reduced to low levels. However, for quantitative analyses at the ng or sub-ng level it is often necessary to prepare less polar, more volatile derivatives.

4. Derivative formation may be necessary to provide a satisfactory separation for both qualitative or quantitative investigation.

5. Derivative formation is useful in confirming tentative identification or in providing structural information of unknown compounds.

6. Derivative formation is usually employed for the analysis of trace-level quantities of compounds with the ECD. These derivatives must exhibit a high electron affinity and have suitable gas-chromatography properties (e.g. perfluoroacyl derivatives).

9.11 PREPARATION OF DERIVATIVES

To be useful for gas-chromatographic analyses derivatives should be formed in quantitative yield, be chemically and thermally stable, and have the required gas-chromatographic properties.

A comprehensive book on preparation of derivatives used in chromatography, which is invaluable to the GC analyst, is already available (Blau and King, 1978). It is not the intention in this chapter to compete with such a work, but instead to select some of the most commonly used methods of derivatisision, together with appropriate examples for their application to capillary GC (see section 9.12).

Reagents for the silylation of organic compounds are probably the most widely used for GC derivatisation. These have been extensively evaluated by Pierce (1968), and more recently by Poole (1978). In silylation, an active hydrogen is replaced by an alkyl silyl group. Silyl derivatisation are generally more volatile, less polar and more thermally stable than their parent compounds. The main application is the silylation of hydroxyl groups to form trimethylsilyl ethers, and the conversion of carboxylic acid groups to form trimethylsilyl esters. Other radicals that are amenable to silylation include amino, sulphydril and, under certain conditions, carbonyl groups. There is a variety of reagents available for silylation and the choice and the conditions of reaction are dependent not only on the radical involved but also on its position within the molecule.

Other common derivatisation methods suitable for capillary GC include acylation and esterification (see Blau and King, 1978; Darbre, 1978). When used with electron-capture detectors, halogenosilyl ethers are highly sensitive for steroids, short-chain acids and alcohols (Eaborn *et al.*, 1969; Thomas, 1971; Brooks *et al.*, 1975; Symes and Thomas, 1976), while fluoroacylation is equally effective for phenols, amides and amines (Blau and King, 1978).

Protective alkylation of amino acids, steroids, organic acids and catacholamines is described by Kovac and Anderle (1978). This is particularly useful for stabilisation of carboxyl groups (e.g. methylation) in preparation of compounds for a second derivatisation (e.g. bile acids) where a further reaction such as silylation is necessary. Methylation of certain drugs (e.g. sulphonamides, narcotics) can actually be carried out by 'flash alkylation', which uses the high temperature of the injection port to rapidly derivatise the sample (Brochman-Hanssen and Olawuyi Oke, 1969; Christophersen and Rasmussen, 1979).

9.12 APPLICATIONS

The problem confronting the analyst in toxicological measurements is whether the toxic compounds themselves can be analysed or whether it is more practical to examine the physiological or biochemical effects caused by exposure to these compounds. We have therefore included examples of both aspects of analysis. Except for methods for the measurement of phenytoin and metranidazole, drugs have purposely been omitted, as analyses of these by capillary GC have already been comprehensively covered (Vandenheuvel and Zweig, 1982; Plotczyk and Larson, 1983; Anderson and Stafford, 1983).

Sometimes the choice of capillary column is determined by what is available to the analyst, so examples using glass and fused-silica WCOT columns and glass SCOT columns have been included, as well as applications involving the use of FID, ECD, nitrogen–phosphorus detection (NPD) and finally mass spectrometry (MS).

9.12.1 Pyrrolizidine alkaloids

Pyrrolizidine alkaloids (PAs) are both liver poisons and carcinogens which occur in various plant species growing throughout the world. They present a hazard to grazing livestock, and sometimes to humans when foodstuff or milk becomes contaminated. Therefore there is a need to identify and measure these compounds in plant, food and animal material.

The toxic alkaloids are esters of amino-alcohols (necines) having the dehydropyrrolizidine ring structure such as in senecionine, which is one of the major PAs contained in the weed tansy ragwort (Figure 9.10). Many of these naturally occurring PAs can be gas-chromatographed without derivatisation on glass or fused-silica columns, as illustrated in Figures 9.11 and 9.12. However, some PAs have to be derivatised to improve their thermal stability or increase their sensitivity of detection (e.g. by ECD or selective ion monitoring MS). A recent study of the GC and MS properties of PAs has recently been made (Farmer *et al.*, 1983).

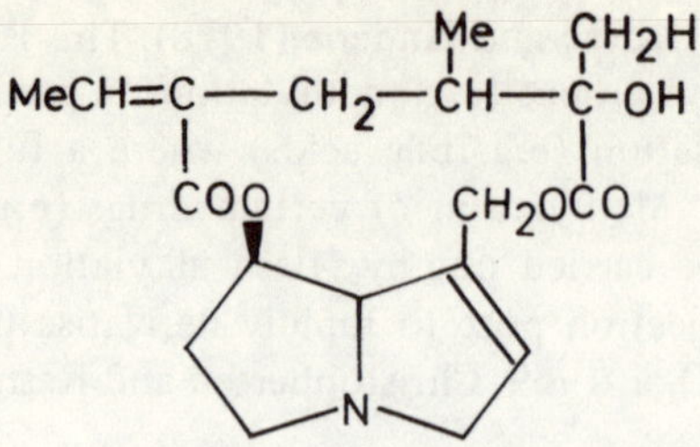

Figure 9.10 Structural formula of the plant pyrrolizidine alkaloid, senecionine.

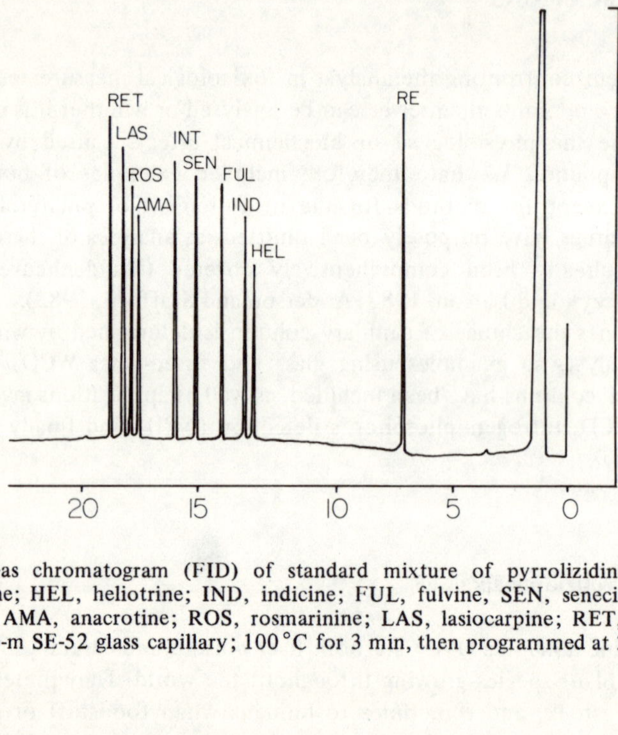

Figure 9.11 Gas chromatogram (FID) of standard mixture of pyrrolizidine alkaloids: RE, retronecine; HEL, heliotrine; IND, indicine; FUL, fulvine, SEN, senecionine, INT, integarrimine; AMA, anacrotine; ROS, rosmarinine; LAS, lasiocarpine; RET, retrorsine. Conditions: 20-m SE-52 glass capillary; 100 °C for 3 min, then programmed at 20 K min^{-1} to 280 °C.

9.12.2 Aromatic and heterocyclic nitro compounds

Aromatic and heterocyclic nitro compounds, of which several have toxic, mutagenic and carcinogenic properties, are widely used in industry, agriculture and medicine. For many of these compounds reduction of the nitro group is necessary for expression of their toxicological properties and the gut microflora are involved in the reduction process. Using high-resolution gas chromatography it has been shown that the reduction rate of several nitro compounds by rat caecal bacteria is strongly influenced by dietary intake (Rowland *et al.*, 1983). For example, 2, 4-

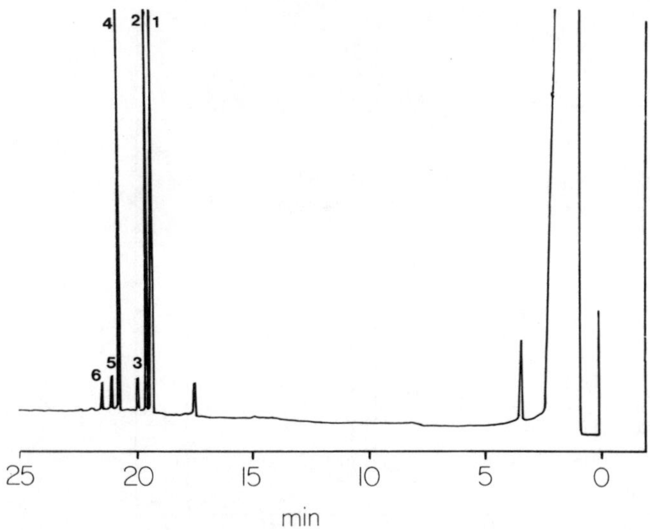

Figure 9.12 Gas chromatogram of tansy-ragwort alkaloids. Conditions: as in Figure 9.11. Peaks identified by GC–MS: (1) senecionine, (2) seneciphylline, (3) integerrimine, (4) jacobine, (5) jacozine and (6) jaconine.

dinitrotoluene (2, 4-DNT), which is a hepatocarcinogen in the rat, is metabolised by rat caecum to 2-amino-4-nitrotoluene (2A4NT), 4-amino-2-nitrotoluene (4A2NT), and 2, 4-diaminotoluene (2, 4-DAT).

Figure 9.13 is a gas chromatogram from the analysis of these metabolites in the caecal contents of a carragheenen-fed rat incubated with 2, 4-DNT. The isomer 2, 6-dinitrotoluene (2, 6-DNT) was added to the incubation mixture as an internal standard just prior to extraction with ethyl acetate. The use of the specific NPD allowed quantitation to be made without any purification of the solvent extract.

A similar gas-chromatograph assay procedure has been used to study the effect of diet on the nitro-reduction rate of metronidazole in rat caecal incubates. This drug (see Figure 9.14), which is used in the treatment of certain anaerobic bacterial infections in humans, can, in high doses, cause tumours in mice and rats. Hence concern has been expressed that it may pose a risk in causing human cancer. The drug was quantitated using the structurally related compound mesonidazole as an internal standard. A typical gas chromatogram from the analysis is illustrated in Figure 9.15.

9.12.3 Pyrethroids

Pyrethroids are an important class of synthetic insecticides possessing low mammalian toxicity. The types most widely used in agriculture are esters of

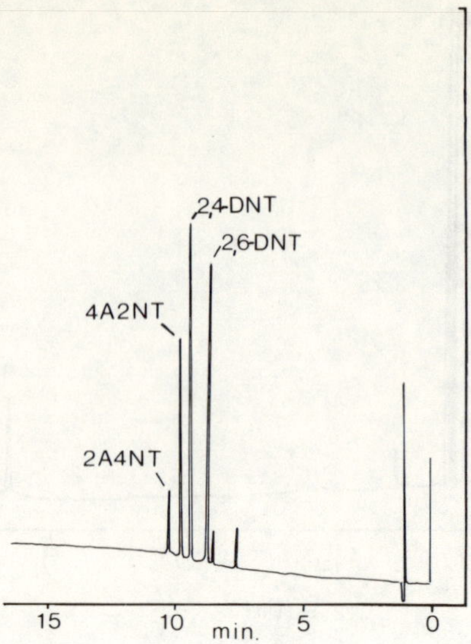

Figure 9.13 Gas chromatogram (NPD) of 2,4-DNT metabolites in rat-caecum extract. Conditions: 20-m cross-linked OV1701 glass capillary, 100 °C for 3 min then programmed at 20 K min^{-1} to 280 °C.

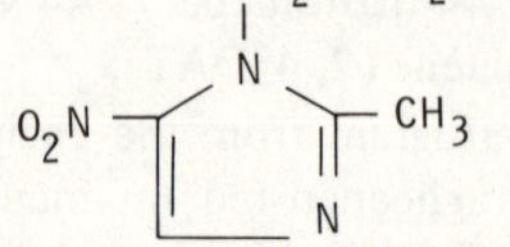

Figure 9.14 Structure of metronidazole.

3-phenoxybenzylalcohol or 2-cyano-3-phenoxybenzyl alcohol and are used either as single isomers (deltamethrin), or as a mixture of stereoisomers (permethrin, fenvalerate, cypermethrin). The *cis-* and *trans-*isomeric forms of these halogen-containing compounds can be separated and quantitated at very low levels using capillary columns with ECD (see Figure 9.16). Thus high-resolution GC is potentially very useful in both residue analysis and metabolic studies in mammalian systems.

9.12.4 Toxicological properties of impurities in the pesticide malathion

Malathion is a widely used organophosphorous pesticide with a low mammalian toxicity. In 1976 during an eradication programme in Pakistan, some 2800 spraymen became poisoned after using this insecticide and five died. The main deter-

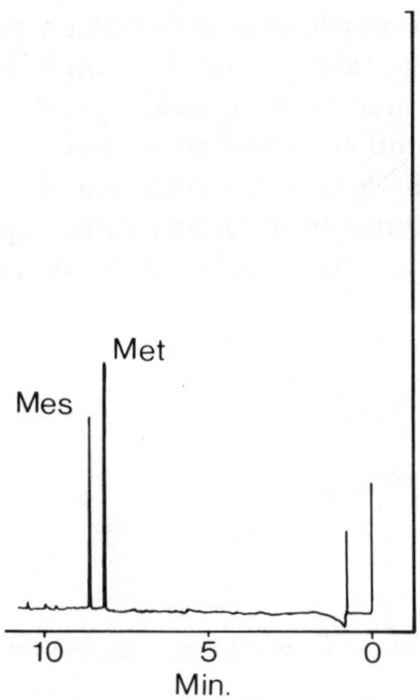

Figure 9.15 Gas chromatogram (NPD) from analysis of the drug metronidazole in a rat-caecum extract. Met, metronidazole; Mes, mesonidazole. For GC conditions see Figure 9.13.

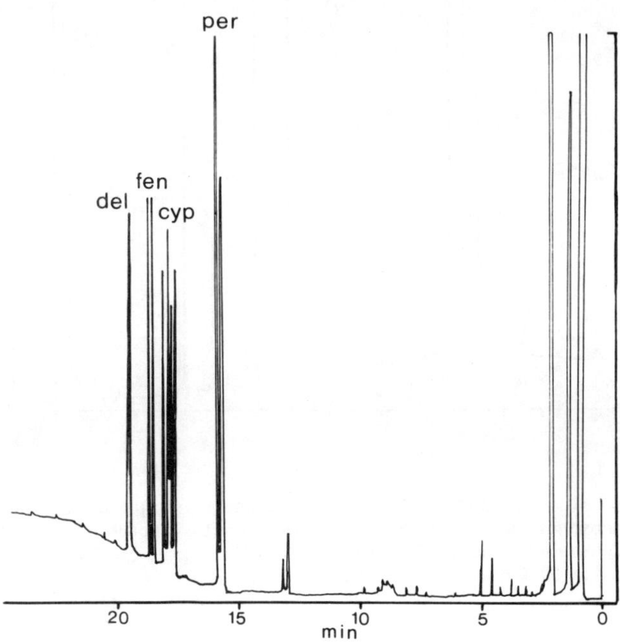

Figure 9.16 Gas chromatogram (ECD) of mixture of authentic pyrethroids (8×10^{-10} g/peak): per, permethrin; cyp, cypermethrin; fen, fenvalerate del, deltamethrin. Conditions: 20-m cross-linked OV-1701 glass capillary, 100 °C for 3 min then programmed at 20 K min^{-1} to 310 °C.

minant of the toxicity was shown to be isomalathion, present as an impurity (the structure of malathion and isomalathion is shown in Figure 9.17). The isomalathion content was also found to increase during storage of the formulated malathion under adverse conditions. Other impurities such as trimethylphosphorothioates also increased the toxicity by inhibition of a carboxylesterase enzyme involved in the detoxification of malathion itself. Capillary GC can be used to separate and measure these toxic impurities in stored-malathion samples (see Figure 9.18).

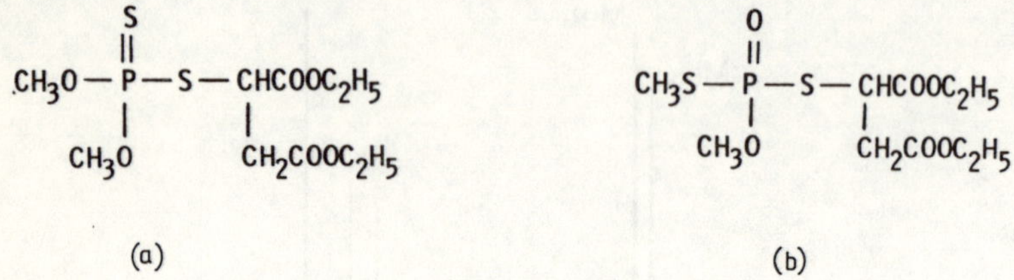

Figure 9.17 Structure of (a) malathion and (b) isomalathion.

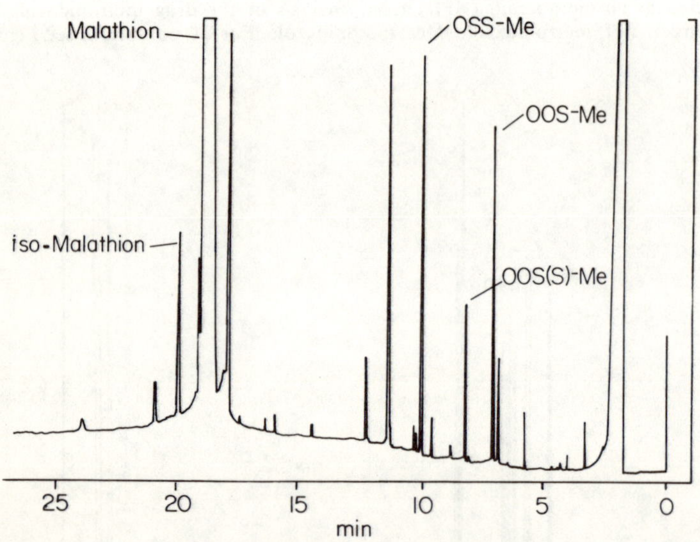

Figure 9.18 Gas chromatogram (FID) of a contaminated sample of malathion; OSS-Me, OSS-trimethylphosphorothioate, OSS(S)-Me, OSS-trimethylphosphorodithioate, OSS-Me, OSS-trimethylphosphorodithioate. Conditions: 20-m SE52 glass capillary, 100 °C for 3 min then programmed at 10 K min^{-1} to 280 °C.

In order to study the pharmacokinetic properties of one of these impurities, OSS-trimethylphosphorodithioate, in the rat, a highly sensitive and specific GC method was developed for quantifying the compound in plasma and tissue samples (Bailey *et al.*, 1981). A capillary GC tracing from the analysis of only a

0.1 ml sample of plasma from a rat dosed with 25 mg kg^{-1} of OSS-trimethylphosphorodithioate is shown in Figure 9.19. The alkali-bead NPD used for this assay is a very stable, sensitive and reliable detector for the measurement of many organophosphorus compounds. When used with a capillary column as little as 1×10^{-12} g of this organophosphorous triester can be detected, with a signal-to-noise ratio of 20 : 1.

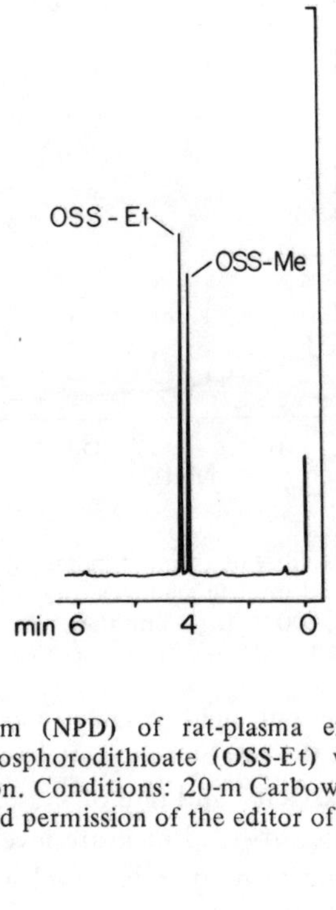

Figure 9.19 Gas chromatogram (NPD) of rat-plasma extract containing 4×10^{-6} g OSS-Me ml^{-1}; OSS-triethylphosphorodithioate (OSS-Et) was added as internal standard prior to ethyl acetate extraction. Conditions: 20-m Carbowax 20M glass capillary at 180 °C isothermal. Reproduced by kind permission of the editor of the *Journal of Chromatography* (Bailey *et al.*, 1981).

9.12.5 Analysis of contaminated cooking oils

Capillary GC with NPD has recently been used to quantitate levels of oleic, linoleic and linolenic fatty-acid anilides in adulterated cooking oils (Bailey *et al.*, 1983a). The compounds have been identified as contaminants associated with the outbreak of poisonings in Spain, which affected over 20 000 people and caused over 300 deaths. Figure 9.20 shows a capillary GC tracing from the analysis of an extracted adulterated cooking-oil sample, which was estimated to contain 123 p.p.m. of these anilides. The oil, spiked with the internal standard oleylorthotoluidide, is extracted with methanol and the dried extract shaken with 2N-KOH–methanol and toluene to transesterify residual triglycerides. The toluene layer is then removed and concentrated for analysis by GC. The ani-

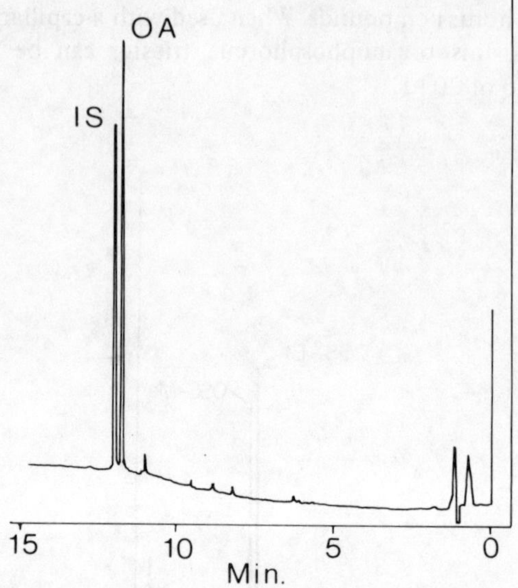

Figure 9.20 Gas chromatogram (NPD) of a contaminated cooking oil. OA, oleylanilide, plus co-eluting anilides of linolenic and linoleic acids; IS, oleylorthotoluidide. Conditions: 20-m cross-linked OV-1 glass capillary; 100 °C for 3 min then programmed to 310 °C.

lides of oleic, linoleic and linolenic acid which co-elute on the nonpolar capillary column can be quantitated in the oils by this method down to a level of 10 p.p.m.

In studies involving the toxicity and fate of these anilides in the rat, capillary GC has also been used to identify and measure levels of the aniline metabolite parahydroxyacetanilide in the urine of rats dosed with oleylanilide (see Figure 9.21) (Cunningham *et al*., 1983).

9.12.6 Analysis of the anticonvulsant drug phenytoin in plasma

Treatment of epilepsy with the drug phenytoin (diphenylhydantoin, Dilantin, Epanutin) requires repeated administration to maintain a steady therapeutic level in the blood. Monitoring of plasma levels in patients is therefore important in determining the correct dosage. As part of a study of the pharmacokinetics of phenytoin during pregnancy and labour, a method using capillary GC has been developed for the measurement of the drug in small plasma volumes (Bailey *et al*., 1983b). The plasma (0.1 ml) is first spiked with the internal standard 5-(*p*-methylphenyl)-5-phenylhydantoin (PTH), extracted into ethyl acetate, and then permethylated by an extractive alkylation technique. High-resolution

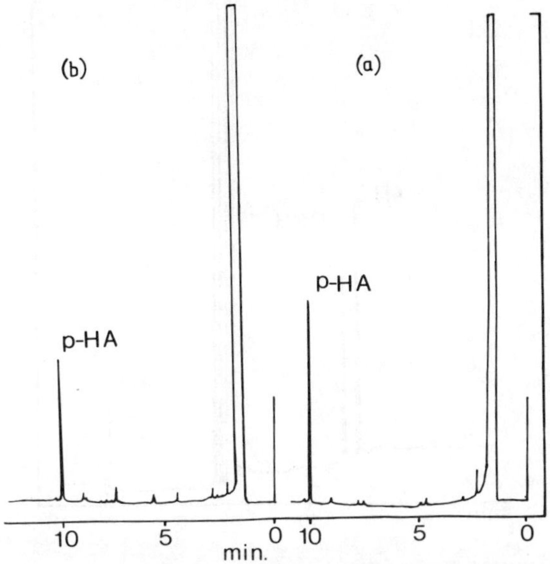

Figure 9.21 Gas chromatogram (FID) from analyses of *p*-HA (parahydroxyacetanilide) in urine extracts from rats dosed with (a) aniline, (b) oleylanilide. Conditions: 20-m cross-linked OV1701 glass capillary, 100 °C for 3 min then programmed at 10 K min^{-1} to 200 °C. Reproduced by kind permission of the editor of the *Archives of Toxicology* (Cunningham *et al.*, 1983).

GC is performed using an NPD. This method, which is both reliable and accurate, is eminently suitable for routine application. Figure 9.22 shows a gas chromatogram of plasma extract from a patient receiving a daily therapeutic dose of phenytoin.

A similar assay procedure has also been developed for quantitation of urinary-conjugated 5-(*p*-hydroxyphenyl)-5-phenylhydantion, which is the major metabolite of phenytion in human urine. A typical GC tracing from this analysis is illustrated in Figure 9.23.

9.12.7 Serum bile-acids

Disturbances in liver function can be monitored by the measurement of serum bile-acids using capillary GC (Paumgartner and Karlaganis, 1982). The analytical method requires 2 ml of serum and involves extraction of the acid conjugate on Amberlite XAD2 (a neutral cross-linked polystyrene resin) followed by separate solvolysis and enzyme (cholyglycine hydrolase) hydrolytic procedures. The free bile-acids (see Figure 9.24) are then subjected to methylation followed by silylation prior to analysis by capillary GC. Figure 9.25 shows a GC separation of bile acids in an extract from the serum of a patient with liver damage.

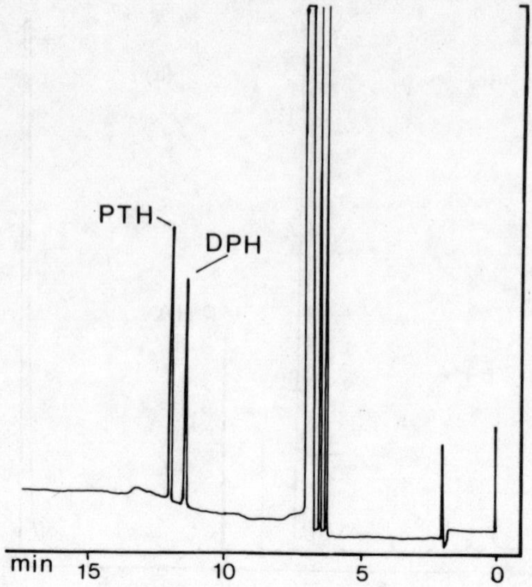

Figure 9.22 Gas chromatogram (NPD) of an extract from a human plasma sample. 5×10^{-6} g ml^{-1} of phenytoin (DPH). Internal standard, 5-(*p*-methylphenyl)-5-phenylhydantoin (PTH). Conditions: 20-m cross-linked OV-1 glass capillary, 100 °C for 3 min then programmed at 30 K min^{-1} to 300 °C.

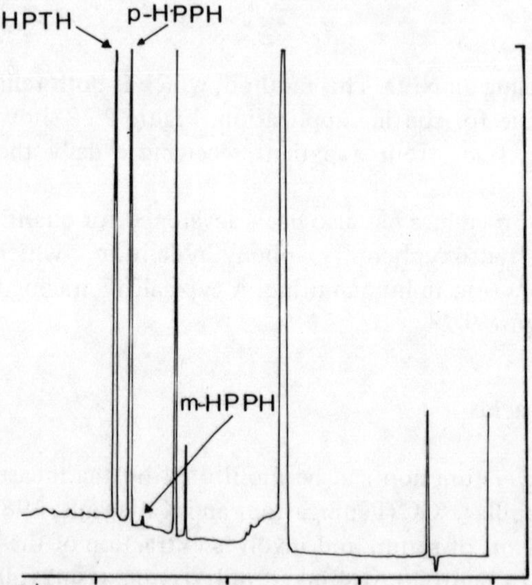

Figure 9.23 Gas chromatogram (NPD) of an extract from a human urine sample 5-(*p*-hydroxyphenyl)-5-phenylhydantoin (*p*-HPPH). Internal standard, 5-(*p*-hydroxyphenyl)-5-(*p*tolyl)hydantoin (HPTH). 5-(*m*-hydroxyphenyl)-5-phenylhydantoin (*m*-HPPH) is a minor urinary metabolite. For conditions see Figure 9.22.

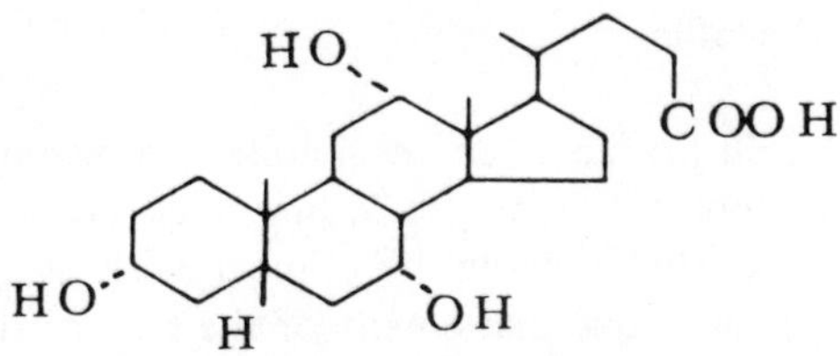

Figure 9.24 Structure of cholic acid.

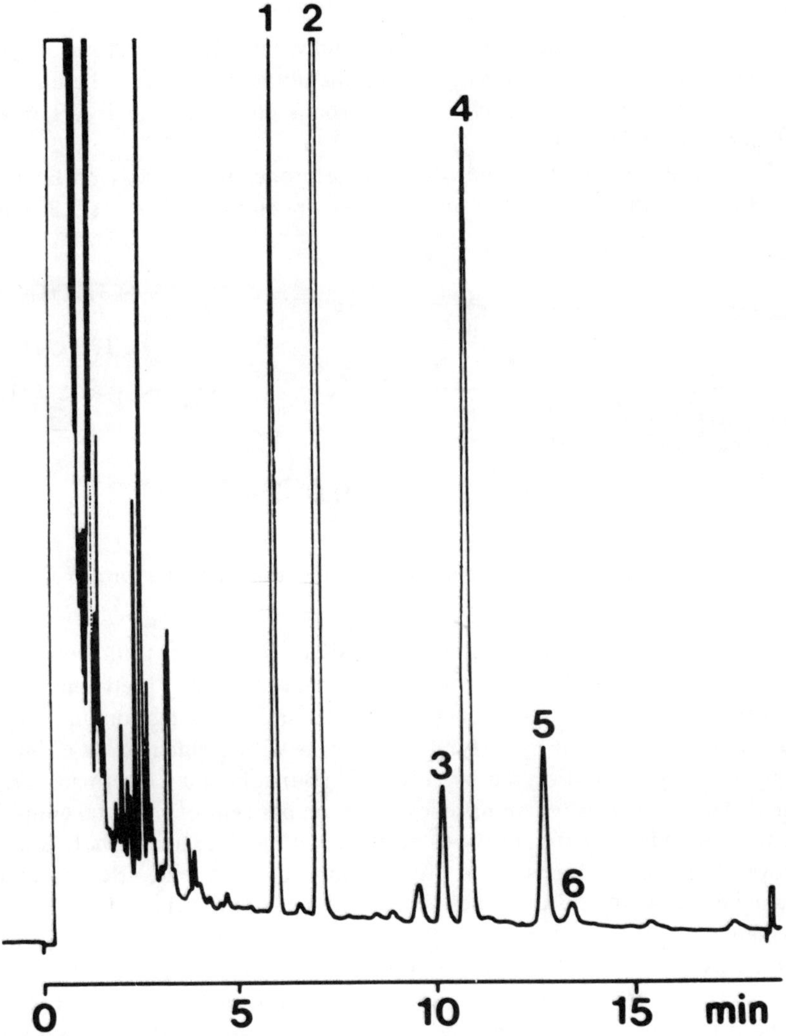

Figure 9.25 Gas chromatogram (FID) of TMS ethers of bile acids extracted from serum from a patient with liver disease: (1) cholesterol; (2) cholic acid; (3) deoxycholic; (4) chenodeoxycholic; (5) hyodeoxycholic (int. std); (6) lithocholic acid. Conditions: 20-m PG 20 000 glass capillary at 230 °C, isothermal. Reproduced by kind permission of Prof. G. Paumgartner, University of Berne, and the editors of *Recent Advances in Capillary Gas Chromatography* (Huthig, Verlag, Heidelberg, 1982).

9.12.8 Urinary steroid profiles

The term 'urinary steroid profiles' denotes a collective measurement of urinary C_{19} and C_{21} neutral steroid metabolites in one single GC assay (Gardiner and Horning, 1966; Horning, 1968). While the original work using packed columns gave at best, a semi-quantitative assessment of the major urinary steroid components, with the advent of capillary columns quantitation with both WCOT and SCOT columns has been shown to be more accurate (e.g. Bailey *et al.*, 1974; Thomas, 1980).

Urinary steroid profiles have not been fully investigated in toxicology, but it is known that changes in corticosteroid metabolism can be mediated by such diverse substances as polycyclic hydrocarbons, pesticides and certain drugs (Chamberlain, 1971).

The formulae of the C_{17} androgen androsterone, and the C_{21} corticosteroid α-cortolone, both major urinary metabolites, are shown in Figures 9.26a and b.

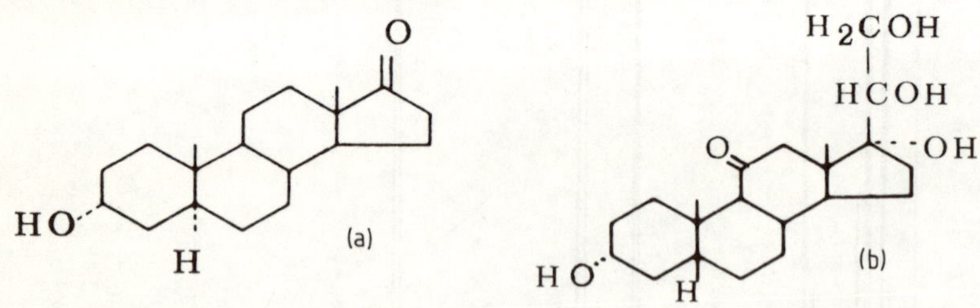

Figure 9.26 Structural formula of (a) androsterone and (b) α-cortolone.

It is usual practice to carry out the analysis of a 24-hour urine collection of which only a 5 to 20 ml aliquot is used. The method involves preliminary extraction of the steroid conjugates (glucuronidates and sulphates) on an Amberlite XAD2 column, followed by enzymic hydrolysis with β-glucuronidase. Sulphate conjugates may be hydrolysed by solvolysis (Burstein and Lieberman, 1958) if desired, but these usually comprise less than ten per cent of the total conjugates. The free steroids are extracted with ethyl acetate and an alkali wash is used to remove acidic compounds. For quantitation, at least one internal standard should be added to the urine before the extraction procedure. In the authors' experience, silylation of the dried extract is best carried out overnight with bistrimethylsilylacetamide-pyridine-trimethylchlorosilane (5 : 5 : 1). Thermolabile steroids with a dihydroxy acetone side chain, such as tetrahydrocortisol, can be quantitatively measured by separate conversion to trimethylsilyl ether-(TMSE-) enolic derivatives (Chambaz *et al.*, 1973). Another method involves the conversion of the C_{20} carbonyl group to the methoxime derivative (C_3 and C_{17} carbonyl groups are also converted) prior to silylation (Fales and Luukkainen,

1965), but in our opinion (B. S. T.) quantitation by this method has not proved so reliable. (See also Ros and Sommerville, 1971.) A urinary steroid profile, using a SCOT column, from a female patient with breast cancer is shown in Figure 9.27.

9.12.9 Estimation of exposure to alkylation agents

Humans are frequently exposed to small traces of alkylating agents and, as many of these compounds are mutagenic and carcinogenic, methods for monitoring such exposure are being investigated. The harmful effects of these substances

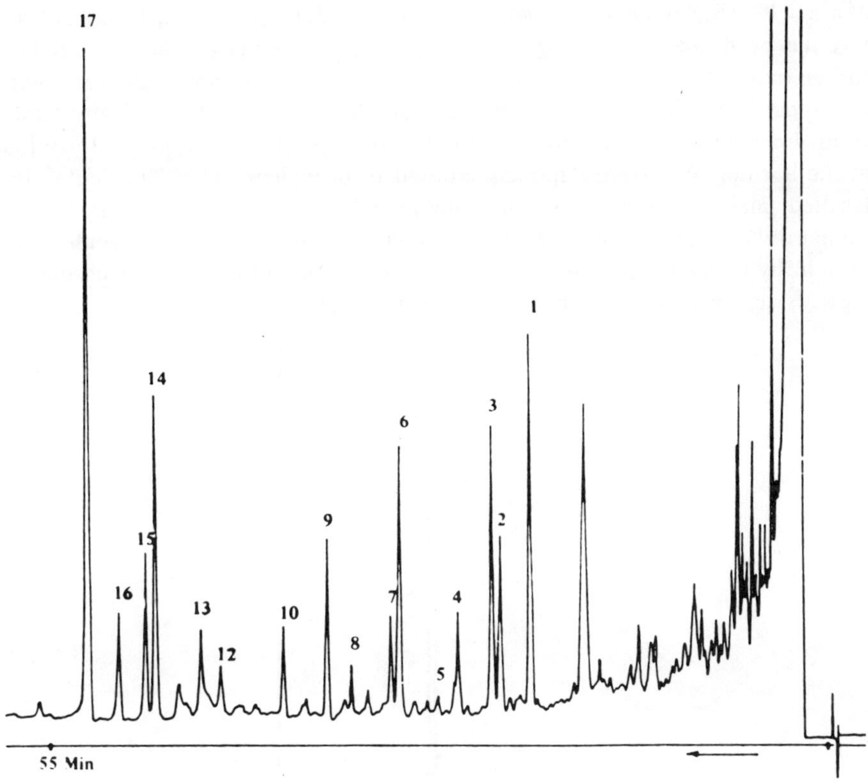

Figure 9.27 Urinary steroid profile: (1) C_{24} alkane (reference standard), (2) androsterone, (3) aetiocholanolone, (4) dehydroepiandrosterone, (5) 11-keto aetiocholanolone, (6) 11β-OH, androsterone, (7) 11β-OH, aetiocholanolone, (8) pregnanediol, (9) 3β-OH, 5α-pregnanediol (internal standard, 1×10^{-10} g), (10) pregnanetriol, (11) pregnanetriolone (not present), (12) tetrahydrocorticosterone, (13) cholesterol, (14) α-cortolone, (15) β-cortolone, (16) β-cortol, (17) C_{34} alkane (reference standard). GC conditions as in Figure 9.7. Reproduced by kind permission of the editor of the *Journal of High Resolution Chromatography and Chromatography Communications* (Thomas, 1980).

are likely to result from the alkylation of DNA, but the monitoring of DNA reactions is difficult. A more practical approach is to measure the exposure by the extent of alkylation of specific amino acids in proteins. Although several proteins could be used, haemoglobin is probably the most suitable because of its long *in vivo* lifetime and its ready availability from humans and from laboratory animals. The amino acids most likely to be alkylated are cysteine and histidine, but the levels of these alkylated amino acids in haemoglobin following exposure are very small ($< 20\ \text{nmol g}^{-1}$). With this in mind, assay procedures have been developed using GC–MS with selected-ion monitoring for the quantitation in haemoglobin of *S*-methylcysteine following exposure to methylating agents, and of *N*-3′-(2-hydroxyethyl)histidine and *N*-3′-(2-hydroxypropyl)-histidine following exposure to ethylene oxide and propylene oxide (Farmer *et al*., 1980; Bailey *et al*., 1980; Bailey *et al*., 1982; Farmer *et al*., 1982). Advantage has been taken of the high resolving power of capillary columns to reduce the amount of sample work-up required, and also to improve assay sensitivity and specificity. Figure 9.28 shows an example of a selected-ion monitor trace from the analyses used to monitor amounts of *N*-3′-(2-hydroxypropyl)histidine in the haemoglobin from a human exposed to propylene oxide. The deuterium-labelled analogue of the alkylated amino acid was employed as an internal standard which was added initially to the globin sample. The amino acids in the protein hydrolysate, after isolation and purification by ion-exchange chromatography, were analysed as *N*-heptafluorobutyrylmethyl esters.

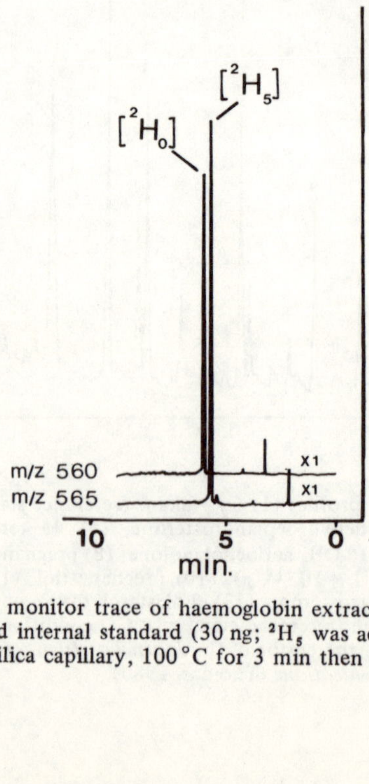

Figure 9.28 Selected ion monitor trace of haemoglobin extract from a human exposed to propylene oxide. Labelled internal standard (30 ng; $^{2}H_5$ was added to globin (1 g). Conditions: 20-m SE52 fused-silica capillary, 100 °C for 3 min then programmed at 32 K min^{-1} to 250 °C.

The original method developed for the measurement of *S*-methylcysteine in haemoglobin by high-resolution GC–MS with multiple-ion detection also employed a deuterated internal standard for quantitation (Farmer *et al.*, 1980). This method was subsequently modified by using the unnatural D-enantiomer of *S*-methylcysteine as an alternative internal standard (Bailey *et al.*, 1980). This allowed the mass spectrometer to be operated in the single-ion rather than the multiple-ion monitor mode, which improved the sensitivity of detection three-fold. The quantitation of amino acids by GC and GC–MS using enantiomer labelling has become feasible with the introduction by Frank *et al.* (1977) of the thermally stable chiral stationary phase Chirasil-Val. Using a capillary column coated with this phase it is possible, after forming suitable esterified acylated derivatives, to resolve almost all the common protein amino acids and their enantiomers in a single programmed GC separation (Frank *et al.* 1978). The separation of a standard racemic mixture of amino acids on a fused-silica column coated with this phase is shown in Figure 9.29.

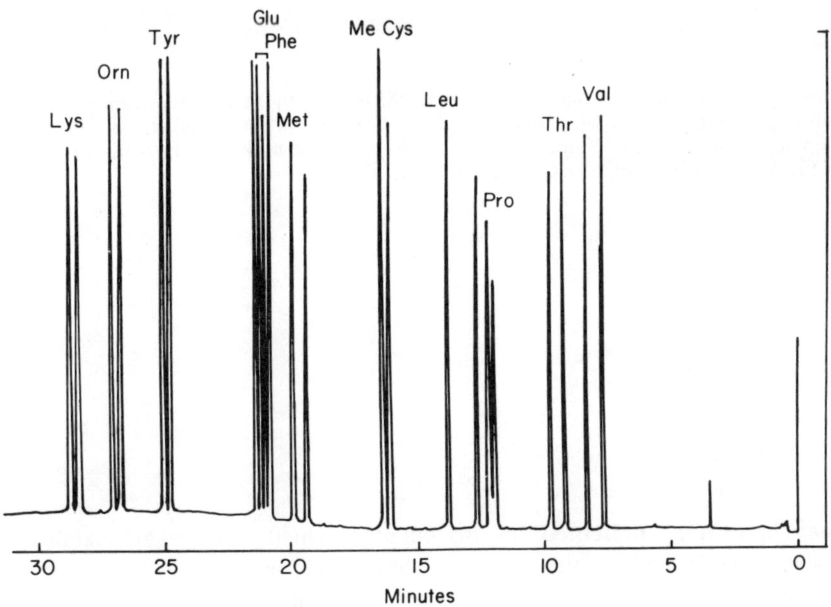

Figure 9.29 Gas chromatogram (FID) of a standard racemic mixture of amino acids as *N*-pentafluoropropionylisopropyl esters. Conditions: 16-m Chirasil-Val fused-silica capillary, 80 °C for 3 min then programmed at 5 K min^{-1} to 190 °C.

The chromatogram illustrated in Figure 9.30 is a single-ion monitor trace of an extract from animal haemoglobin for the estimation of *S*-methyl-L-cysteine, using the *S*-methyl-D-cysteine as an internal standard.

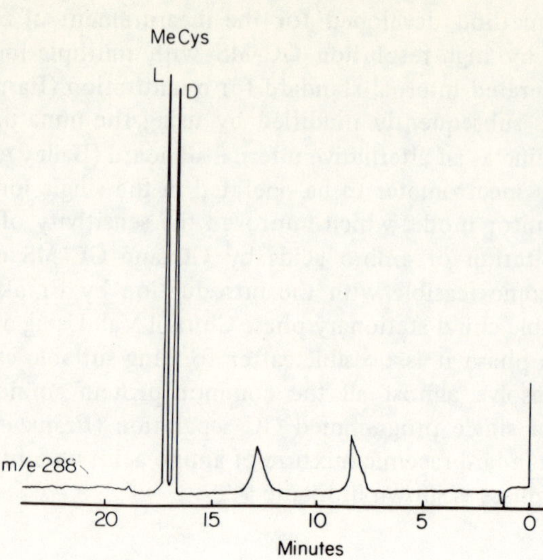

Figure 9.30 Single ion monitor trace (m/z 288) of methyl-L-cysteine from an extract of guinea-pig haemoglobin. GC conditions: 20-m Chirasil-Val glass capillary, 80°C for 3 min then programmed at 5 K min^{-1} to 180°C. Reproduced by kind permission of the editor of the *Journal of Chromatography* (Bailey *et al.*, 1980).

9.13 CONCLUSIONS

The applications presented in this chapter, which were taken mainly from analyses performed in the authors' laboratories, are intended to show how capillary GC can be used to study toxicological problems. It is not always possible to detect toxic compounds in samples from mammalian systems previously exposed to hazardous materials, as often only the physiological effects remain. These physiological changes in metabolism may therefore be the only means by which such effects can be measured, for example liver damage, which can be caused by many compounds, or changes in DNA structure produced by certain carcinogenic alkylating agents. Capillary GC is, of course, not the only method of analysis in toxicology studies, but it is a very powerful and sensitive tool, especially when linked to MS. However, alternative analytical techniques, e.g. high-performance liquid chromatography and thin-layer chromatography, may often be more appropriate. We have tried to put a case for capillary GC as a vital weapon in the toxicologist's armoury.

REFERENCES

Anderson, W. H., and Stafford, D. T. (1983). Applications of capillary gas chromatography in routine toxicological analyses. *J. High Res. Chromatogr. Chromatogr Comm.* **6**, 247–54.

Bailey, E., Fenoughty, M., and Chapman, J. R. (1974). Evaluation of a gas–liquid chromatographic method for the determination of urinary steroids using high resolution open-tubular glass capillary columns. *J. Chromatogr.* **96**, 33–46.

Bailey, E., Farmer, P. B., and Lamb, J. H. (1980). The enantiomer as internal standard for the quantitation of the alkylated amino acid *S*-methyl-L-cysteine in haemoglobin by GC–Cl-MS with single ion detection. *J. Chromatogr.* **200**, 145–52.

Bailey, E., Peal, J. A., and Verschoyle, R. D. (1981). The determination of *O*, *S*, *S*-trimethylphosphorodithioate in the plasma and various tissues of rats using high-resolution gas chromatography with nitrogen–phosphorus detection. *J. Chromatogr.* **219**, 285–90.

Bailey, E., Farmer, P. B., and Campbell, J. B. (1982). Determination of alkylated amino acids in haemoglobin by capillary gas chromatography–mass spectrometry. Recent advances in gas chromatography–mass spectrometry. *Analyt. Proc.* **19**, 239–41.

Bailey, E., Peal, J., and Brooks, A. G. F. (1983a). Determination of fatty acid anilides in contaminated cooking oils using high resolution capillary gas chromatography. *J. High Res. Chromatogr. Chromatogr. Comm.* **6**, 452–3.

Bailey, E., Farmer, P. B., Hoskins, J. A., Lamb, J. H. and Peal, J. A. (1983b). To be published.

Blau, K., and King, G. (1978). Acylation. In Blau and King (eds), *Handbook of Derivatives for Chromatography*. Heydon, London and Philadelphia, pp. 104–51.

Blomberg, L., Buijten, J., Markides, K., and Wannman, T. (1983). Some aspects of cross-linked silicone stationary phases for gas chromatography. In Rijks, J. (ed.), *Fifth International Symposium of Capillary Chromatography. Riva del Garde, Italy*. Elsevier, Amsterdam, pp. 99–107.

Bouche, J., and Verzele, M. (1968). A static coating procedure for glass capillary columns. *J. Gas Chromatogr.* **6**, 501–5.

Bremner, N. (1967). Basic knowledge of gas chromatography and gas chromatographic instruments. In Ettre, L. S., and Zlatkis, A. (eds.), *The Practice of Gas Chromatography*. Wiley, New York and London, pp. 1–50.

Brochmann-Hanssen, E., and Olawuyi Oke, T. (1969). Gas chromatography of barbiturates, phenolic alkaloids and xanthine bases: flash heater methylation by means of trimethylanilinium hydroxide. *J. Pharm. Sci.* **58**, 370–1.

Brooks, J. B., Liddle, J. A., and Alley, C. C. (1975). Electron capture gas chromatography and mass spectral studies in iodomethyl–dimethylsilyl ethers of some short-chain acids, hydroxy acids, and alcohols. *Analyt. Chem.* **47**, 1960–5.

Burstein, S., and Liberman, S. (1958). Hydrolysis of ketosteroid conjugates by solvolysis procedures. *J. Biol. Chem.* **233**, 331–5.

Chambaz, E. M., Defaye, G., and Madani, C. (1973). Trimethylsilyl ether-enol-trimethylsilyl ether–a new type of derivative for the gas phase study of hormonal steroids. *Analyt. Chem.* **45**, 1090–8.

Chamberlain, J. (1971). Determination of urinary 6-oxygenated cortisol in evaluating liver function. *Clin. Chim. Acta.* **34**, 269–71.

Christophersen, A. S., and Rasmussen, K. E. (1979). Glass capillary column gas chromatography of narcotic drugs after flash heater trimethylsilylation. *J. Chromatogr.* **174**, 454–60.

Cropper, F. R., and Heywood, A. (1953). The analysis of fatty acids and fatty alcohols by vapour phase chromatography. In Destý, D. H. (ed.), *Vapour Phase Chromatography*, Academic, New York, pp. 316–28.

Cunningham, V. J., Tucker, S. P., and Bailey, E. (1983). Hydrolysis of oleylanilide in the rat. *Arch. Toxicol.* **54**, 157–62.

Dandeneau, R. D., and Zerenner, E. H. (1979). An investigation of glasses for capillary chromatography. *J. High Res. Chromatogr. Chromatogr. Comm.* **2**, 351–6.

Darbre, A. (1978). Esterification. In Blau, F., and King, G. (eds), *Handbook of Derivatives for Chromatography* Heyden, London and Philadelphia, pp. 39–103.

Desty, D. H. (1965). Capillary columns–trials, tribulations and triumphs. *Adv. Chromatogr.* **1**, 199–229.

Desty, D. H., Goldup, A., and Whyman, B. H. F. (1958). The potentialities of coated capillary columns for gas chromatography in the petroleum industry. *J. Inst. Petrol.* **45**, 287–97.

Desty, D. H., Haresnape, J. N., and Whyman, B. H. F. (1960). Construction of long lengths of coiled glass capillary. *Analyt. Chem.* **32**, 302–4.

Eaborn, E., Holder, C. A., Walton, D. R. M., and Thomas, B. S. (1969). Gas chromatographic assay at nanogram levels of steroid (halogenomethyl)-dimethylsilyl ethers. *J. Chem. Soc. (c)*, 2502–3.

Fales, H. M., and Luukainen, A. A. (1965). *O*-Methyloximes as carbonyl derivatives in gas chromotography, mass spectrometry, and nuclear magnetic resonance. *Analyt. Chem.* **37**, 955–9.

Farmer, P. B., Bailey, E., Lamb, J. H., and Connors, T. A. (1980). Approach to the quantitation of alkylated amino acids in haemoglobin by gas chromatography–mass spectrometry. *Biomed. Mass Spectrom.* **7**, 41–6.

Farmer, P. B., Gorf, S. M., and Bailey, E. (1982). Determination of hydroxypropylhistidine in haemoglobin as a measure of exposure to propylene oxide using high resolution gas chromatography–mass spectrometry. *Biomed. Mass Spectrom.* **9**, 69–71.

Farmer, P. B., Bailey, E., and Mattocks, A. R. (1983). Gas chromatographic and mass spectrometric properties of pyrrolizidine alkaloids (to be published).

Frank, H., Nicholson, G. J., and Bayer, E. (1977). Rapid gas chromatographic separation of amino acid enantiomers with a novel chiral stationary phase. *J. Chromatogr. Sci.* **15**, 174–6.

Frank, H., Nicholson, G. J., and Bayer, E. (1978). Enantiomer labelling, a method for the quantitative analysis of amino acids. *J. Chromatogr.* **167**, 187–96.

Frigerio, A. (1978). The Seveso Case: TCDD in animals from contaminated areas. In Reid, E. (ed.), *Blood, Drugs and Other Analytical Challenges*. Ellis Horwood, Chichester, pp. 161–6.

Gardiner, W. L., and Horning, E. C. (1966). Gas–liquid chromatography separation of C_{19} and C_{21} human steroids by a new procedure. *Biochim. Biophys. Acta* **115**, 524–32.

Golay, M. J. E. (1958). In Desty, D. H. (ed.), *Gas Chromatography*. Butterworths, London, pp. 36–55.

Grob, K. (1978). Everyday problems of glass-capillary GC. In Reid, E. (ed.), *Blood, Drugs and Other Analytical Challenges*. Ellis Horwood, Chichester, pp. 89–96.

Grob, K., and Grob, K., Jun. (1978). On-column injection onto glass capillary columns. *J. Chromatogr.* **151**, 311–20.

Grob, K., Jun., Grob, G., and Grob, K. (1978). Comprehensive standardised quality test for glass capillary columns. *J. Chromatogr.* **156**, 1–20.

Grob, K., and Grob, G. (1979). Further evidence for the silica layer as produced by acid leaching. *J. High Res. Chromatogr. Chromatogr. Comm.* **2**, 527–8.

Grob, K., Grob, G., and Grob, K., Jun. (1979). Deactivation of glass capillaries by persilylation. 2: Practical recommendations. *J. High Res. Chromatogr. Chromatogr. Comm.* **2**, 677–8.

Grob, K., and Grob, G. (1982). Preparation of inert glass capillary columns for gas chromatography. A revised comprehensive description. *J. Chromatogr.* **244**, 197–208.

Horning, E. C. (1968). Gas phase analytical methods for the study of steroid hormones and their metabolites. In Eik-Nes, K. B. and Horning, E. C. (eds), *Gas Phase Chromatography of Steroids.* Springer Verlag, Berlin and New York, pp. 1–71.

Jennings, W. G. (1978). *Gas Chromatography with Glass Capillary Columns*. Academic, New York.

Kovac, P., and Anderle, D. (1978). Protective alkylation. In Blau, K., and King, G. (eds),

Handbook of Derivatives for Chromatography. Heyden, London, pp. 201–33.

Kovats, E. (1958). Gas-chromatographische charakterisierung organischer verbindungen. 1: Retentionindices aliphatischer Halogenide, Alkohole, Aldehyde unde Ketone. *Helv. Chim. Acta* **41**, 1915–30.

McReynolds, W. O. (1970). Characterisation of some liquid phases. *J. Chromatogr. Sci.* 8, 685–91.

Markides, K., Blomberg, L., Buijten, J., and Wannman, T. (1983). Cyano silicones as stationary phases in gas chromatography. 2: Gum and rubber phases on fused silica. In Rijks, J. (ed.), *Fifth International Symposium on Capillary Chromatography, Riva del Garde, Italy*. Elsevier, Amsterdam, pp. 117–26.

Paumgartner, G., and Karlaganis, G. (1982). Capillary gas liquid chromatography of bile acids: improvement with on-column injections. In Bertsch, W., Jennings, W. G., and Kaiser, R. E. (eds), *Recent Advancements in Capillary Gas Chromatography*. Huthig, Heidelberg, pp. 361–7.

Pierce, A. E. (1968). *Silylation of Organic Compounds*. Pierce Chemical, Rockford, Illinois.

Plotczyk, L. L., and Larson, P. (1983). Advances in fused-silica column technology for the analysis of underivatised drugs. *J. Chromatogr.* **257**, 211–6.

Poole, C. F. (1978). Recent advances in silylation of organic compounds for GC. In Blau, K., and King, G. (eds), *Handbook of Derivatives for Chromatography*, Heyden, London, pp. 152–200.

Poy, F., Visani, S., and Terrosi, F. (1981). Automatic injection in high-resolution gas chromatography: a programmed temperature vaporiser as a general purpose injection system. *J. Chromatogr.* **217**, 81–90.

Richter, B. E., Kuei, J. C., Shelton, J. I., Castle, L. W., Bradshaw, J. S., and Lee, M. L. (1983). Cross-linking of moderately polar stationary phases for capillary column gas chromatography. In Rijks, J. (ed.), *Fifth International Symposium on Capillary Chromatography, Riva del Garde, Italy*. Elsevier, Amsterdam, pp. 108–26.

Rohrschneider, I. (1966). Eine methode zur charackterisierung von gas-chromatographischen trennflussigkeiten. *J. Chromatogr.* **22**, 6–22.

Ros, A., and Sommerville, I. F. (1971). Gas–liquid chromatography with high resolution gas capillary columns for the simultaneous determination of urinary steroids. *J. Ob. Gyn. Brit. Comm.* **78**, 1096–1107.

Rowland, I. R., Mallett, A. K., Wise, A., and Bailey, E. (1983). Effect of dietary carragheenan and pectin on the reduction of nitro-compounds by the rat caecal microflora. *Xenobiotica* **13**, 251–6.

Stark, T. J., Dandeneau, R. D., and Mering, L. (1980). Pittsburgh Conference on Analytical Chemistry and Applied Spectroscopy, Atlantic City, NJ, *Abstr. 2*.

Symes, E. K., and Thomas, B. S. (1976). Method for the measurement of plasma dehydroepiandrosterone by gas–liquid chromatography with electron capture detection. *J. Chromatogr.* **116**, 163–7.

Thomas, B. S. (1965). The specificity of a gas chromatographic method for the determination of urinary androsterone, aetiocholanolone and dehydroepiandrosterone. In Lipsett, M. (ed.), *Gas Chromatography of Steroids*. Plenum, New York, pp. 1–9.

Thomas, B. S., and Walton, D. R. M. (1967). The use of haloalkylsilyl ether steroid derivatives for analysis by gas–liquid chromatography. In Grant, J. K. (ed.), *Memoirs of the Society for Endocrinology*. Cambridge University Press, pp. 199–209.

Thomas, B. S. (1980). Steroid analysis by gas chromatography with SCOT and wide-bore ether by gas–liquid chromatography. *J. Chromatogr.* **56**, 37–50.

Thomas, B. S. (1980). Steroid Analysis by gas chromatography with SCOT and wide-bore WCOT columns. *J. High Res. Chromatogr. Chromatogr. Comm.* **3**, 241–7.

Van Boven, M., and Sunshine, I. (1979). Capillary gas chromatography for drug analysis. *J. Analyt. Toxicol.* **3**, 174–6.

Van den Berg, P. M. I., and Cox, T. (1972). All glass sampling device for open tubular columns in gas chromatography. *Chromatographia* **5**, 16–21.

Vandenheuvel, W. J., and Zweig, J. A. (1982). Analysis of drugs and related compounds by capillary GC. In Bertsch, W., Jennings, W. G., and Kaiser, R. E., (eds), *Recent Advances in Capillary Gas Chromatography*. Huthig, Heidelberg, pp. 25–62.

Verzele, M., Van Roelenbosch, M., Diricks, G., and Sandra, P. (1983). In situ gummification of methylphenylsilicones in fused silica capillary columns. In Rijks, K., (ed.), *Fifth International Symposium on Capillary Chromatography, Riva del Garde, Italy*. Elsevier, Amsterdam, pp. 94–8.

Wright, B. W., Peaden, P. A., and Lee, M. L. (1982). Free radical cross-linking in the preparation of non-extractable stationary phases for capillary chromatography. *J. Chromatogr.* 248, 17–34.

GLOSSARY

ECD Electron capture detector
FID Flame ionisation detector
GC Gas chromatography
MS Mass spectrometry
ME Methyl ester
ME–TMSE Methyl ester–trimethylsilyl ether
m.u. Methylene unit
MO–TMSE Methyloxime–trimethylsilyl ether
NPD Nitrogen phosphorus detector
PLOT Porous-layer open tubular column
tr, rel Relative retention time
tr Retention time
SCOT Support-coated open tubular column
TMSE Trimethylsilyl ethers
WCOT Wall-coated open tubular columns

10
Analysis of the cannabinoids

D. J. HARVEY

10.1 INTRODUCTION

Cannabis preparations, derived from the hemp plant, *Cannabis sativa* L., have been used by man for their euphoric effects for over four thousand years (Nahas, 1973) and represent the most widely used of all illicit drugs. The active constituents, which are found mainly in the resin associated with the flowering tops of female plants, belong to a group of compounds classified as cannabinoids and which are unique to *Cannabis*. To date, over sixty of these compounds have been identified (Turner *et al.*, 1980a) with the structure of the major active constituent, Δ^1-tetrahydrocannabinol (Δ^1-THC, Figure 10.1a), being elucidated as recently as 1964 (Gaoni and Mechoulam, 1964). Two numbering systems are in use for this compound, the monoterpene system (Figure 10.5a) used in this chapter, and the benzopyran system (Figure 10.5b) under which THC is named Δ^9-THC. Other major cannabinoids are shown in Figures 10.2 to 10.4. Of these, cannabidiol (CBD, Figure 10.2a), a biochemical precursor of Δ^1-THC, and cannabinol (CBN, Figure 10.3a), a chemical degradation product, are generally the most abundant. Both of these compounds are devoid of psychotomimetic properties although they do show other pharmacological activities.

The ratio of these compounds varies considerably with both the source and, particularly, the geographical origin of the plant. Resin from high-THC strains may contain as much as five per cent of the drug whereas in other strains, particularly the fibre type, little or no Δ^1-THC is present and the major cannabinoid is usually CBD. On the other hand, CBD is absent from some strains (Turner and Hadley, 1973a). The concentration of CBN generally increases as the result of oxidation as the sample ages.

In fresh plant material, most if not all of the cannabinoids are present as their carboxylic acid derivatives. These are of two types, as shown in Figure 10.6a and b,

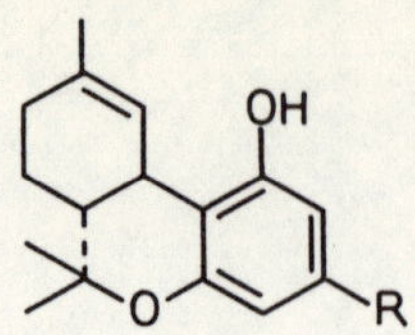

Figure 10.1 (a) R = n-C_5H_{11} (Δ^1-THC); (b) R = n-C_3H_7; (c) R = CH_3; (d) R = n-C_4H_9.

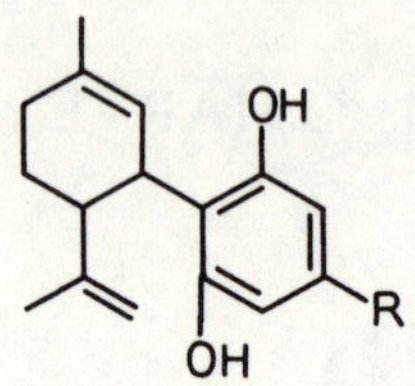

Figure 10.2 (a) R = n-C_5H_{11} (CBD); (b) R = n-C_3H_7; (c) R = CH_3; (d) R = n-C_4H_9.

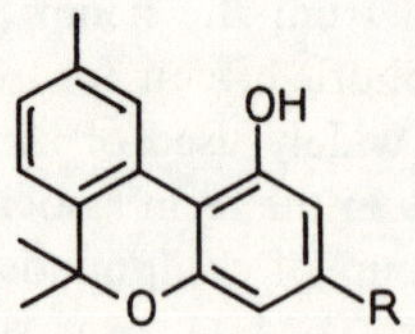

Figure 10.3 (a) R = n-C_5H_{11} (CBN); (b) R = n-C_3H_7; (c) R = CH_3; (d) R = n-C_4H_9.

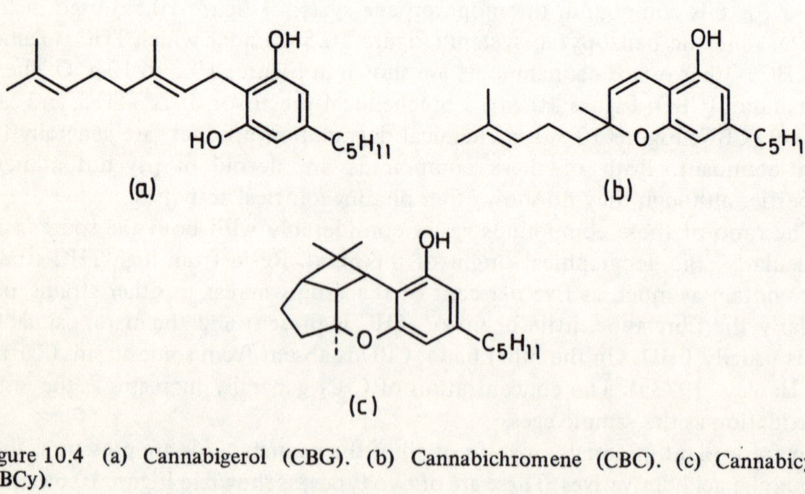

Figure 10.4 (a) Cannabigerol (CBG). (b) Cannabichromene (CBC). (c) Cannabicyclol (CBCy).

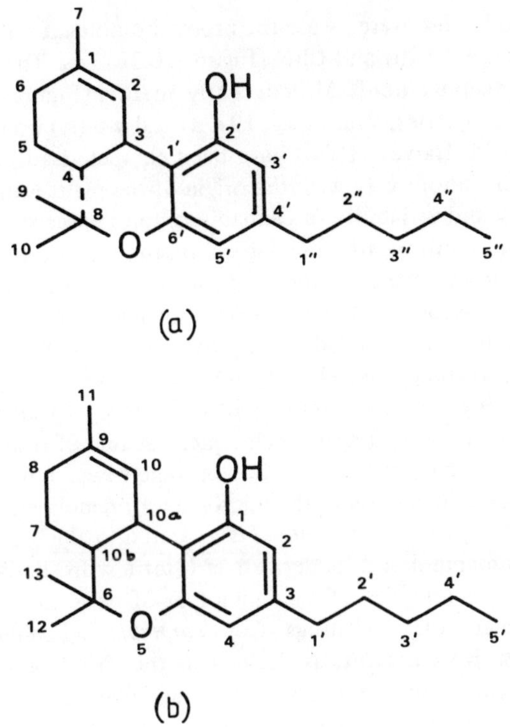

Figure 10.5 (a) Δ^1-THC, monoterpene numbering. (b) Δ^1-THC, dibenzpyran numbering (Δ^9-THC).

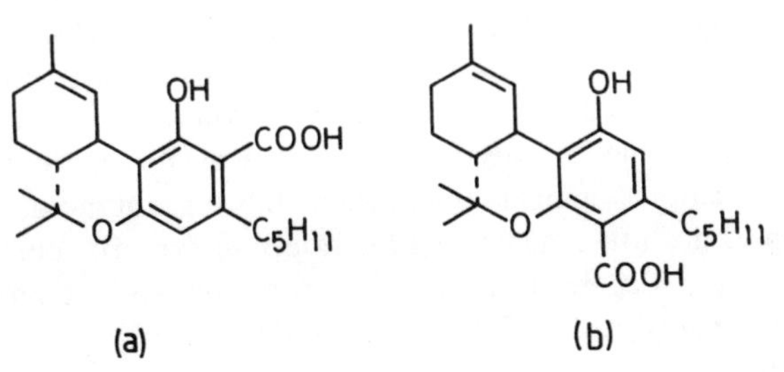

Figure 10.6 (a) Δ^1-THC acid A. (b) Δ^1-THC acid B.

for Δ^1-THC. These compounds undergo slow spontaneous decomposition at room temperature to release the neutral cannabinoids, but at the high temperatures associated with smoking, decarboxylation is rapid and complete.

Complicating the cannabinoid profile still further is a series of homologues whose relative abundance also seems to reflect the geographical origin of the plant. The first to be discovered were the propyl homologues of Δ^1-THC (Figure 10.1b), CBD (Figure 10.2b) and CBN (Figure 10.3b) (see Turner *et al.*, 1980a) and various minor cannabinoids. More recently, methyl (Figures 10.1c, 10.2c and 10.3c, cannaborcinol series; Vree *et al.*, 1972a) and *n*-butyl homologues (Figures 10.1d, 10.2d, 10.3d, Harvey, 1976) have been characterised, but the extent to which their concentrations vary with the origin of the plant is unknown.

The complexity and variability of cannabis samples poses several problems for the analyst and the solutions to these depend on the type of information sought. For forensic purposes, demonstration of the presence of one or more major cannabinoids in a suspect sample is often sufficient, whereas for botanical investigations, methods are needed which enable each of the many constituents to be separated and quantified. The correlation between cannabinoid content and geographical origin of the sample is of obvious significance for tracing the source of seized material, and again techniques capable of resolving compounds such as the propyl homologues are useful. In some cases, only small samples are available, necessitating detection at the microgram or nanogram level.

The law in the UK relating to *Cannabis* as stated in the Misuse of Drugs Act 1971 separates cannabinol and its derivatives ('tetrahydro derivatives of cannabinol and 3-alkyl homologues of cannabinol or of its tetrahydro derivatives'), which are designated 'Class A' drugs, from *cannabis* and *cannabis* resin which are listed as 'Class B'. *Cannabis*, as defined in the Criminal Law Act 1977, is '(except in the expression "*cannabis* resin") any plant of the genus *Cannabis* or any part of any such plant (by whatever name designated) except that it does not include *cannabis* resin or any of the following products after separation from the rest of the plant, namely (a) mature stalk of any such plant, (b) fibre produced from mature stalk of any such plant and (c) seed of any such plant'. *Cannabis* resin. To some extent this is reflected by the content of CBD; as all obtained from any plant of the genus *Cannabis*'. For forensic purposes, therefore, the analyst is not concerned with the strain of the plant producing the material in question but he is concerned with whether or not the material is *Cannabis* resin. To some extent this is reflected by the content of CBD, as all *Cannabis* resin samples appear to contain this cannabinoid, whereas many *Cannabis* samples do not, a negative TLC response for CBD enables the analyst to state, with a fair degree of confidence, that the suspect material does not derive from *Cannabis* resin (Baker and Phillips, 1983). The converse is, of course, not true.

Baker and Phillips (1983) in their recent review on the forensic analysis of drugs of abuse, state that for forensic purposes, analysis can be divided into four operations: (1) screening for the presence of *Cannabis* products, (2) identification of the products, (3) quantitation of the products and (4) quantitation of specific cannabinoids. The complexity of the analysis generally increases from (1) to (4) and thus (4) is rarely used. Much of the analysis classified under (1) is simple and can be performed 'in-field', but the simplicity of many such tests often produces erroneous results, necessitating confirmatory laboratory investigations which preferably employ an independent technique. Baker and Phillips (1983) in fact state that in their opinion 'criminal prosecutions relating to *Cannabis* products where the only evidence is a positive field test are dangerous and should not be pursued'. On the other hand, a combination of simple tests generally gives unambiguous identification of the material under test and is both quicker and cheaper than the more complex but highly specific techniques such as mass spectrometry which, if available, are reserved for confirmatory purposes only.

The most widely used of the more simple tests are usually based on a microscopic examination of the cystolith hairs (Nakamura, 1969) which are particularly characteristic (Stearn, 1970), on simple colour reactions, or on thin-layer chromatographic (TLC) examination of extracts of the material. Although it has been estimated that a trained microscopist can provide unequivocal identification of a botanical specimen of *Cannabis* (Stearn, 1970), the majority of forensic samples have undergone gross distortion to the original plant morphology, thus disguising many of the characteristic features. In these cases, colour reactions or chromatographic examination are mandatory. An elegant combination of microscopic examination and a colour reaction involving staining of the cystolith hairs with Fast Blue B (3, 3′-dimethoxybiphenyl-4, 4′-*bis*-diazonium chloride) (Segelman, 1973; Segelman *et al.*, 1973) has recently been reported to give greatly improved selectivity over direct microscopy.

In a typical examination of suspect material, three tests are generally employed, namely microscopic examination for the detection of cystolith hairs, a colour test, usually a modified Duquenois–Levine test (see below), and examination of an extract by TLC. Coutts and Jones (1979) have confirmed the validity of this three-parameter approach by comparative analysis of 100 samples using gas–liquid chromatography (GLC, PC-3210 and Ultrabond columns) and combined gas chromatography–mass spectrometry (GC–MS). It was concluded that the identification of Δ^1-THC and one other, unspecified, cannabinoid was sufficient to establish a *Cannabis* preparation as the source of the suspect material. Liu *et al.* (1979) have claimed that mass spectrometry using direct probe introduction and multiple regression analysis gives sufficient specificity for use with out any additional test.

With more detailed analysis it is possible to obtain considerable information on the age and geographical origin of a sample. Aged samples have low levels of cannabinoid acids and high levels of CBN. Geographical origin is reflected to a large extent in the proportion of propyl homologues but more importantly (De Faubert Maunder, 1976) in the relative amount of CBD. Even the more simple procedures, however, can give considerable information on this point. Baker *et al.* (1980a), for example, after examination of a large number of samples, have concluded that careful visual inspection and comparative TLC can enable the analyst to offer an opinion as to the geographical origin of most samples. Although techniques such as TLC can give considerable detail on many aspects relating to geographical origin (Baker *et al.*, 1980a), the complexity of many samples dictates the use of more selective techniques such as GLC. For a meaningful analysis using any of these techniques, care must be exercised in the treatment of material as conditions such as drying time and temperature have been reported to affect cannabinoid content (Coffman and Genter, 1974).

Analytical requirements for the detection of cannabis use and for investigations of metabolism and pharmacokinetics are very different on account of the low concentrations of drug usually encountered in body fluids and tissues. In general, only the most sensitive techniques, usually based on electron-capture GLC, GC-MS or radioimmunoassay (RIA), are appropriate. Many of the available methods have been included in the proceedings of three recent symposia (Willette, 1976; Vinson, 1979; Hawks, 1982). The low drug-concentrations in blood are the result of both the high psychoactivity and the high lipophilicity of the drug, the latter property resulting in considerable uptake of the drug into tissues, particularly fat (Kreuz and Axelrod, 1973). Typical concentrations of Δ^1-THC in blood during intoxication are in the low-ng ml^{-1} range and these rapidly fall to the pg ml^{-1} range within a few hours of drug ingestion. These levels are too low to be measured by most existing techniques and even today, early 1984, the half-life of Δ^1-THC in humans is not known with certainty. Estimates of 56 hours for nonusers and 28 hours for users have been obtained by Lemberger *et al.* (1970) using radiolabelled THC, and values of 33.2 ± 4.7 and 27.7 ± 4 hours for male and female subjects respectively have been found by Wall and Perez-Reyes (1981) using GC-MS after intravenous injection of the drug. It is not certain from these studies if the elimination phase of the plasma concentration–time curve had been reached, thus giving an underestimation of even impossible to use a single measurement of plasma drug concentration to predict presumptive intoxication at a given time. This is unlike the case of alcohol, which is cleared from the body rapidly and for which blood levels can readily be used to determine intoxication.

Accumulation of Δ^1-THC in tissues produces elevated plasma levels of the drug for some time (days or even weeks) after ingestion ceases. Plasma concentrations of Δ^1-THC in chronic users will therefore be much higher after a given dose than those measured in the blood of infrequent users, making it difficult or even impossible to use a single measurement of plasma concentration to predict presumptive intoxication at a given time. This is unlike the case of alcohol, which is cleared from the body rapidly and for which blood levels can readily be used to determine intoxication.

Analysis of the drug in other biological media may prove to be a better basis for a reliable forensic test. For example, although Δ^1-THC does not appear to cross the blood–saliva barrier, it can be detected in saliva and breath for several hours after smoking, probably as the result of the slow release of the drug sequestered in the mouth or lungs. As the drug is cleared from these sites much more rapidly than from the plasma, saliva or breath analysis may be a better method for the determination of recent drug use than analysis of blood. Hackel (1972) has detected cannabinoids in saliva by TLC for up to an hour after cannabis smoking and Just *et al.* (1972, 1974) have reported detection for up to two hours using a two-dimensional TLC system and mass spectrometry. Candela and Marino (1979), using TLC and GLC, report a positive reaction for up to four hours in this medium and for up to 12 hours in finger washings from people smoking or handling cannabis. Dental deposits have also been used (Noirfalise and Lambert, 1978) to yield samples for TLC analysis and Grlic (1974) has concluded after an extensive review of the literature that dental deposits and finger washings are the only practical media to use for the detection of cannabis use. Expired air contains residual cannabinoids for some time after smoking, as shown by Hauck and Moll (1974), who detected Δ^1-THC and CBD for 8 and 14 minutes respectively in the breath of a user after termination of smoking; and by McCarthy and Van Zyl (1972) who were able to detect the drug for up to two hours.

Another aspect of the analysis of cannabinoids in body fluids and tissues relates to metabolism. This is rapid and extensive (Harvey *et al.*, 1979), with some 100 metabolites of Δ^1-THC having so far been identified in a number of species (Figure 10.7). Several of these metabolites show pharmacological activities comparable with Δ^1-THC itself. The major site of biotransformation is at

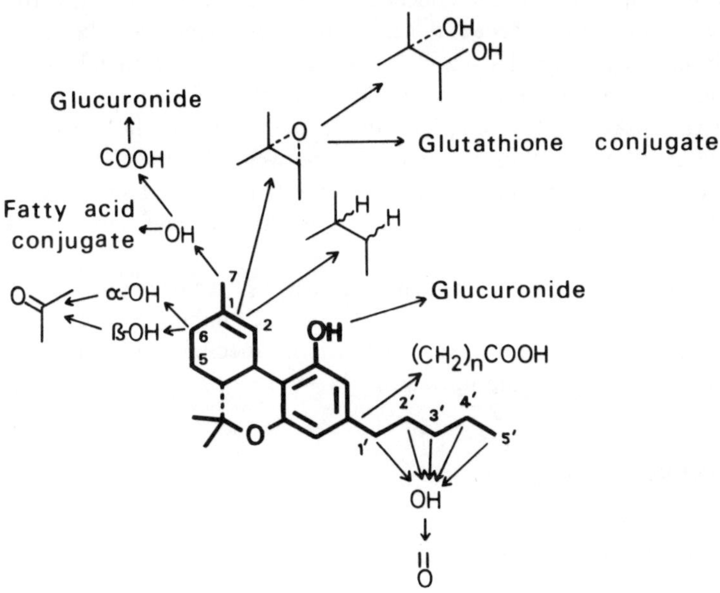

Figure 10.7 Summary of the metabolic pathways shown by Δ^1-THC.

C-7 to produce initially 7-hydroxy-Δ^1-THC (Figure 10.8a). This compound is oxidised to Δ^1-THC-7-oic acid (Figure 10.8b) via the aldehyde and is conjugated, mainly through the acid group, with glucuronic acid to produce the major urinary excretion product in man (Williams and Moffat, 1980). Hydroxylation

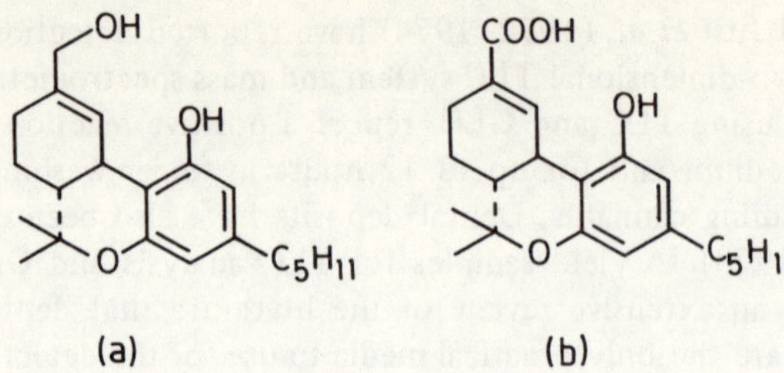

Figure 10.8 (a) 7-hydroxy-Δ^1-THC. (b) Δ^1-THC-7-oic acid.

and oxidation occur at other positions, particularly at C-6 and in the side chain, and polysubstituted metabolites in various oxidation states are common. Excreted materal is almost entirely in the form of metabolites, with the faeces being the preferred route for elimination in most species except the rabbit. In urine, only a minute amount of unchanged Δ^1-THC is present; Hollister *et al*. (1974) have measured this to be 0.01–0.005% of the administered dose, and this was detectable for only a few hours after drug administration. In blood, although Δ^1-THC levels initially fall rapidly, the concentrations of Δ^1-THC-7-oic acid rise for the first hour, when they exceed the Δ^1-THC levels. Thus, for the detection of cannabis use using blood or urine, the measurement of metabolite levels is often more appropriate and sensitive than detection of the natural cannabinoids themselves. However, the long half-life of the drug and the consequent slow excretion result in little or no correlation between urinary and faecal levels of the metabolites and the time of cannabis use. Other cannabinoids such as CBD and CBN appear to be metabolised along similar pathways and to show similar pharmacokinetics.

Several general reviews of cannabinoid analysis have been published in recent years (Willinsky, 1973; Mechoulam *et al*., 1976; Crombie, 1976; Harvey, 1981a; Fishbein, 1982; Gough and Baker, 1982). More specific reviews are listed in the following sections where appropriate.

10.2 GENERAL FEATURES

10.2.1 Stability of the cannabinoids

Several of the natural cannabinoids have been reported to be unstable to varying degrees. Analyses should thus be conducted under conditions which minimise decomposition and the results should be interpreted so as to allow for any derived artefacts.

CBN is the main decomposition product of aged samples of Δ^1-THC and appears to be produced through oxidation (Turner and Elsohly, 1979) involving free radicals (Miller *et al.*, 1982). Disproportionation into CBN and hexahydrocannabinol has also been reported (Garrett and Tsau, 1974). Acidic cannabinoids are less stable and decompose even in the dark (Smith and Vaughan, 1977). Exposure of neutral cannabinoids to light causes considerable decomposition (Turner and Henry, 1975; Fairbairn *et al.*, 1976), and is responsible for much loss of pharmacological activity in old resin and plant samples. Under acidic conditions, but above pH 4, Δ^1-THC isomerises to Δ^6-THC (Figure 10.9a) with an equilibrium favouring the Δ^6-isomer by 97% : 3%. 9-Hydroxyhexahydrocannabinol is also found in this pH range and Garrett *et al.* (1978) have proposed a mechanism involving formation of the tertiary carbonium ion (Figure 10.9b). Below pH 4 the oxygen in the pyran ring is protonated, causing ring

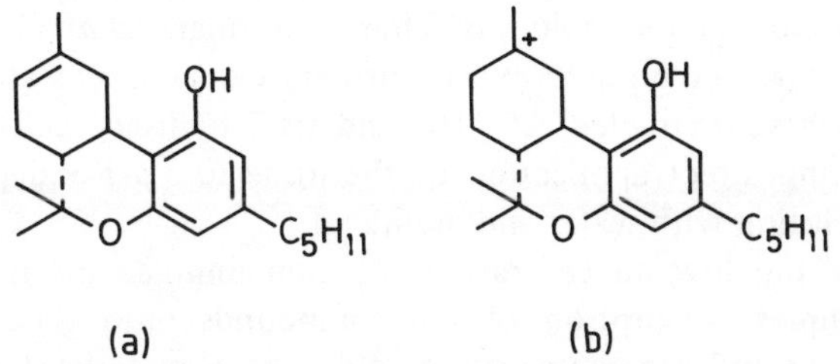

Figure 10.9 (a) Δ^6-THC. (b) Tertiary carbonium ion of Δ^6-THC.

cleavage and the formation of various substituted CBDs (Garrett and Tsau, 1974; Garrett *et al.*, 1978). Various solvents, particularly chloroform (Turner and Henry, 1975), also catalyse decomposition of a number of cannabinoids, CBD being particularly susceptible (Parker *et al.*, 1974).

Although Δ^1-THC appears to be reasonably stable in blood, Wong *et al.* (1982) have reported that measured levels of the drug in stored samples drop suddenly after about 17 weeks. This, however, was attributed to decomposition of bound proteins rather than to initial decomposition of the drug itself.

10.2.2 Extraction of the cannabinoids

Most organic solvents can be used to extract cannabinoids from plant and resin samples. Light petroleum has been reported to extract 98 to 99% of the THC present in cannabis samples following double extraction (Fairbairn and Liebman, 1973) and is reasonably selective; solvents such as ethanol additionally remove much more noncannabinoid material. Ethyl acetate is an excellent solvent for all the cannabinoids and their metabolites and is also nontoxic. Chloroform is also very efficient (Turner *et al.*, 1973; Fairbairn and Liebman, 1973) but is toxic, causes some decomposition, and should be avoided if possible.

Extraction of natural cannabinoids from body fluids has traditionally been accomplished with Brodie's solvent (1.5% isoamyl alcohol (3-methylbutan-1-ol) in hexane); but in recent publications (Rosenthal *et al.*, 1978; Foltz *et al.*, 1979; Harvey *et al.*, 1980) it has been shown that hexane alone extracts natural cannabinoids very efficiently and gives extracts which in some cases are clean enough for direct analysis by gas-phase techniques. Hexane also extracts monohydroxy metabolites to a limited extent. Ether, a more polar solvent, extracts many more metabolites (Kanter *et al.*, 1974a) and has been shown to extract acids and conjugates of neutral metabolites and weakly polar acids from urine (Kanter *et al.*, 1982a). Ethyl acetate can be used to extract a wide range of metabolites and their conjugates from both fluids and tissues (Harvey *et al.*, 1977).

Extractions have also been performed using direct application of body fluids to various chromatography columns. Thus Scherrmann *et al.* (1980) have used a diatomaceous earth column to extract urinary cannabinoids at pH 3 and Foltz *et al.* (1979) have extracted Δ^1-THC and its 7-hydroxy and acid metabolite from urine using direct application of the urine to a μ-Bondapak-C_{18} column and gradient elution with water and methanol.

Because of the low concentrations of cannabinoids often encountered in biological samples, adsorption of the compounds onto glassware is often a significant factor and can cause considerable loss of material (Garrett and Hunt, 1974). The best method to prevent this appears to be silanisation of all glassware (Garrett and Hunt, 1976).

As an alternative to solvent extraction of cannabinoids from plant or resin samples prior to detection by techniques such as TLC, several methods involving heat treatment have been reported for recovery of cannabinoids. Although these cause decarboxylation of cannabinoid acids, the resulting increase in the proportion of neutral cannabinoids can give rise to increased sensitivity. For example, Chiesa *et al.* (1973) have heated samples of marihuana in sealed glass cartridges for 2 minutes at 250 °C and detected cannabinoids in the volatile fraction using silica gel–TLC, and Martone and Della Casa (1975) have reported improved TLC detection following combustion of samples in tinfoil tubes and extraction of the condensed vapour with petroleum ether.

10.3 SPECIFIC ANALYTICAL TECHNIQUES

10.3.1 Colour tests

Of the many colour tests developed for the detection of cannabinoids in plant and resin samples, those developed by Beam (1911), Chamrawy (1937) and Duquenois and Moustapha (1938) (see Willinsky, 1973; Crombie, 1976) have received particular attention. The Beam test is relatively specific and relies on the oxidation by air and a 5% ethanolic solution of potassium hydroxide of the diphenolic cannabinoids CBD and CBG to quinones (Figure 10.10) the anions of which are violet (Mechoulam *et al.*, 1968). Weak positive reactions are also

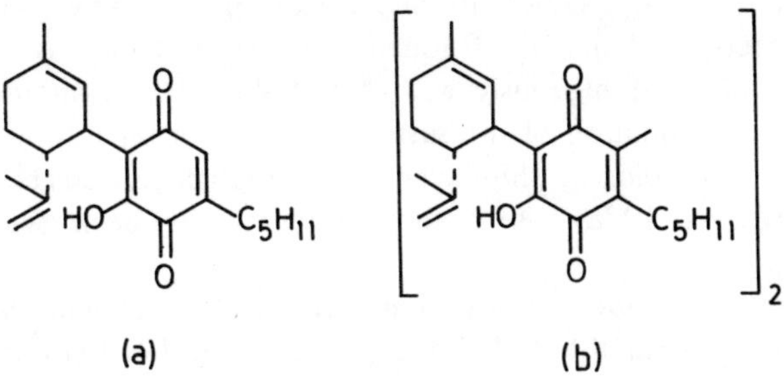

Figure 10.10

given by *Salvia officinalis* and *Rosmarinus oficinalis* and interference by extracts of tobacco have also been reported (Nickolls, 1936). As the test relies on the presence of one of the diphenolic cannabinoids and not Δ^1-THC, false negatives may arise from samples lacking these cannabinoids.

A violet colour is also a positive result in the Duquenois test in which a petroleum–ether extract of the suspect material is evaporated to dryness and the residue treated with vanillin, acetaldehyde, ethanol and concentrated hydrochloric acid. The colour develops through green and blue over about 10 minutes. Although reported to be less specific than the Beam test, the Duquenois test is more sensitive and has been improved by Levine (Butler, 1962), who recommends shaking the mixture with chloroform to extract the compounds producing the purple colour if this is derived from a cannabinoid. The chemical basis for the test is unclear. A resorcinol structure appears to be necessary for a positive reaction but is not the sole prerequisite (Pitt *et al.*, 1972). The coloured species are believed to be produced by the action of concentrated acids on intermediates of the type shown in Figure 10.11 (see Willinsky, 1973). False positives have been reported for several Indian essential oils including patchouli, clove, river tea tree and spearmint oils (Goutam and Agnihotri, 1981), and for coffee

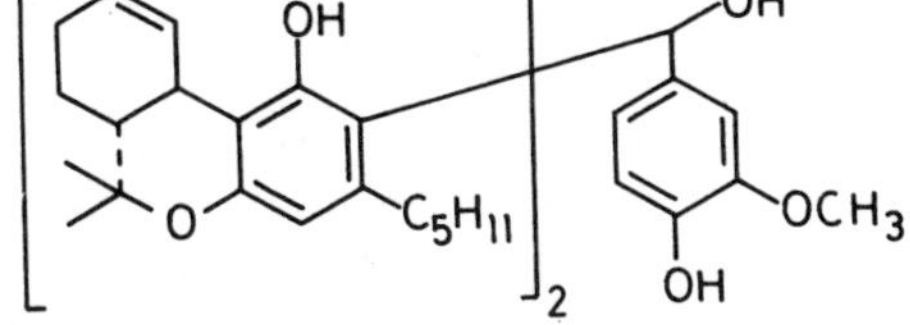

Figure 10.11

(Fochtman and Winek, 1971; Lau-Cam, 1978). To overcome the interference by coffee the Meta-Duquenois test (De Faubert Maunder, 1969a), in which metaldehyde is used in place of the acetaldehyde, has been further modified by the addition of *p*-dioxane. This produces a stable blue-violet colour, extractable with chloroform and not subject to false positive reactions by coffee. It seems to be generally recognised that the Duquenois-Levine test alone is not sufficient to identify cannabis unambiguously and that it should be combined with either morphological examination of the suspect material or separation and identification of the cannabinoids by thin-layer chromatography (TLC) (Pitt *et al*., 1972; Hughes and Warner, 1978). Use of the test has recently been reviewed by Bailey (1979).

Another recently modified test (Lau-Cam and McDonnell, 1978) is the furfural test developed in the 1940s and published in 1970 (Fulton, 1970). For this, a petroleum-ether extract of the material is treated with ethanol, furfural and hydrochloric acid. This is dried and treated with ethanolic sulphuric acid to give a purple-red residue which dissolves on swirling. In the modified test, chloroform is added and the mixture is shaken vigorously. A positive reaction is the appearance of purple-red layers of different intensity. Although this test is stated to be more sensitive than the Duquenois-Levine test, it is not as specific as the Beam test and is subject to false positives by anethole and thymol.

Included in a number of other recent tests is one (Tewari and Sharma, 1979) involving a reaction with *p*-aminophenol which is claimed to distinguish between different cannabis preparations. Thus, following reaction with the chromogen, bhang, ganja and charas gave stable green, blue, and pink-violet colours respectively.

Possibly the most specific colour reaction, and the one preferred for TLC work, involves the reaction of the cannabinoids with an alkaline solution of Fast Blue B (De Faubert Maunder, 1969b). Colour differentiation between the cannabinoids is obtained; thus Δ^1-THC gives scarlet, CBN gives violet and CBD gives orange. The colours are retained by the homologous cannabinoids and by the acids (Crombie and Crombie, 1975). Colour differences are also produced by some metabolities of Δ^1-THC. Thus introduction of hydroxylation at C-6α or C-7 produces a slight bathochromic shift towards red-violet and the introduction of a ketone function at C-6 gives a more pronounced shift towards violet. No change is observed with hydroxylation at C-6β, C-3$''$, C-4$''$ (Binder and Meisenberg, 1978). The reagent is very sensitive and allows the cannabinoids to be detected to the 10 to 50 ng level (Korte and Sieper, 1964), compared with the 0.5 to 1 μg range achieved by other reagents. A few plants such as nutmeg (*Myristica fragrans* Houtt) have been reported to give false positive reactions, but by combining this colour reaction with a simple chromatographic separation using either columns (Lau-Cam and Pizzitola, 1979) or thin-layer plates, very specific tests can be produced. For example, out of 562 samples from 427 plant species recently examined by TLC, coupled with detection by Fast Blue B and preheating the sample with chloral hydrate (the 'Rutgers Identification for

Marihuana' or 'RIM' test; Segelman and Segelman, 1976), only cannabis gave a positive result. The sensitivity of detection achieved with Fast Blue B is such that it has been used in a breath test to detect cannabis use for up to two hours after smoking (McCarthy and van Zyl, 1972). The suspect is required to blow into a filter-paper or tissue bag freshly dampened with an aqueous solution of Fast Blue B. An orange–pink colour is obtained up to 15 minutes after smoking and the test is still positive for two hours, although colour development is sometimes slow. False positives are obtained with certain brands of South African toasted tobacco, and the test is not quantitative.

Caution should be exercised in the use of Fast Blue B, as it is suspected of being a carcinogen. An alternative dye, Fast Blue BB (4-benzoylamino-2, 5-diethoxybenzene diazonium chloride) has thus been proposed (De Faubert Maunder, 1974a) but this dye is not as stable as Fast Blue B and only fresh solutions should be used (Hughes and Kessler, 1979). Because of its toxic properties, Fast Blue B has recently been applied to TLC plates before addition of the cannabinoids and development, in order to avoid spraying. It was found that under these conditions each cannabinoid gave several spots, corresponding either to different reaction products or to the possibility that the dye was not homogeneous (Pranitis and Kornfield, 1982). The dyes Fast Corinth 5 and 1-diazo-4-benzoylamino-2,5-diethoxybenzene have also been reported to have the same specificity as Fast Blue B (De Faubert Maunder, 1974b).

10.3.2 Use of fluorescent derivatives

Methods for improving sensitivity in the more simple assays usually involve the production of fluorescent derivatives or adducts. Heating of the sample has been reported to produce fluorescence at 420 nm (excitation at 370 nm) (Dionyssiou-Asteriou and Miras, 1974) and a fluorescent derivative can also be produced by irradiation with u.v. light (Twitchett *et al.*, 1978). De Clercq *et al.* (1973) have induced fluorescence by dissolving petroleum-ether extracts of the plant or resin in sulphuric acid, heating briefly on a water-bath and treating the resulting mixture with ammonia. Dansyl (5-dimethylaminonaphthyl-1-sulphonate A, Table 10.1) derivatives produce an intense fluorescence and have been used in combination with both TLC (Just *et al.*, 1972; Friedrich-Fiechtl *et al.*, 1973; Forrest *et al.*, 1971; Scherrmann *et al.*, 1977; Nojima and Shoyama, 1980) and HPLC systems (Abbott *et al.*, 1975; Johnson *et al.*, 1977). Melikian and Forrest (1973) have studied the physical properties of these derivatives and have found a slow change in their TLC characteristics after exposure to u.v. light at 350 or 254 nm and have reported that they are unstable in ethanol. Fluorescence has also been produced by conversion of the cannabinoids into *o*,*o*'-dihydroxyazo compounds which form chelates with gallium. Fluorescence in these experiments was measured at 595 nm after excitation at 515 nm (Bourdon, 1976) and less than 30 ng ml^{-1} of the cannabinoids could be measured in urine.

Table 10.1 Derivatives used for the analysis of Δ^1-THC

No.	Structure	Name
A	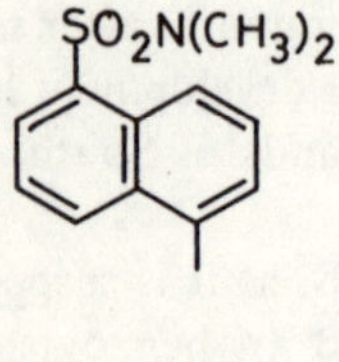	Dansyl
B	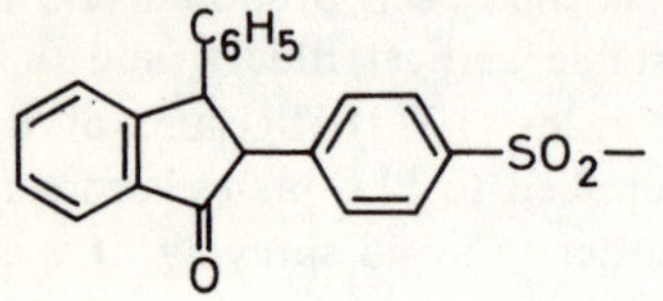	
C	$-PO(OC_2H_5)_2$	diethylphosphate
D	$-Si(CH_3)_2$-*tert*-C_4H_9	*tert*-butyldimethylsilyl (TBDMS)
E	$-COCH_2-OSi(CH_3)_3$	trimethylsilylacetyl
F	$-Si(CH_3)_3$	trimethylsilyl (TMS)
G	$-Si(C_2H_5)_3$	triethylsilyl
H	$-Si(C_3H_7)_3$	tripropylsilyl
I	$-Si(C_4H_9)_3$	tri-*n*-butylsilyl
J	$-COCH_2Cl$	chloracetyl
K	$-COC_6H_5$	pentafluorobenzoyl (PFB)
L	$-COCF_3$	trifluoroacetyl (TFA)
M	$-COC_2F_5$	pentafluoropropionyl (PFP)
N	$-COC_3F_7$	heptafluorobutyryl (HFB)
O	$-CH_2C_6F_5$	pentafluorobenzyl
P	$-COC_6H_4CF_3$	*p*-trifluoromethylbenzyl
Q	$-Si(CH_3)_2CH_2Cl$	chloromethyldimethylsilyl (CMDMS)
R	$-Si(CH_3)_2CH_2-CH=CH_2$	allyldimethylsilyl
S	$-COCH_3$	acetyl
T	$-C^2H_3$	trideuteromethyl
U	$-CH_3$	methyl
V	$-C_2H_5$	ethyl

10.3.3 Paper and thin-layer chromatographic methods

10.3.3.1 Paper chromatography

Paper-chromatographic methods have largely been superseded by thin-layer methods, but several paper-based systems were investigated in the early 1960s. De Ropp (1960) isolated 8 compounds including Δ^1-THC from the phenolic fraction of cannabis in 1960 and Korte and Sieper (1960) identified Δ^1-THC in the same year using paper impregnated with silicone resin. Kolsek *et al.* (1962) separated several Fast Blue B-positive compounds from both acid and phenol fractions of *cannabis* using paper impregnated with dimethylformamide but the compounds were not identified. Separation of THC, CBD and CBN has been achieved on Dowex silicone paper by Schultz and Mohrmann (1962) using solvent mixtures of toluene, methanol and water.

10.3.3.2 Separation of natural cannabinoids

Separation of cannabinoids by TLC is difficult because of the close similarity in structure between the different compounds. Much of the earlier work has been reviewed (Parker and Fiske, 1972; Willinsky, 1973; Crombie, 1976; Mechoulam *et al.*, 1976; Gough and Baker, 1982). Although alumina has been used (Tewari *et al.*, 1974), silica gel is the most widely used absorbent together with, in the simplest situation, single or mixed solvents of low polarity. Separation of individual compounds, and particularly of the propyl homologues, is often poor under these conditions, but has been considerably improved by the addition of a base to either the solvent or plate, or by the impregnation of the plate with silver nitrate or a buffer. Two-dimensional chromatography also gives improved separation.

Plates impregnated with dimethylformamide were developed by Korte and Sieper (1964), Miras *et al.* (1964), Betts and Holloway, (1967) and Merkus (1971) in combination with various spray reagents of which Fast Blue B gave the most sensitive detection. Compounds of low polarity migrate fastest with cannabigerol and cannabidiolic acid remaining at the origin. Reproducible R_f-values are, however, difficult to obtain; this has been attributed to the moisture content of the dimethylformamide (Aramaki *et al.*, 1968) and to ambient humidity (Nielson, 1970). Impregnation of silica-gel sheets with either di- (Grlic, 1970) or tri-ethylamine (Vinson and Hooyman, 1975) has been reported to give good separation of the major cannabinoids and the sheets are usable several weeks after treatment. CBD runs fastest, followed by Δ^1-THC and then CBN. Both systems utilised a single solvent, toluene in the former and benzene in the latter, and thus had some advantage over systems using mixed solvents. Addition of diethylamine to the solvent has also been employed with untreated plates; thus Aramaki *et al.* (1968) separated all three major cannabinoids on silica gel using benzene–hexane–diethylamine (25 : 10 : 1). De Faubert Maunder (1970), however, has cautioned against the use of diethylamine-containing solvents on account of their tendency to cause streaking.

Impregnation of plates or silica-gel sheets with silver nitrate, which has the effect of complexing with double bonds of the cannabinoids, has been investigated by several groups as a method of separating the major cannabinoids (Hively *et al*., 1966; Caddy and Fish, 1967; Turk *et al*., 1969; Patterson and Stephens, 1970; Grlic, 1971). Either mixed- or single-solvent systems can be employed, with the migration order of the major cannabinoids generally being the reverse of that found with the tertiary-amine-treated plates. The major disadvantage appears to be the plate's instability to light which produces darkening and loss of contrast.

Many studies have been performed with unmodified plates and with the availability of highly consistent commercial plates and sheets this method is now preferred (Gough and Baker, 1982). Mixed solvents, usually consisting of hexane or another low-polarity liquid together with a small amount of a polar solvent such as ether or ethyl acetate, are the most common. Generally, cannibicyclol and THC migrate ahead of the more polar cannabinoids such as CBD or CBG, although some variation is found. Examples include the use of petroleum-ether-ether (Machata, 1969; Paris and Paris, 1973), hexane-dioxane (Parker *et al*., 1968), pentane-ether (Gaoni and Mechoulam, 1971) and pentane-dioxane (Parker and Fisk, 1972). Single solvents have also been used; thus De Faubert Maunder (1969c) has separated the major cannabinoids on silica-gel sheets using toluene and has emphasised the need for small spot-areas to prevent loss of resolution.

Cannabinoid acids often streak and do not usually migrate satisfactorily in the same solvents that are used to examine the neutral cannabinoids, and must therefore be examined separately. Thus Mechoulam *et al*. (1969) have investigated benzene-methanol-acetic acid (88 : 10 : 2) and Masoud and Doorenbos (1973) have used hexane-ether-acetic acid. Good resolutions of the three major cannabinoid acids have been achieved using the system described by Parker *et al*. (1968) with hexane-diethyl ether as the solvent (Verwey and Witte, 1972). Streaking of the acids is probably caused by polar interactions or decomposition and can be reduced by derivatisation. This technique involving the formation of methyl esters has been adopted by Krejci and Hanus (1976) to identify the three major acids, using silica gel with hexane-dioxane-methanol as the solvent.

Considerable improvement in resolution can be achieved using two-dimensional TLC. Mobarak *et al*. (1974) for example have used this technique for the separation of twenty-seven constituents of the resin and Mobarak *et al*. (1978) have used silica-gel plates developed first in pentane-diethyl ether (9 : 1) and then pentane-acetone (9 : 1) to achieve similar separations. CBD and its propyl homologue could be differentiated by the use of 2-hydrazono-2, 3-dihydro-3-methylbenzothiazole hydrochloride (HMBT) as the spray reagent. Bertulli *et al*. (1976), using silica gel with chloroform as the developing solvent, noted that CBN could not be separated from THC but that by spraying the developed plate with a mixture of dimethylformamide and carbon tetrachloride (1 : 1), and developing in the second direction with cyclohexane, separation could be achieved. Fowler *et al.* (1979) have recently developed a method in which the cannabinoids were run in one direction on unmodified silica gel using chloroform-1, 1-dichloroethane (3 : 2) and then in a second direction using xylene-1, 4-dioxane (19 : 1) after spraying the plate with diethylamine. The method separated all of the major cannabinoids together with their propyl homologues and the cannabinoid acids would be detected following thermal decarboxylation after the first development.

In addition to the Fast Blue salts, a number of other spray reagents have been used for TLC visualisation. Diazotised benzidine has been used by Krejci and Hanus (1976) and by Aramaki *et al.* (1968) but would appear to be as hazardous as Fast Blue B. HMBT, which gives brown spots, as used in the two-dimensional TLC method reported by Mobarak *et al.* (1978), is not very sensitive. It has also been investigated by Baggi (1980) as a replacement for Fast Blue B. 1-Nitroso-2-naphthol, which gives colours in the blue-violet range, has been proposed by Rao (1977) and anisaldehyde which also gives a variety of colours has been used by El-Feraly *et al.* (1977). An advantage of the latter reagent is that it gives colours with cannabinoid methyl ethers, unlike Fast Blue B, which appears to require the presence of a free phenol group. In spite of the work on alternative reagents. Fast Blue salts still appear to be the best reagents for cannabinoid detection. De Faubert Maunder (1974a) has discussed the preservation of TLC plates once the spots have been developed. Spraying the plate with diethylamine both before and after spraying the colour reagent was proposed for improving the storage properties of the plate.

10.3.3.3 Detection and measurement in physiological media

Detection and measurement of cannabinoids in biological fluids by TLC is more difficult than from plant or resin samples on account of the much lower concentrations involved and the presence of other compounds extracted from the medium. In 1973, Salaschek *et al.* (1973) examined fifty urine samples from marihuana-treated subjects and after finding cannabinoids in only four of them concluded that 'reliable detection of hashish in urine by means of the methods reported in the literature proved impossible'. Since then there has been much improvement in sensitivity and an emphasis on the detection of metabolites such as Δ^1-THC-7-oic acid (Kaistha and Tadrus, 1982; Kanter *et al.*, 1982b). In the procedure described by Kaistha and Tadrus, Gelman silica-gel–glass-fibre sheets (250 μm) were developed in chloroform–methanol–ammonium hydroxide (85 : 15 : 2) for 55 to 60 minutes. Visualisation was with Fast Blue RR which gave a pink spot and quantitation was achieved by densitometric scanning. In Kanter's procedure a silica-gel plate was used and developed first with acetone–chloroform–triethylamine (80 : 20 : 1) and then with petroleum-ether–ether–acetic acid (50 : 50 : 1.5). The spray was Fast Blue B, giving a detection limit in the 20 to 50 ng ml^{-1} range. The amount of acetic acid in the second solvent was critical; 1% caused little movement whereas 2% caused the acid to migrate into the zone containing endogenous material.

Cannabis metabolites, with their wide range of chemical structures, appear to be more easily separated by TLC than are the natural cannabinoids. Kanter *et al.* (1974b) have separated 6β-hydroxy-Δ^1-THC from the 7-hydroxy metabolite on silica gel using petroleum-ether–ether–acetic acid (50 : 50 : 1) and, by using chloroform and methanol (87 : 13) as the developing solvent, have also separated these compounds from Δ^1-THC-6β, 7-dihydroxy (Kanter *et al.*, 1975). In a further publication by these investigators (Lombrozo *et al.*, 1976) a sequential TLC system using three solvents was developed for separating nonpolar, basic and acid metabolites respectively. The first development was with petroleum-ether–ether (85 : 15) to separate nonpolar compounds; the spot was then moved to the next plate which was developed in chloroform–acetone–triethylamine (80 : 20 : 1), and finally to a third system where petroleum-ether–ether–acetic acid (50 : 50 : 1) was used to identify acidic components. Separation of several hydroxy and oxo-metabolites of Δ^1-, Δ^6-THC, CBD and CBN has been investigated (Fonseka *et al.*, 1976; Agurell *et al.*, 1976a) using silica-gel F plates developed in ether–petroleum-ether (3 : 2), as shown in Figure 10.12.

Fast Blue salts are the preferred visualising agents in much of the reported work involving TLC examination of biological fluids but, as noted above, increased sensitivity has been achieved by use of fluorescent derivatives. Vinson

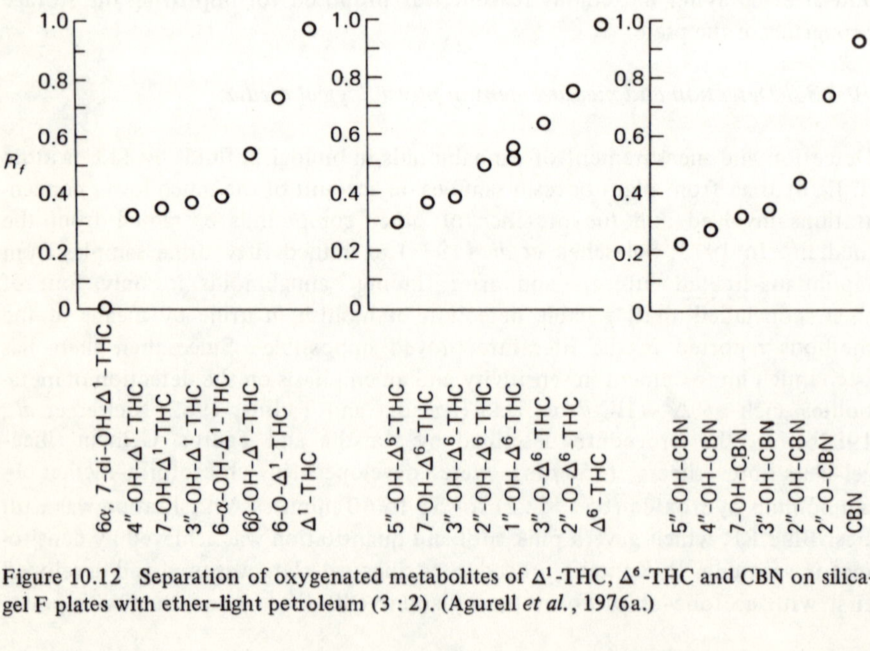

Figure 10.12 Separation of oxygenated metabolites of Δ^1-THC, Δ^6-THC and CBN on silica-gel F plates with ether–light petroleum (3 : 2). (Agurell *et al.*, 1976a.)

et al. (1977) have developed a method in which THC extracted from serum was derivatised with 2-*p*-chlorosulphonylphenyl-3-phenylindone to give the derivative B (Table 10.1) prior to TLC. The developed plate was sprayed with an alkoxide to produce the fluorescent derivative and a detection limit of 0.2 ng ml^{-1} was claimed. Dansyl derivatives appear to be the most widely used derivatives for fluorescent detection. Forrest *et al.* (1971) investigated the separation of 9 cannabinoids in 4 solvent systems using these derivatives and reported the best resolution with a mixture of cyclohexane and ethyl acetate (5 : 1), although the best detection was achieved using benzene–acetone (9 : 1). Detection limits using this derivative can be in the low-picogram range. Scherrmann *et al.* (1977), in a related method, have derivatised urinary extracts with [methyl-^{14}C] dansyl chloride prior to TLC separation. Detection of the spots was achieved by their fluorescence but quantitation was by radiodensitometric scanning using tritiated THC as the internal standard.

10.3.4 Column chromatography

In contrast to TLC, column chromatography is generally used as a preparative rather than an analytical technique and has not been exploited so extensively for examination of resin and plant samples. Silica-gel columns provide separations similar to those obtained with TLC using the same adsorbant. Thus Shoyama *et al.* (1970), using solvent mixtures of hexane–ethyl acetate ((5 : 1) : (3 : 1)), separated all of the major cannabinoids and their acids, the elution order being cannabicyclol, CBD, CBC and THC and ending with the more polar CBN and CBG. Fractions were stained with diazotised benzidine which gave colour differentiation in the orange–red–violet region. In a further study with the same solvent system the cannabinoid acids were eluted in the order, CBCy-A, THC-A, CBD-A, CBC-A and CBG-A (Shoyama *et al.*, 1972). Good separations of several minor cannabinoids have also been achieved on these columns as exemplified by isolations of (+)-cannabitriol and (−)-10-ethoxy-9-hydroxy-$\Delta^{6a(10a)}$-tetrahydrocannabinol (Elsohly *et al.*, 1977) and propyl-cannabinoids (Mole and Turner, 1974). Silica gel modified by the addition of silver nitrate has been used for separation of major cannabinoids (Turk *et al.*, 1971; Mechoulam *et al.*, 1976) and THC isomers (Razdan *et al.*, 1972). Petcoff *et al.* (1971) have published a method whereby centrifugal force was used to accelerate chromatography of cannabinoids on microparticulate silica gel. The columns were extruded after a given time and treated with Fast Blue Salt B to reveal the presence of the cannabinoids. Modification of the method by Ribi *et al.* (1973) enabled cannabinoids to be isolated in milligram quantities and resolution was claimed to be better than that achieved by GLC at that time.

Florisil has been used quite extensively for column chromatography, particularly in early studies on the isolation of the natural cannabinoids (Gaoni and Mechoulam, 1964, 1966; Davis *et al.*, 1970). Synthetic methods for Δ^1-THC invariably produce mixtures of isomers and Florisil has also found application in their separation (Razdan *et al.*, 1974) and in the isolation of metabolites (see for example Nordqvist *et al.*, 1979a, b).

Purification of cannabinoids has been achieved by gel filtration on Sephadex LH 20 using chloroform–ethyl acetate and methanol as the eluting solvents; the compounds eluted in the order CBN-C_3, THC-C_5, CBN-C_5, CBD-C_5, CBD-C_3, THC-C_3 and THC-A (Straight *et al.*, 1973). The system is interesting in that it achieves separation of propyl homologues as well as the major cannabinoids and their acids. Several examples are given in this chapter of the use of Sephadex LH 20 columns for isolating Δ^1-THC and its metabolites from biological fluids and tissues. Complex lipids such as triglycerides are eluted ahead of the cannabinoids and can thus easily be removed (Harvey *et al.*, 1977). Separation of neutral cannabinoids from their metabolites and fractionation of these into groups of varying oxidation level has been performed using chloroform as solvent (Harvey *et al.*, 1977). The behaviour of several monohydroxy metabolites of various cannabinoids on these columns has been studied and is outlined in Figure 10.13 (Fonseka *et al.*, 1976; Agurell *et al.*, 1976a).

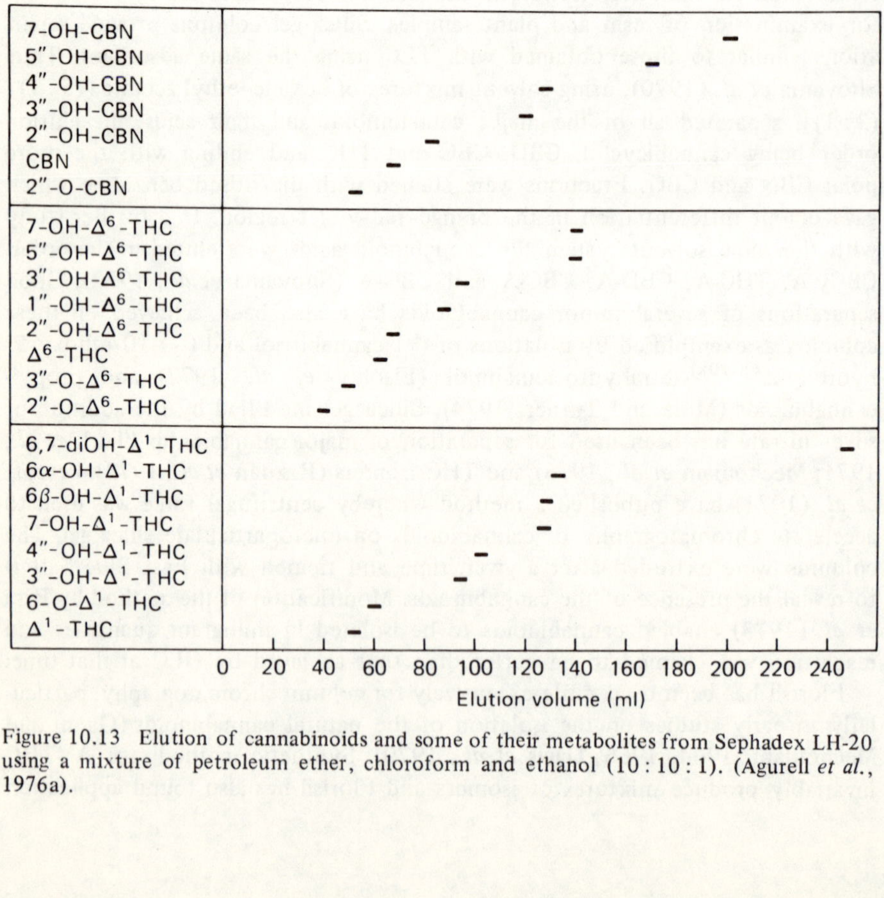

Figure 10.13 Elution of cannabinoids and some of their metabolites from Sephadex LH-20 using a mixture of petroleum ether, chloroform and ethanol (10 : 10 : 1). (Agurell *et al.*, 1976a).

A chromatographic system involving Amberlite XAD-2 has recently been reported for separating both neutral and acidic cannabinoids and for fractionation of the latter compounds using a different solvent system (Hendricks *et al.*, 1981). The method was reported not to catalyse decarboxylation of the acids as has been reported with other systems and it was able to produce good separation of the major cannabinoids from their propyl homologues. Acids and neutrals were separated using graded elution with 0.5M tris buffer in 30% ethanol at pH 10 with the ethanol content rising to 70%, and neutral cannabinoids were fractionated using graded elution with 0.5M lithium chloride in 60 to 90% ethanol.

10.3.5 High-pressure liquid chromatography (HPLC)

10.3.5.1 Natural cannabinoids

Extension of column chromatography into the analytical field has been made possible by the advent of HPLC. Separations are comparable to those achieved by packed-column gas–liquid chromatography (GLC) but the technique has not been used to the same extent as GLC as it would appear to offer no particular advantage except perhaps for the separation of the cannabinoid acids; these must be derivatised for examination by gas-phase methods. Both reversed- and normal-phase systems are in use with detection usually being by u.v. absorption.

An early reversed-phase system is that of Wheals and Smith (1975) in which the column was prepared by reacting microparticulate silica with octadecyltrichlorosilane. Methanol containing 0.02N sulphuric acid (4 : 1) was used as the eluting solvent and u.v. detection was at 254 nm. Eight major peaks were observed and identified later by GC–MS as CBD, CBD-A, CBN, Δ^9-THC, CBC, CBN-A, Δ^9-THC-A and CBC-A (Smith, 1975). Quantitative analysis of these compounds was achieved with the same system in the following year (Smith and Vaughan, 1976). Precision was between 2 and 3%, except for CBN which was 4 to 6%, and it was noted that recording at a wavelength of 220 nm gave a better response for CBN than the signal at 254 nm.

In a recent modification to the original system, Turner and Mahlberg (1982) have noted that the cannabinoid acids can be separated from the neutral cannabinoids by changing the pH of the eluting solvent from 2.7 to 6.0. An Altex octadecylsilyl reversed-phase column was used with a gradient elution employing acetonitrile and water as the solvents. At pH 6.0 the acids were eluted ahead of the neutral cannabinoids.

Baker *et al.* (1980b) have described a system based on a spherisorb S5ODS column with methanol–acetonitrile–sulphuric acid (8 : 9 : 7) as the elutant and u.v. detection at 220 nm. All the major cannabinoids and cannabinoid acids, including several propyl homologues, were separated, although not all peaks were completely resolved. Spherisorb S5 has also been used by Kanter *et al.*

(1978, 1979) for quantitative measurements of Δ^1-THC, but in this case the column was run in the normal-phase mode with hexane–3% methanol in dichloromethane (97 : 3) as the solvent. Detection was by u.v. absorption at 215 nm. Other systems include the use of a Lichrosorb RP-18 column with methanol–0.02 N sulphuric acid (4 : 1) to separate the major cannabinoid acids (Yotoriyama *et al.*, 1980), a system using 5% THF in hexane to separate Δ^1 from Δ^6-THC (Garrett and Hunt, 1977b) and the use of a μ-Bondapak-C_{18} column with methanol–water as the solvent to achieve a similar separation (Knaus *et al.*, 1976). Diethyl phosphate (C, Table 10.1) and various silyl derivatives (D, E) were investigated in the latter study in order to reduce possible losses through oxidation and isomerisation. However, most authors find no evidence of decomposition with the reported systems.

10.3.5.2 Cannabinoids and metabolites in physiological media

Low sensitivity has generally limited the use of HPLC assays for cannabinoids in biological fluids using ultraviolet detection, but several assays have been reported in which HPLC separations have been followed by more sensitive detection methods such as radioimmunoassay or GC–MS. U.V. detection at shorter wavelengths to increase sensitivity has been used by Valentine *et al.* (1979a) to detect Δ^1-THC and its acid metabolite to 2 ng ml^{-1} in plasma. Using the same wavelength, Valentine and Psaltis (1979) detected CBN as a fluorescent derivative produced by u.v. irradiation to 1 ng ml^{-1} in saliva. Kanter *et al.* (1978) have found that 220 nm gave the best sensitivity for Δ^1-THC and its metabolites in urine. The compounds were isolated by TLC and separated by HPLC using a 250 x 3 mm column of Spherisorb with hexane–methanol (3%) and dichloromethane (97 : 3) as the solvent. The system gave good separation of THC, CBD and CBN. In another technique (Borys and Karler, 1981), for the measurement of cannabinoids in tissues and plasma, a reversed-phase system was used followed by an on-line post-column derivatisation technique with Fast Blue B and spectrophotometric detection at 490 nm. Sensitivity was reported to be better than 50 ng. Detection to the low-picogram range has been reported for Δ^6-THC and its 7-hydroxy metabolite using fluorescence detection of their dansyl derivatives (A, Table 10.1) (Abbott *et al.*, 1975). Twitchett *et al.* (1978) have used post-column u.v. irradiation of the effluent to give a u.v.-absorbing derivative capable of detecting 1 ng of CBN. An electrochemical detector was used by Masoud and Wingard (1979) in combination with a Lichrosorb RP 18 silica column to separate CBD, Δ^6- and Δ^1-THC. The solvent was methanol–0.05 M phosphoric acid and the detection limit was 2 ng of Δ^1-THC.

10.3.6 Gas–liquid chromatography

10.3.6.1 Natural cannabinoids

1. Qualitative aspects The most versitile methods for cannabinoid analysis are based on GLC and GC–MS. The techniques yield both quantitative and qualitative information and all major and minor cannabinoids can be separated with a suitable choice of column. For forensic detection, it has been argued that GLC offers little over TLC and with flame-ionisation detection it is less sensitive (Gough and Baker, 1982); however, for detailed analysis of cannabinoid profiles, gas-phase methods provide much more information, particularly on the nature of minor compounds.

Many stationary phases have been used for packed-column GLC separations and much of the early work has been reviewed (Fish, 1974; Parker and Stembal, 1974; Crombie, 1976; Mechoulam *et al.*, 1976). More recent reviews include those of Fishbein (1982) and Gough and Baker (1982). Conventional packed columns afford separation of all of the major cannabinoids and many of the minor ones, although the cannabinoid acids require derivatisation to prevent on-column decarboxylation. The low-polarity methylsilicone phases SE-30 (De Zeeuw *et al.*, 1972; Harvey, 1976) and OV-1 (Vree *et al.*, 1972b; Hoffman and Yang, 1972) were used in much of the early work but the phenyl-methylsilicone polymer, OV-17, seems to be the phase of choice with most investigators (see for example Gaoni and Mechoulam, 1971; Fetterman *et al.*, 1971a, b; Stromberg, 1971; Rasmussen *et al.*, 1972; Bercht, *et al.*, 1973; Fairbairn and Liebman, 1973; Vree *et al.*, 1973; Waller, *et al.*, 1976; Grote and Spiteller, 1978). Better separations of Δ^1- and Δ^6-THC have been claimed for this phase (Parker and Stembal, 1974). Other phases include Apiezon L (Vree *et al.*, 1972b), Apiezon M (Martin *et al.*, 1961), Carbowax 20M (Heaysman *et al.*, 1967; Crombie and Crombie, 1975), SE-52 (Merkus, 1971), OV-7 (Willinsky and Di Simone, 1973), OV-210 (Hoffman and Yang, 1972), OV-225 (Hoffman and Yang, 1972; Crombie and Crombie, 1975), XE-60 (Schou *et al.* (1971; Vree *et al.*, 1972b) and CDMS (Patterson and Stevens, 1970). The elution order from the low-polarity silicone phases is CBD, Δ^1-THC and then CBN with the propyl homologues eluting in the same order ahead of CBD. Derivatised acids elute after CBN. Retention indices have been found to increase in equal increments with increasing side-chain length above C-3 (Bailey *et al.*, 1973). The less-polar phases such as SE-30 do not retain the cannabinoids to the same extent as the more polar phases such as OV-17 and thus enable them to be separated from long-chain *n*-hydrocarbons (C_{27} and C_{29}) which have also been reported in some cannabis extracts (De Zeeuw *et al.*, 1973). Glass columns have been recommended in preference to stainless-steel ones (Turner *et al.*, 1974), which can cause up to 30% losses. Silanisation of the steel only reduces this loss to 15% (Turner *et al.*, 1973a). Loss of material has also been reported (Hoffman and Yang, 1972) with columns containing 3% or less of either OV-1 or OV-210. However, with silanised supports and the use of a suitable derivative such as the trimethylsilyl (TMS) ether (F, Table 10.1) (Harvey *et al.*, 1980), this effect is not observed. On-column decomposition of underivatised CBD and CBG to give olivetol has recently been reported (Bailey, 1978). The effect is not observed for the cyclic cannabinoids Δ^1-THC or CBN.

Rasmussen *et al.* (1972) have described a method of GLC analysis which avoids extraction of the sample prior to chromatography. Instead, a 1 mg sample was introduced directly into the chromatograph where the cannabinoids vaporised. In a later modification an SE-30 column was used to prevent interference by alkanes (Rasmussen, 1975a) and in another the cannabinoids were converted into their TMS derivatives by injection of *bis*-(trimethylsilyl) acetamide into the chromatograph where it reacted with the cannabinoids which were cold-trapped at the top of the column (Rasmussen, 1975b). Spots removed from TLC plates have also been examined in the same way (Rasmussen and Aaro, 1977). Fairlie and Fox (1976) have used a related method to determine Δ^1-THC to an accuracy of better than 5%.

Because of the large number of cannabinoids present in many samples, capillary GLC can be used to advantage as demonstrated by Novotny *et al.*, 1976, 1982). Samples were concentrated on a pre-column and the resulting chromatograms could be used to 'fingerprint' samples of marihuana. The major cannabinoids have also been identified in the smoke from a room using a 60-m SF-96 glass capillary column. Preconcentration of the sample was achieved by passing a known volume of air through poly-*p*-2,6-diphenyloxide polymer. The use of OV 255 support-coated open tubular (SCOT) columns has been investigated by Crombie and Crombie (1975) and found to provide good separations of a wide range of cannabinoids belonging to several homologous series.

Although good separations of the major neutral cannabinoids can be achieved on most phases, superior results can usually be obtained after derivatisation, particularly as TMS ethers (Turner *et al.*, 1974); peak shapes are generally improved, tailing is reduced and much higher sensitivities can be obtained. Small changes in relative retention times introduced by the derivative frequently improve separation between cannabinoids of dissimilar structure. Thus CBD and CBC, which are difficult to separate in their underivatised state (Waller *et al.*, 1976), separate well when chromatographed as TMS (Turner and Hadley, 1973b) or as methyl ethers (Bailey and Gagne, 1975). Δ^1- and Δ^6-THC also separate better as TMS ethers than as the free alcohols (Claussen *et al.*, 1966a). The major cannabinoids, CBD, THC and CBN, are eluted in the same order both as underivatised compounds and as their TMS ethers (Figure 10.14). Higher trialkylsilyl derivatives (G–I, Table 10.1) have been used to achieve differential separations between mono- and di-hydroxylated cannabinoids because of the greater retention increment imparted to the dihydroxy compounds such as CBD and CBG by the large silyl substituents (Harvey and Paton, 1975). The cannabinoid acids must, as mentioned above, be derivatised prior to GLC assay in order to prevent thermal decarboxylation. TMS esters (Davis *et al.*, 1970;

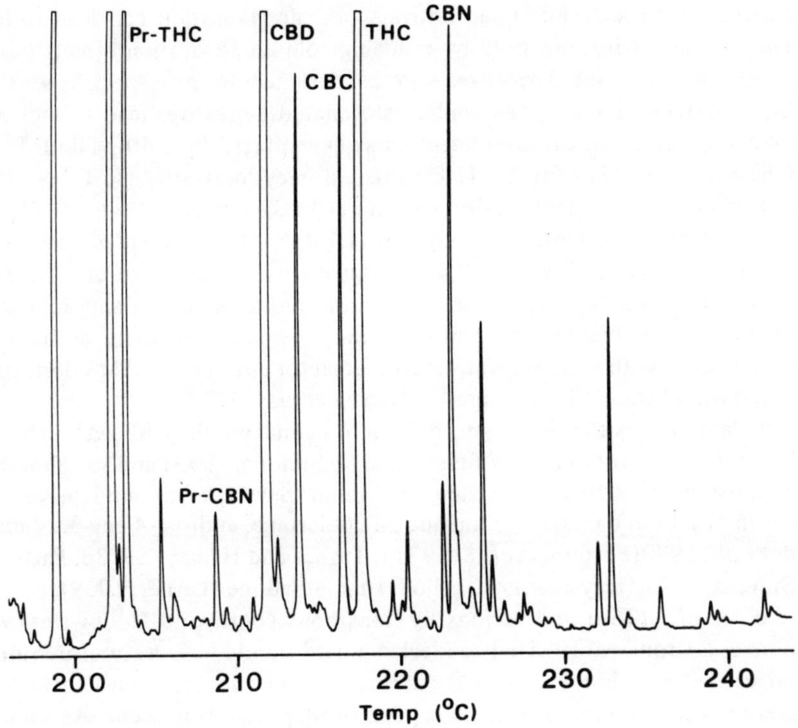

Figure 10.14 GLC separation of the TMS derivatives of cannabinoids from a sample of Pakistani cannabis (Cannabis tincture, BPC 1949) on a 30-m OV-1 support-coated open tubular column.

Fetterman *et al.*, 1971b; Turner and Hadley, 1973b; Turner *et al.*, 1974) or methyl esters prepared either by on-column methylation using trimethylanilinium hydroxide (Skinner, 1971; Bjorkman, 1982) or reaction with diazomethane (Mechoulam, 1970) have both been used successfully.

Derivatisation of cannabinoids in general has been criticised as it adds a further stage to the analysis. However, on balance, the advantages would appear to outweigh the disadvantages. Reactions are often very quick and require little more than mixing the sample and reagents. In many cases the mixture can be injected directly into the chromatograph, and with TMS derivatives this has the advantage of keeping the column and other parts of the system well silanised and thus nonpolar. Though some contamination of the flame-ionisation detector is produced, this can usually be removed quickly. Extraction of TMS derivatives of THC into, for example hexane, prior to chromatography appears to lead to some decomposition, possibly due to traces of moisture.

2. Quantitative aspects For quantitative work, derivatisation can lead to large increases in sensitivity, not only by reducing column adsorption effects but by virtue of the fact that derivatives can be designed to suit specific sensitive detection systems. Thus, for example, halogenated derivatives lead to increased response from electron-capture detectors as exemplified by a 40-pg limit found by Schou *et al.* (1971) for Δ^1-THC as its chloracyl derivative (J, Table 10.1), 5 pg of Δ^1-THC as its pentafluorobenzoate (K) (Garrett and Hunt, 1973), and 1 pg of Δ^1-THC as its heptafluorobutyrate (HFB, N) (Fenimore *et al.*, 1973). Of eight derivatives (J–Q, Table 10.1) investigated by Fenimore *et al.*, the HFB derivative gave the best response. Detection limits with a flame-ionisation detector are generally in the low-nanogram range. Greater sensitivity, as discussed later, is achieved with a mass-spectrometric detector but here the TMS derivatives have been found to be the most useful (Harvey *et al.*, 1979).

With flame-ionisation detection, the major cannabinoids, CBD, Δ^1-THC and CBN give different responses (Willinsky and Di Simone, 1973) and so calibration curves must be constructed for each compound. Several compounds have been used as internal standards; these include 5α-cholestane, androst-4-ene-3,17-dione (Davis *et al.*, 1970; Fetterman *et al.*, 1971a; Turner and Hadley, 1973b, Patterson and Stevens, 1970; Heaysman *et al.*, 1967) DL-methadone (Lerner, 1969), cocaine (Aramaki *et al.*, 1968) and various hydrocarbons (Betts and Holloway, 1967; Crombie and Crombie, 1975). The ideal standard should have a structure similar to that of the cannabinoids, so that extraction properties are equivalent, and be sufficiently separated from them that peak overlap does not occur. As some of the above compounds have substantially longer retention times than the major cannabinoids, on low-polarity phases in particular, more rapid analysis can be achieved under temperature-programmed conditions but at the expense of some precision. The steroid androst-4-ene-3,17-dione seems to have found the widest application, as it is well separated from the cannabinoids. Although it has been used both for underivatised samples and TMS ethers, some caution should be exercised with the latter method because of the possibility of TMS-enol formation. With underivatised samples a precision of 1.4% was obtained by Fetterman *et al.* (1971a) with this standard. External standards generally give less-precise assays, for example 13% reported by Lerner (1969), although Chiesa *et al.* (1973b) have reported a precision of 2.9% with Δ^1-THC as the external standard.

10.3.6.2 Measurements in physiological media

As with most chromatographic methods for cannabinoid quantitation, the sensitivity achieved with GLC for measurements of Δ^1-THC in body fluids and tissues is limited by the signal-to-noise ratio achieved at the chromatographic detector. Although detection limits in the low-picogram range are readily attainable with sensitive detectors when pure compounds are measured, the 'biological noise' arising from coextracted lipids severely reduces the sensitivity in the 'real' situation. Reductions in the order of a thousand fold are not uncommon. Consequently, most assays employing GLC and GC–MS contain at least one clean-up stage between the extraction of the cannabinoids from the biological matrix and their ultimate measurement. This, of course, considerably lengthens the analysis time and cost and in some cases tends to reduce the usefulness of these assays. On the other hand, the high specificity and sensitivity that can be obtained, especially with GC–MS, more than justify their use if the necessary apparatus is available.

Sensitive electron-capture GLC procedures have been described by several laboratories. Fenimore *et al.* (1973) have used the HFB derivative (N, Table 10.1) to measure THC in blood with a detection limit of 100 pg ml^{-1}. Hexahydrocannabinol was used as the internal standard, the cannabinoids were extracted with 1.5% isoamyl alcohol in heptane, purified by base–acid partition, and the HFB derivatives were prepared and analysed on a dual-column chromatograph to minimise interference from co-extracted material. The column effluent from a 6-ft (1.83-m), 5% SE-30 column was monitored with a flame-ionisation detector and only the effluent containing the cannabinoids was diverted to the second analytical column, which was a 280-ft (85.34-m) capillary coated with OV-17. This system reduced baseline drift at the electron-capture detector, as the capillary column could be run under isothermal conditions. It also accommodated large injection volumes, and enabled stationary phases of differing polarity to be used. In a later publication (Fenimore *et al.*, 1976) the use of the same GLC system, but fitted with a 10% OV-101 packed column and a 100-ft (30.48-m) Poly I-110 capillary column, was reported in an assay for THC sensitive to 500 pg ml^{-1}. A simpler extraction method was employed and THC was analysed by electron-capture detection as its pentafluoropropionyl ester (M, Table 10.1). Jones *et al.* (1981) have recently described an assay for CBD in plasma using extraction methods similar to those above. The compound was analysed as its PFB derivative by electron-capture to 50 ng ml^{-1}.

Garrett and Hunt (1973) have used an OV-225 packed column and the pentafluorobenzoates (K, Table 10.1) of Δ^1- and Δ^6-THC in their electron-capture method for THC measurement. Sample clean-up was by HPLC. Although a detection limit of 40 to 125 pg ml^{-1} was found, it would appear from the authors' later work (Garrett and Hunt, 1977a) that 0.5 to 1 ng ml^{-1} is a more realistic limit for this assay and the fact that this was obtained for plasma levels of THC in fasted dogs emphasises the detrimental effects of plasma lipids. In the nonfasted animals the limit was 5 to 10 ng ml^{-1}. Fenimore *et al.* (1976) have found that samples extracted from human blood are usually more contaminated then those from animals, again reflecting dietary influences.

TLC was used by Bachmann *et al.* (1979) to isolate THC from plasma prior to assay by electron-capture GLC. In this case, however, the HFB derivative (N, Table 10.1) was formed prior to TLC separation. A detection limit of 8 pg was found for the pure compound, but this was reduced to 1 ng ml^{-1} when the compound was assayed in plasma.

As an alternative to electron-capture detection, McCallum (1973) has used flame-photometric detection of the diethylphosphate derivative (C, Table 10.1) to give a detection limit of 2 ng ml^{-1} on a 3% OV-1 column. The method has recently been extended to measurements in both blood and brain (McCallum *et al.*, 1978; McCallum and Shaw, 1981) where 10 ng g^{-1} could be measured in brain. The limit in blood was 0.5 ng ml^{-1}.

10.3.7 Mass spectrometry and combined gas chromatography–mass spectrometry

This represents the most sensitive and selective of all analytical techniques for cannabinoid analysis, but the complexity of the equipment has restricted its use in forensic studies. It is, however, extensively used for metabolite identification and for pharmacokinetic analysis and the subject has been reviewed (Gudzinowicz and Gudzinowicz, 1980; Gudzinowicz *et al.*, 1980).

10.3.7.1 Mass spectrometry

The mass spectra of the cannabinoids (Budzikiewicz *et al.*, 1965; Claussen *et al.*, 1966b; Terlouw *et al.*, 1974; Vree and Nibbering, 1973; Boeren *et al.*, 1976; Vree, 1977) and in particular their TMS derivatives (Figure 10.15) (Billets *et al.*, 1976; Harvey, 1981b) are very characteristic and often contain abundant molecular ions. Many of the fragment ions are the result of considerable rearrangement (Boeren *et al.*, 1976). At low electron-energies, the relative intensity of these ions varies in a characteristic way with the energy of the electron beam and this has been used as a method for characterising cannabinoids in small samples (Vree *et al.*, 1971; Turner *et al.*, 1980b). The spectra of the TMS derivatives of THC acids of type A are not very informative, as they are dominated by a cyclic $[M\text{-}15]^+$ ion (Figure 10.16a) formed by elimination of a methyl group from a derivatised function as shown by the preparation of [$^2H_9$]TMS derivatives. Formation of the methyl ester–TMS ether derivative, however, prevents this and leads to a more informative spectrum (Bjorkman, 1982). Better spectra are also produced by the cyclic alkane boronates (Figure 10.16b) (Harvey, 1977) on account of the transfer of ionisation from the TMS groups to the pyran oxygen. The resulting spectra are thus similar to that of the TMS derivatives of Δ^1-THC itself, which ionises at the same site. Δ^1-THC acids of type B (Figure 10.6b) can easily be distinguished from the type-A acids (Figure 10.6a) using TMS derivatives as, on electron impact, they are unable to form cyclic ions of the type shown in Figure 10.16a and so the abundance of this ion is very much less (Billets *et al.*, 1976).

Fragmentation patterns of most substituted silyl derivatives of Δ^1-THC are similar to that of the TMS derivative, as fragmentation is directed mainly by charge localisation on the pyran oxygen. However, silyl ethers having substituents capable of forming stable radicals following electron impact, for example *tert*-butyldimethylsilyl (D, Table 10.1) and allyldimethylsilyl ethers (R in the table) produce additional ions representing loss of these radicals (Harvey, 1978).

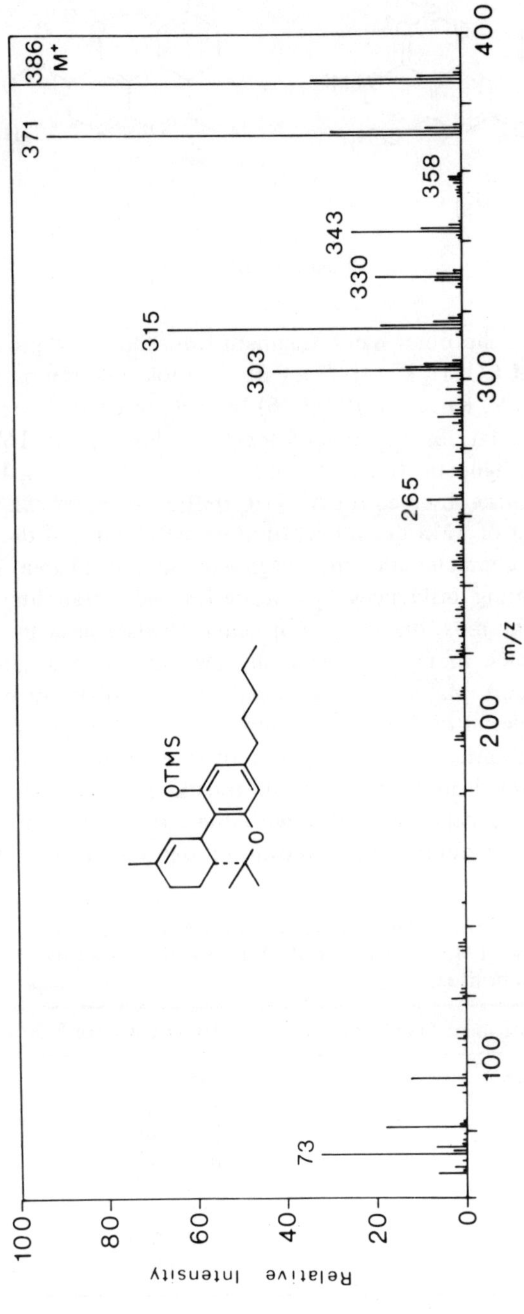

Figure 10.15 25-eV mass spectrum of the TMS derivative of Δ^1-THC.

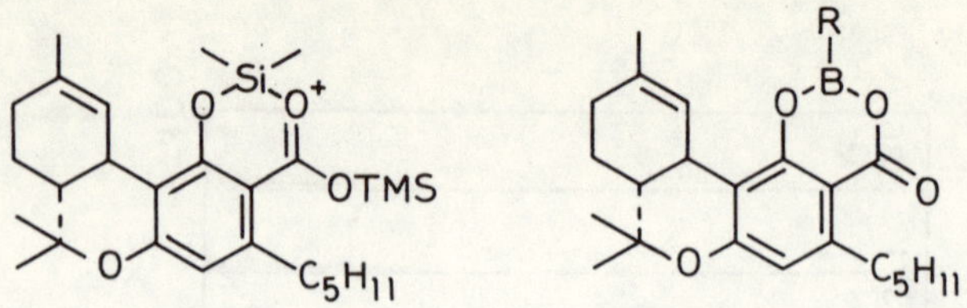

(a) (b)

Figure 10.16

The acetates (S), on the other hand, fragment from the acetyl group to produce abundant ions at $[M\text{-}COCH_3]^+$ (100%), with the molecular ion having an abundance of 15% at 25 eV. Knaus *et al.* (1976) have reported that the TMS acetate (E) gives no molecular ion because of the facile loss of the TMS-CH_2-CO$\cdot$ radical. However, diagnostic fragment ions were still produced, but at masses one unit less than those observed for Δ^1-THC itself.

The mass spectra of TMS derivatives of most metabolites of the major cannabinoids give very characteristic and diagnostic spectra (Table 10.2). Strong fragmentation-directing influences by the derivatised-metabolite function frequently result in the most diagnostic ion being the base peak in the spectrum. Di- and tri-substituted metabolites generally give the same diagnostic ions for each functional group. Major fragment ions were described by Wall and Brine (1976) and by Binder *et al.* (1974), who reported the mass spectra of side-chain hydroxylated metabolites in both their derivatised and underivatised states. Detailed mechanisms leading to these diagnostic ions for Δ^6- and Δ^1-THC (Harvey, 1981d) have been elucidated with the aid of deuterium labelling. A technique involving stereospecific removal of deuterium from the 3 (axial)

Table 10.2 Diagnostic ions in the mass spectra of the TMS derivatives of hydroxylated Δ^1-THC metabolites.

Position of OTMS group	Diagnostic ion*
1″	$[M-57]^+$
2″	*m/z* 145
3″	$[M-144]^+$
4″	*m/z* 117
5″	*m/z* 315
6α	$[M-90]^+$
6β	$[M-131]^+$
7	$[M-103]^+$

*100% relative abundance in all cases except that of the 4″-OTMS derivative.

position during electron-impact-induced loss of trimethylsilanol has been used to deduce the stereochemistry of several trimethylsilyloxy and acid groups substituted on the terpene ring (Harvey, 1980). The mass spectra of acetate derivatives of cannabinoid metabolites are generally not as diagnostic as those of the TMS derivatives and are frequently dominated by losses of acetic acid or ketene (Inayama *et al.*, 1976).

10.3.7.2 GC–MS studies of natural cannabinoids

GC–MS has found its greatest application in the area of natural cannabinoid identification. Among the many examples are the characterisation of the methyl (Vree *et al.*, 1972a), propyl (Fetterman and Turner, 1972; Turner *et al.*, 1973b) and butyl homologues (Harvey, 1976) of various cannabinoids by packed-column GC–MS and the studies by Novotny *et al.* (1982) using capillary-column methods. In a related technique, Karasek *et al.* (1975) have used plasma chromatography to detect less than 100 ng of Δ^1-THC; a strong MH^+ ion was produced with nitrogen serving both as carrier and reagent gas.

10.3.7.3 Identification of metabolites by GC–MS

For GC–MS identification of metabolites, some pre-GLC clean-up and separation stages are necessary to remove lipids; these are usually performed by column chromatography using Porisil or Sephadex LH-20 (Jones *et al.*, 1974; Nordqvist *et al.*, 1979a, b; Harvey *et al.*, 1977). Some laboratories use several separation stages in order to obtain samples for other physical techniques such as NMR. However, in the case of many metabolites, concentrations are not sufficient unless very large samples are processed. Here, direct GC–MS analysis of crude metabolite fractions can give more information by reducing losses of the minor compounds. For example, Harvey *et al.* (1977) have extracted livers of drug-treated animals with a polar solvent (ethyl acetate), separated lipids by chromatography on Sephadex LH-20 and then proceeded directly to GC–MS. Functional groups in the metabolites were identified by the formation of group-specific derivatives such as methyl esters for fatty acids and methyloximes for ketones. Differentiation of metabolites from lipids which sometimes give similar mass spectra, for example the TMS derivatives of 7-hydroxy-Δ^1-THC and 1-monopalmitin (Harvey and Paton, 1980), has been achieved using stable-isotope labelling. A 1 : 1 molar mixture of the cannabinoid whose metabolism was being studied and a deuterated analogue were administered to the experimental animal and the resulting spectra were examined for the presence of ion doublets from the metabolites.

10.3.7.4 Quantification of cannabinoids in physiological media

GC–MS assays are undoubtedly the most selective and sensitive for quantification of cannabinoids in biological media and are often used as a standard with which to compare other procedures. Detection limits of pure THC injected into a GC–MS instrument operating under electron-impact conditions are in the upper-picogram range (Harvey *et al*., 1979) but, as with simple GLC assays, these can be considerably improved by derivatisation of the phenol group as, for example, its TMS ether (Harvey *et al*., 1979; Ohlsson *et al*., 1979). Detection limits as low as 500 fg (5×10^{-13} g) have been obtained in this way (Harvey *et al*., 1980). However, ions commonly monitored for the TMS derivatives of THC (*m/z* 386 and 371) and its 7-hydroxy and acid metabolites (*m/z* 371, base peaks) have been reported to be subject to interference (Bergman *et al*., 1981) from compounds co-extracted from blood, and in this case the pentafluoropropionate derivative (M, Table 10.1) was recommended and a detection limit of 1 ng ml^{-1} was achieved. The most sensitive GC–MS technique reported to date employs detection of the pentafluorobenzoyl ester (K, Table 10.1) with electron-capture negative-ion mass spectrometry. As little as 10 fg could be detected but the method was not developed into an assay technique for the measurement of THC in biological samples (Hunt and Crow, 1978).

The first GC–MS method based on selected-ion monitoring was published by Agurell *et al*. (1973). Clean-up was by Sephadex LH-20 column chromatography and THC was measured to 1 ng ml^{-1} in plasma in the underivatised state using $[1'', 1''\text{-}^2H_2]\,\Delta^1$-THC as the internal standard. Other deuterated standards have been investigated for this assay by Ohlsson *et al*. (1976a) and $[1'', 1'', 2'', 2''\text{-}^2H_4]\,\Delta^1$-THC has been adopted. It was emphasised in this work that deuterated standards prepared by a nonexchange method were superior to standards produced by exchange techniques, as greater incorporation of deuterium could be achieved. $[^2H_3]\,\Delta^1$-THC has also been used in recent assays (Ohlsson *et al*., 1976b; Agurell *et al*., 1979). The method was extended to Δ^6-THC in 1976 (Agurell *et al*., 1976b) and the use of TMS derivatives (F, Table 10.1), introduced in 1979 (Ohlsson *et al*., 1979). An interesting modification of this technique for determining the pharmacokinetics of Δ^1-THC in cases where the drug is already present in the body as the result of earlier use was recently reported (Ohlsson *et al*., 1982). Deuterium-labelled $[5'', 5'', 5''\text{-}^2H_3]\,\Delta^1$-THC was given as a 'pulse' bolus injection and because of the difference of three mass units between its molecular weight and that of natural Δ^1-THC, it could be monitored independently by mass spectrometry using $[1'', 2'', 3'', 4'', 5'', 5'', 5''\text{-}^2H_7]$ THC as the internal standard. CBN and CBD have also been measured against deuterated internal standards by slight modifications of the original method for Δ^1-THC (Ohlsson *et al*., 1976b; Agurell *et al*., 1981) and further modifications have led to a semi-quantitative assay for THC-7-oic acids (Nordqvist *et al*., 1976).

The poor availability of standards and reference material has been one of the limiting factors in the development of assays of this type. One method for partially overcoming this (Rosenfeld *et al.*, 1974) has been the use of the [$^2H_3$] methyl ether (T, Table 10.1) as the internal standard. THC was extracted from the plasma using Brodie's solvent, purified with Claisen's alkali and methylated by an on-column technique to give U (Table 10.1). The molecular ions from the labelled and unlabelled forms of the drug were monitored and a 300pg ml^{-1} detection limit was reported. A possible difficulty with assays of this type where the internal standard contains the label as part of the derivative rather than the basic molecule, is loss of label through hydrolysis or exchange reactions. However, no loss seemed to arise in this assay. In a modification to the method (Rosenfeld, 1977), both Δ^1-THC and its 7-hydroxy metabolite were measured. Extractive ethylation to give V (Table 10.1) rather than methylation was used to overcome possible interference by metabolically produced THC methyl ether. The corresponding [$^2H_5$] ethyl derivative was used as the internal standard and the detection limits were 1 ng ml^{-1} of the metabolite and 5 ng ml^{-1} of Δ^1-THC. Rosenfeld and Taguchi (1976) have also assayed 7-hydroxy-Δ^1-THC in plasma to 3 ng ml^{-1} using extractive ethylation and TMS derivatisation of the 7-hydroxy group. Rosenfeld (1979) has also discussed in some depth various parameters related to assays of this type.

Several approaches to GC–MS quantitation have been investigated by Wall *et al.* (1976), at the Research Triangle Institute, for simultaneous measurements of Δ^1-THC, 7-hydroxy-Δ^1-THC, and CBN in plasma. In the first of these, [5″, 5″, 5″-$^2H_3$] analogues were used as the internal standards, extraction was by Brodie's solvent and clean-up by chromatography on Sephadex LH-20. TMS derivatives were then prepared from the 7-hydroxy-Δ^1-THC fraction only and the compounds were monitored by electron-impact GC–MS using a 1% SE-30 column. Derivatisation of THC and CBN was not adopted, in order to 'simplify procedure and eliminate potential sources of error' (Rosenthal *et al.*, 1978). Detection limits were around 0.5 ng ml^{-1} for THC. Hexane extraction was later used in this assay (Rosenthal *et al.*, 1978) to give cleaner extracts than those obtained with Brodie's solvent. This did not improve sensitivity but did enable the LH 20 chromatographic step to be dispensed with. In a parallel assay with comparable sensitivity, hexane extracts of THC and CBN were purified by acid–base partition and analysed as their pentafluoropropionate derivatives (M, Table 10.1) by chemical-ionisation mass spectromety with hexahydrocannabinol as the internal standard. The measurement of Δ^1-THC-7-oic acid was later added to this assay (Wall *et al.*, 1979); purification was by HPLC and the acid was measured by electron-impact mass spectrometry as its di-methyl derivative with [5″, 5″, 5″-$^2H_3$] Δ^1-THC-7-oic acid as the internal standard. Pharmacokinetic studies in man using these techniques were reported in these and several other recent papers (Wall and Brine, 1979; Wall and Perez-Reyes, 1981).

Hexane was also used as the extraction solvent in the GC–MS method described by Detrick and Foltz (1976) and the noise level was reduced further by the use of chemical-ionisation mass spectrometry using methane and ammonia as the reagent gas. Some clean-up was necessary, however, this being achieved by acid–base partition. THC was measured in plasma as its TMS derivative to 0.5 ng ml^{-1}, with [$^2H_3$] THC as the internal standard. In an extension to this assay, Foltz *et al.* (1979) have also been able to measure 7-hydroxy-Δ^1-THC and Δ^1-THC-7-oic acid in plasma. The cannabinoids were extracted and partially purifed by reversed-phase HPLC following direct injection of the plasma onto the column and elution with a water–methanol gradient. The quantification step used a 25-m SE-30 capillary column for chromatography of the TMS derivatives and again the [$^2H_3$] analogues of the compounds were used as internal standards. In 1982, Foltz and Hidy reported that a related assay in which Δ^1-THC could be measured to 0.2 ng ml^{-1} of plasma against [$^2H_3$] Δ^1-THC by positive ammonia chemical ionisation mass spectrometry had been in use for four years at Batelle Columbus Laboratories and that over two-thousand samples had been processed. One person could complete the analysis of thirty-six samples in two eight-hour days.

Foltz *et al.* (1983) have recently published another GC–MS method based on negative chemical-ionisation mass spectrometry for the measurement of Δ^1-THC, 7-hydroxy-Δ^1-THC and Δ^1-THC-7-oic acid in blood, plasma and urine samples with sensitivities of 0.2, 0.5 and 0.1 ng ml^{-1} for the three cannabinoids respectively. Samples were deproteinised with acetonitrile, the THC and its 7-hydroxy metabolite were extracted at high pH with a 9 : 1 mixture of hexane–ethyl acetate and the acid metabolite was subsequently extracted with the same solvent after acidification. The neutral cannabinoids were converted into their TFA derivatives and the acid was methylated with BF_3 before formation of TFA derivatives. GC–MS measurement involved a 15-m fused-silica capillary column with hydrogen as the carrier gas and methane as the chemical-ionisation reagent gas. As examples of the utility of the method, four cases were described in which THC was implicated as the presumptive intoxicant in various fatal accidents.

Another method sensitive to 0.5 ng ml^{-1} is that described by Pirl *et al.* (1979). Δ^1-THC, CBN and CBD were extracted from post-mortem samples with chloroform and purified by paper chromatography. Eight ions were monitored using a data system and the method was thus able to give partial mass spectra, useful for forensic confirmation of the presence of cannabinoids.

Using mass-spectrometic detection of cannabinoids eluting from an HPLC column of silica gel, Valentine *et al.* (1977) have detected Δ^1-THC in plasma to 2.5 ng ml^{-1} with [$^2H_3$] Δ^1-THC as the internal standard. The double-focusing mass spectrometer was adjusted to a resolution of 2500 and ions at *m/z* 314 and 317 were monitored. Valentine *et al.* (1979b) later used the same assay method for the analysis of Δ^1-THC in human breath, following trapping of the compound with either a polyethylene-foam wafer or a cryogenic trap containing ethanol.

The most sensitive assay reported to date for the measurement of Δ^1-THC in plasma and tissues is that developed by Harvey *et al.* (1980) with a detection limit of 5 pg ml^{-1}. Extraction was again with hexane to minimise the amount of coextracted lipid; measurement of THC as its TMS derivative was achieved with a double-focusing mass spectrometer tuned to a metastable ion rather than to the molecular or fragment ion. This gave greatly increased selectivity and hence sensitivity and additional clean-up was not necessary. Focusing of the mass spectrometer was achieved as follows. The magnet was set to record *m/z* 371, the $[M\text{-}CH_3]^+$ ion, with the accelerating voltage at its normal setting of 4 kV. This voltage was then raised until *m/z* 371 formed from *m/z* 386 (M^+) in the first field-free region was brought into focus. Ions at *m/z* 371 formed from endogenous lipids do not, in general, originate from a species of mass 386 and so are not transmitted through the electrostatic analyser under these conditions. As these are the ions causing the high background-noise, the selectivity and hence sensitivity of the system was increased considerably. Residual interfering ions from fatty acids were eliminated by methylation of the sample prior to TMS formation, leaving an almost clean background against which Δ^1-THC could be measured to 5 pg ml^{-1}. The internal standard was $[1'', 1'', 2'', 2''\text{-}^2H_4]$ CBN, a compound giving a metastable ion at the same mass as that from THC and which could be separated by GLC. For measurements of Δ^1-THC in tissues, an additional clean-up stage using Sephadex LH-20 column chromatography was necessary before derivatisation (Harvey *et al*., 1982).

A different approach to detection and quantification has been taken by Green and co-workers (Green, 1976; Green *et al*., 1979). Urine samples were processed with an extraction technique including several solvents, TLC and HPLC, and the residues, as TMS derivatives, were examined with a computer-based GC–MS system using probability-based matching. Ions from THC and several of its metabolites were matched against library spectra using a reverse-search procedure. Although the sensitivity was not as great as could be obtained by other GC–MS techniques, the method allowed unambiguous identification of several metabolites in a single experiment.

10.3.8 Immunoassay methods

Sensitive immunoassay techniques generally have the advantage over methods such as GC–MS in that they are more rapid and simpler to operate and do not require such complex equipment. Cross-reactivity, however, can be a serious disadvantage and can reduce both the selectivity and sensitivity of an assay. Specificity within the cannabinoid group is usually poor, as Δ^1-THC antisera often cross-react with several other cannabinoids and with THC metabolites. Although this is of little consequence for simple detection of the presence of cannabinoids and even leads to increased overall sensitivity, immunodetection of THC alone using nonspecific antisera requires a cannabinoid separation stage before measurement. With specific antisera, it is possible to measure Δ^1-THC directly.

10.3.8.1 Detection by fluorescence

The first of these immunodetection methods appears to be that published by Grant *et al.* (1972), who used rabbits to produce antibodies to Δ^1-THC bound to keyhole limpet haemocyanin via an azo-coupling reaction and condensation with cyclohexylcarbodiimide (I, Table 103). Detection was by an immunofluor-

Table 10.3 THC haptens used for conjugation to proteins for immunoassay studies

No.	Position of substitution	Link group
I	3′ or 5′	–N=N–
II	phenol	–COOH
III	phenol	$-CO-CH_2-CH_2-COOH$
IV	phenol	$-CO-(C_2)_4COOH$
V	phenol	$-CO-(CH_2)_8COOH$
VI	5′	$-CH_2OOH$
VII	5′	–COOH
VIII	5′	$-C_2H_4COOH$
IX	phenol	$-CH_2COOH$
X	10-iodine, 9-	–NHCOOH
XI	5″	–COOH
XII	5′	–COOH
XIII	6	–COOH

escent technique using the reduced azobenzoyl-THC. Although the method was not applied to the measurement of THC in physiological media it was anticipated that detection limits in the region of 10^{-11} to 10^{-14} mol ml^{-1} could be obtained.

10.3.8.2 Detection by radiolabelling

In an extension to the above technique (Gross *et al.*, 1974), antibodies were raised in goats using the same THC hapten and measurement was by radioimmunoassay using [^{3}H] Δ^6-THC. A detection limit of 25 to 50 ng ml^{-1} was determined and low cross-reactivity to CBD (0.5% and Δ^1-THC-7-oic (2.6%) was found. 7-Hydroxy-Δ^1-THC, however, cross-reacted to a much greater (47%) extent. In a further extension of this technique, an antiserum specific for Δ^1-THC-7-oic acid has been prepared, thus enabling Δ^1-THC and its acid metabolite to be measured in blood and urine (Gross and Soares, 1976; Soares and Gross, 1976). Measurements in urine could be made directly, but those in plasma required extraction of the cannabinoids with ether. In a later study (Yeager *et al.*, 1981) the goat antiserum to Δ^1-THC was used for direct measurements in haemolysed blood and serum and the validity of the assay was checked by GC–MS. Correlation coefficients of 0.94 and 0.88 were found for blood and serum respectively, with detection limits in the 3 ng ml^{-1} range. A solid-phase version of this assay having comparable sensitivity to the liquid-phase version has also been developed (Soares *et al.*, 1982). The antiserum had a high avidity for Δ^1-THC and Δ^6-THC (100.0) and for the 7-hydroxy- (97.6) and 7-carboxylic acid (96.5) metabolites of Δ^1-THC, whereas cross-reactivity with CBN (15.5) and CBD (0.1) was low. It was reported to be useful for small saliva, breath or dried-blood samples and it was emphasised that detection of the 7-substituted metabolites was probably a good indicator of acute cannabis use.

Antibodies raised in sheep to THC bound to bovine serum albumin (BSA) via the phenol group are the basis of an assay reported in 1974 by Teale *et al.* (1974a, b). Coupling to BSA was by formation of the chlorocarbonate (II, Table 10.3) by reaction with phosgene and conjugation with the protein using a Schotten–Baumann reaction. About 12 hapten molecules were found to be bound to each protein molecule, and radioimmunoassay was conducted using the commercially available [^{3}H] Δ^6-THC following separation of free and bound THC by precipitation with dextran-coated charcoal. Like the above assay, measurements could be made in urine directly, but plasma required deproteinisation with ethanol. The detection limit was about 6 ng ml^{-1}. In a later assay developed by the same group (Teale *et al.*, 1975), antibodies were raised in sheep to Δ^1-THC linked, again through the phenol, to BSA, but this time from Δ^1-THC hemisuccinate (III, Table 10.3). Triton X-405 was used as a solubilising detergent to reduce nonspecific binding and the assay was capable of detecting 7.5 ng ml^{-1} of THC in plasma and 1.0 ng ml^{-1} in urine. Considerable cross-reactivity occurred between cannabinoids containing three rings (Marks *et al.*, 1976) but none was reported for CBD, cannabichromene or cannabicyclol. A number of other THC-protein links were investigated (IV–VIII, Table 10.3) (Marks *et al.*, 1976; Teale *et al.*, 1979) but none proved to be as immunogenic as the THC-hemisuccinate-BSA (III) complex.

As with any immune method, antibody selectivity is greatest for those parts of the hapten furthest from the link to the protein, a feature which has prompted the synthesis of a range of THC-protein links (Tsui *et al.*, 1974) (I, III, IX, X, Table 10.3). Cook and co-workers (Cook *et al.*, 1976; Cook, 1979) have argued that the best link to expose the tricyclic THC structure would be by the pentyl chain and have thus coupled Δ^6-THC to BSA via an amide link to C-5″ (XI, Table 10.3). Comparative cross-reactivity studies were then made between antibodies to this hapten and to those produced from succinoyl- (Teale *et al.*, 1975) and azobenzoyl- (Gross *et al.*, 1974) linked haptens. CBN showed a fourfold decrease in cross-reactivity with the amyl and azobenzoyl-linked antibody compared with the succinoyl-linked THC. The 7-hydroxy and, to a greater extent, the 7-acid metabolite showed much less cross-reactivity with the azobenzoyl- and amyl-linked antibodies. Cook *et al.* (1972) have also developed a highly specific assay for Δ^1-THC-7-oic acid, again based on antibodies raised against the hapten, Δ^1-THC-7-oic acid, bound to BSA via an amide link at the end of the pentyl chain. Cross-reactivity with Δ^1-THC and its 7-hydroxy metabolite was extremely low (less than 0.1%) and the acid metabolite could be measured to between 20 and 50 pg. Cross-reactivity with other polar acid metabolites was not determined.

Another reported radioimmunoassay is that of Chase *et al.* (1976), which gave a sensitivity of 0.25 ng to antibodies of *O*-carboxymethyl-linked Δ^1-THC (IX, Table 10.3) raised in rabbits. Cross-reactivity was high with Δ^6-THC and with a number of metabolites, and detection was again with [^{3}H] THC.

Tritiated tracers are not ideal for RIA techniques for several reasons. As tritium is a β-emitter, detection has to be by liquid scintillation counting and is thus difficult to automate and its theoretical specific activity is lower than for tracers such as iodine-125. Iodine also has the advantage of measurement by γ-counting, but its bulk usually inhibits binding when incorporated into small drug molecules (Robinson *et al.*, 1975). Several successful assays have, however, been reported in which THC labelled in the 5$''$-position (alkyl chain) has been used as the tracer. Cook (1979) detected THC to 50 pg using the iodinated tracer of 3.7 TBq mmol^{-1} specific activity prepared by Pitt *et al.* (1980). Using the same antiserum, Owens *et al.* (1981) have developed a related assay with ^{125}I-Δ^6-THC as tracer and have measured THC to 0.3 ng ml^{-1} in plasma and 1.1 ng ml^{-1} in haemolysed blood. The ^{125}I-tracer had a specific activity five times that of the available [^{3}H] THC. This assay differs from most of the others in that precipitation of the bound radioactivity was achieved by a specific immunogenic method involving the use of goat anti-rabbit immunoglobulins bound to microspheres. The assay has also been shown to work equally well in methanol (Owens *et al.*, 1982), thus allowing rapid partial purification of blood samples by alcohol precipitation prior to RIA analysis. Law *et al.* (1982a) have recently synthesised a highly active (81.4 TBq mmol^{-1}) tracer in which iodinated histamine was bound to the phenol group of Δ^6-THC-7-oic acid. Cook (1979) has pointed out however that in cases where the label is attached to the drug in such a manner, it is possible for antibodies to recognise the drug–iodine link rather than the drug itself and thus cause a reduction in assay specificity.

To overcome problems of cross-reactivity in measurements of specific cannabinoids by RIA, Williams *et al.* (1978) have introduced a reversed-phase HPLC stage before measurement by RIA. The Teale antiserum (Teale *et al.* 1975) was used and the method was capable of measuring Δ^1-THC to 0.1 ng ml^{-1} in plasma. In a later publication by the same group (Williams *et al.*, 1979) this assay has been extended to the measurement of Δ^1-THC-7-oic acid in human urine. Separation prior to RIA enabled a sensitive but relatively nonspecific antiserum to be used (Moffat *et al.*, 1982).

10.3.8.3 Detection by electron-spin resonance

A third immunoassay technique for cannabinoids is that of free-radical immunoassay (Cais *et al.*, 1975). Here several carboxylic acid derivatives (IX, XII, XIII, Table 10.3) were coupled to ovalbumin or BSA with iso-butylchloroformate and tracers were synthesised by coupling the same acids to the stable free-radical 3-amino-2, 2, 5, 5-tetramethylpyrrolidine-1-oxyl. The competitively displaced labelled hapten was then monitored using electron-spin resonance.

10.3.8.4 EMIT techniques

Related to the simple immunoassay techniques are the EMIT (enzyme-multiplied immunoassay technique) methods. These rely on the observation that certain enzymes can be inhibited by antihapten antibodies when the hapten is covalently bound to the enzyme. In the assay developed by Rowley *et al.* (1976), Δ^7-THC (Figure 10.17) was converted into the carboxymethyloxime derivative (Table 10.3) and this was bound with *N*-hydroxysuccinimide either to malate dehydro-

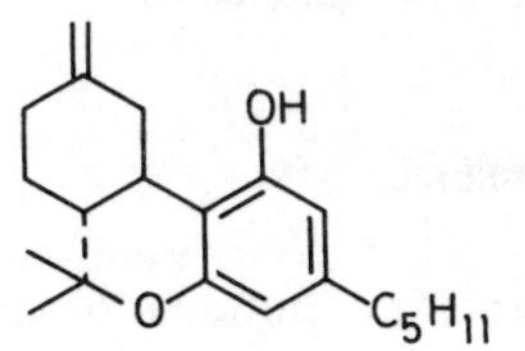

Figure 10.17 Δ^7-THC.

genase or to bovine-γ-globulin using the condensing agent *N*-dimethylamino-propyl-*N*′-ethyl carbodiimide. The protein complex was used to raise antibodies in sheep, and malate dehydrogenase activity was measured spectrophotometrically. 0.5 ng ml^{-1} of Δ^1-THC and Δ^1-THC-7-oic acid could be measured using this technique but a 25 ng ml^{-1} cut-off value was recommended in order to eliminate false positives (Rogers *et al.*, 1978). Antibodies to a second immunogen prepared from Δ^6-THC-7-al bound to BSA were also investigated and found to give a very good response with Δ^1-THC-7-oic acid and 7-hydroxy-Δ^1-THC (Rogers *et al.*, 1978; Rubenstein, 1979). EMIT assays are generally rather insensitive when compared with RIA (e.g. O'Connor and Rejent, 1981) and at best must be regarded as semiquantitative techniques. Law *et al.* (1982b) have found that twenty-five per cent of their assays performed by this technique give false negative results and have also commented that the method is relatively more expensive than RIA.

An EMIT technique developed at Syva Research Institute and also based on pig-heart mitochondrial malate dehydrogenase has been reported to detect

Δ^1-THC and its metabolites to 20 ng ml^{-1} of urine in a one-minute spectrophotometric measurement (De Laurentis *et al.*, 1982). An evaluation of this assay, now supplied in kit form, together with the tritiated RIA developed by Gross *et al.* at Receptor Research Institute, has recently been reported by Peat *et al.* (1982). Evaluation of the results of the immunoassays was subsequently made by GC–MS using the Battelle and Research Triangle methods described above. The tritiated-RIA method proved rather difficult to use and detection by ^{125}I was recommended as a preferable alternative. Correlation between GC–MS and the RIA method was reported as being 'far from adequate'. Six false positives (1.9% of the total or 13.9% of the presumptive positives) were found. Although regression coefficients (GC–MS against RIA) for the results from participating laboratories were usually greater than 0.93, one laboratory achieved only 0.46. Comparable results were found for the EMIT procedure. Several samples providing positive results by EMIT had levels of cannabinoids that were undetectable by GC–MS even after enzymatic hydrolysis. Similarly, some samples producing negative results by EMIT contained measurable amounts of cannabinoids when examined by GC–MS. Clearly, results from immunoassay techniques, particularly when low levels of Δ^1-THC or its metabolites are involved, must still be treated with some caution.

10.3.9 Nuclear magnetic resonance

A considerable amount of structural information on both natural cannabinoids and their metabolites has been obtained using NMR techniques. Chemical shifts were assigned to the protons of Δ^1- and Δ^6-THC by Gaoni and Mechoulum (1964) using a 60-MHz instrument and a detailed analysis of the 220-MHz spectra of Δ^1- and Δ^6-THC, CBN and HHC was reported by Archer *et al.* (1970). Conformational analysis was preformed by this group using Westheimer and extended Huckel molecular orbital calculations and it was shown that the cyclohexane ring (C) adopts a half-chair conformation, with the dihedral angle between the A- and C-rings being 19°. On the other hand, following studies at 90 MHz (Binder *et al.*, 1979), the C-ring of Δ^7-THC is thought to adopt the chair conformation, and studies on HHC suggest a similar conformation for the C-ring in this compound (Archer *et al.*, 1970). The B-ring of Δ^1-THC adopts a conformation so that the C-8 methyl group is axial with a C-3 : C-8 : 0 dihedral angle of 56° (Archer *et al.*, 1970). Steric interaction between the C-2 proton and the phenol group forces the latter out of the plane of the benzene ring. Interactions between the substituents on the A- and C-rings of CBD force the aromatic ring out of the plane of the terpene ring (see Binder *et al.*, 1979). NMR data for most naturally occurring cannabinoids have been listed by Mechoulam and Gaoni (1967).

^{13}C-NMR spectra of several THC isomers (Wenkert *et al.*, 1972; Hawkins and Roberts, 1973) and of other cannabinoids (Archer *et al.*, 1977; Binder *et al.*,

1982) have been reported and assignments made for all the carbon atoms in the molecule.

Proton magnetic resonance studies of side-chain hydroxy metabolites of the cannabinoids have been reported by Binder *et al.* (1974); these can be used diagnostically to determine the substituent position providing that sufficient material is available.

REFERENCES

Abbott, S. R., Abu-Shumays, A., Loeffler, K. O., and Forrest, I. S. (1975). High pressure liquid chromatography of cannabinoids as their fluorescent dansyl derivatives. *Res. Commun. Chem. Pathol. Pharmacol.* **10**, 9–19.

Agurell, S., Gustafsson, B., Holmstedt, B., Leander, K., Lindgren, J.-E., Nilsson, I., Sandberg, F., and Asberg, M. (1973). Quantitation of Δ^1-THC in plasma from cannabis smokers. *J. Pharm. Pharmacol.* **25**, 554–558.

Agurell, S., Binder, M., Fonseka, K., Lindgren, J.-E., Leander, K., Martin, B., Nilsson, I. M., Nordqvist, M., Ohlsson, A., and Widman, M. (1976a). Cannabinoids: Metabolites hydroxylated in the pentyl side-chain. In Nahas, G. G. (ed.), ***Marihuana: Chemistry, Biochemistry and Cellular Effects***. Springer, New York, pp. 141–57.

Agurell, S., Levander, S., Binder, M., Bader-Bartfai, A., Gustafsson, B., Leander, K., Lindgren, J.-E., Ohlsson, A., and Tobisson, B. (1976b). Pharmacokinetics of Δ^8-tetrahydrocannabinol in man after smoking: relations to physiological and psychological effects. In Braude, M. C., and Szara, S. (eds), ***Pharmacology of Marihuana***. Raven, New York, 49–61.

Agurell, S., Lindgren, J.-E., and Ohlsson, A. (1979). Introduction to quantification of cannabinoids and their metabolites in biological fluids. In Nahas, G. G., and Paton, W. D. M. (eds), ***Marihuana: Biological Effects***. Pergamon, Oxford, 3–13.

Agurell, S., Carlsson, S., Lindgren, J.-E., Ohlsson, A., Gillespie, H., and Hollister, L. (1981). Interactions of delta-1-tetrahydrocannabinol with cannabinol and cannabidiol following oral administration in man. Assay of cannabinol and cannabidiol by mass fragmentography. ***Experientia*** **37**, 1090–2.

Aramaki, H., Tomiyasu, N., Yoshimura, H., and Tsukamoto, H. (1968). Forensic chemical study on marihuana. 1. *Chem. Pharm. Bull.* **16**, 822–6.

Archer, R. A., Boyd, D. B., Demarco, P. V., Tyminski, I. J., and Allinger, N. L. (1970). Structural studies of cannabinoids. A theoretical and proton magnetic resonance analysis. *J. Amer. Chem. Soc.* **92**, 5200–6.

Archer, R. A., Johnson, D. W., Hagaman, E. W., Moreno, L. N., and Wenkert, E. (1977). Carbon-13 nuclear magnetic resonance spectroscopy of naturally occurring substances. 47. Cannabinoid compounds. *J. Org. Chem.* **42**, 490–5.

Bachmann, E. W., Hofmann, A. A., and Waser, P. G. (1979). Identification of Δ^9-tetrahydrocannabinol in human plasma by gas chromatography. *J. Chromatogr.* **178**, 320–3.

Baggi, T. R. (1980). 3-Methylbenzthiazolinone-2-hydrazone (MBTH) as a new visualisation reagent for the detection of cannabinoids on thin-layer chromatography plates. *J. Forens. Sci.* **25**, 691–4.

Bailey, K. (1978). Formation of olivetol during gas chromatography of cannabinoids. *J. Chromatogr.* **160**, 288–91.

Bailey, K. (1979). The value of the Duquenois test for cannabis–A survey. *J. Forens. Sci.* **24**, 817–41.

Bailey, K., and Gagne, D. (1975). Distinction of synthetic cannabidiol, cannabichromene and cannabivarin by GLC using on-column methylation. *J. Pharm. Sci.* **64**, 1719–20.

Bailey, K., Legault, D., and Verner, D., (1973). Identification of synthetic cannabinoids by gas chromatography. *J. Chromatogr.* 87, 263–6.

Baker, P. B., and Phillips, G. F. (1983). The forensic analysis of drugs of abuse. A review. *Analyst* **108**, 777–807.

Baker, P. B., Gough, T. A., and Taylor, B. J. (1980a). Illicitly imported *cannabis* products: some physical and chemical features indicative of their origin. *Bull. Narcot.* **32**(2), 31–40.

Baker, P. B., Fowler, R., Bagon, K. R., and Gough, T. A. (1980b). Determination of the distribution of cannabinoids in cannabis resin using high-performance liquid chromatography. *J. Analyt. Toxicol.* **4**, 145–52.

Beam, W. (1911). Fourth report of the Wellcome Tropical Research Laboratories, B, 25–6. Gordon Memorial College, Khartoum, p. 25.

Bercht, C. A. L., Lousberg, R. J. J. Cl., Kuppers, F. J. E. M., Salemink, C. A., Vree, T. B., and van Rossum, J. M. (1973). Cannabis. 7: Identification of cannabinol methyl ether from hashish. *J. Chromatogr.* **81**, 163–6.

Bergman, R. A., Lukaszewski, T., and Wang, Y. S. S. (1981). The detection of tetrahydrocannabinol in blood: a comparative study. *J. Analyt. Toxicol.* **5**, 85–9.

Bertulli, G., Mosca, L., and Pedroni, G. (1976). Rapid method for the detection and identification of cannabinoids in cannabis. *Boll. Chim. Farm.* **115**, 714–9.

Betts, T. J., and Holloway, P. J. (1967). Chromatographic identification of cannabis. *J. Pharm. Pharmacol.* **19**, 97S–102S.

Billets, S., El-Feraly, F., Fetterman, P. S., and Turner, C. E. (1976). Constituents of *Cannabis sativa* L. 12: Mass spectral fragmentation patterns of some cannabinoid acids as their TMS derivatives. *Org. Mass Spectrom.* **11**, 741–51.

Binder, M., Agurell, S., Leander, K., and Lindgren, J.-E., (1974). Zur Identifikation potentieller Metabolite von Cannabis-inhaltstoffen: Kernresonanz und Massenspektroskopische untersuchungen und Seitenketten-hydroxylierten Cannabinoiden. *Helv. Chim. Acta* **57**, 1626–41.

Binder, M., Edery, H., and Porath, G. (1979). Δ^7-Tetrahydrocannabinol, a non-psychotropic cannabinoid: structure–activity considerations in the cannabinoid series. In Nahas, G. G., and Paton, W. D. M. (eds), *Marihuana: Biological Effects*. Pergamon, Oxford, pp. 71–80.

Binder, M., Franke, I., Schmidt, B., and Dietrich, W. (1982). C-13-NMR spectra of natural and semi-synthetic cannabinoids. *Helv. Chim. Acta* **65**, 807–11.

Binder, M., and Meisenberg, G. (1978). Microbial transformation of cannabinoids. 2: a screening of different microorganisms. *Eur. J. Appl. Microbiol. Biotechnol.* **5**, 37–50.

Bjorkman, S. (1982). Gas chromatography of cannabis constituents, including cannabinoid acids, with on-column alkylation and esterification. *J. Chromatogr.* **237**, 389–97.

Boeren, E. G., Heerma, W., and Terlouw, J. K. (1976). The use of labelled analogues for the determination of mass spectrometric fragmentation mechanisms of cannabinoids. A re-investigation of the formation of the most abundant fragment ion $[C_{15}H_{19}O_2]^+$ in $\Delta^{1(6)}$-tetrahydrocannabinol. *Org. Mass Spectrom.* **11**, 659–63.

Borys, H. K., and Karler, R. (1981). Post column derivatization procedure for the colorimetric analysis of tissue cannabinoids separated by high-performance liquid chromatography. *J. Chromatogr.* **205**, 303–23.

Bourdon, R. (1976). Identification and quantification of cannabinoids in urine by gallium chelate formation. In Nahas, G. G., and Paton, W. D. M. (eds), *Marihuana: Biological Effects*. Pergamon, Oxford, pp. 111–21.

Budzikiewicz, H., Aplin, R. T., Lightner, D. A., Djerassi, C., Mechoulam, R., and Gaoni, Y. (1965). Massenspektroskopie und Ihre Anwendung auf Strukturelle und Stereochemische Probleme. 68: Massenspektroskopische Untersuchung der Inhaltstoffe von Hashische. *Tetrahedron* **21**, 1881–8.

Butler, W. P. (1962). Duquenois–Levine test for marihuana. *J. Assoc. Official. Analyt. Chemists* **45**, 597–9.

Caddy, B., and Fish, F. (1967). A screening technique for Indian hemp (*Cannabis sativa* L.). *J. Chromatogr.* **31**, 584–7.

Cais, M., Dani, S., Josephy, Y., Modiano, A., Gershon, H., and Mechoulam, R. (1975). Cannabinoid metabolites. Free radical immunoassay. *FEBS Letters* **55**, 257–60.

Candela, R. G., and Marino, C. (1979). Determination of cannabinols in biological fluids. *Boll. Soc. Ital. Biol. Sper.* **55**, 32–7. (*Chem. Abstr.* **91** (1979) 118070e.)

Chase, A. R., Kelley, P. R., Taunton-Rigby, A., Jones, R. T., and Harwood, T. (1976). Quantitation of cannabinoids in biological fluids by radioimmunoassay. In Willette, R. E. (ed.), *Cannabinoid Assays in Humans*. Res. Monogr. Ser. No. 7. NIDA, Rockville, pp. 1–8.

Chiesa, E. P., Rondina, R. V. D., and Coussio, J. D. (1973a). A rapid thermomicro/thin-layer chromatography procedure for the identification of cannabinoids in marihuana. *J. Chromatogr.* 87, 298–9.

Chiesa, E. P., Rondina, R. V. D., and Coussio, J. D. (1973b). Chemical composition and potential activity of Argentine marihuana. *J. Pharm. Pharmacol.* **25**, 953–6.

Claussen, U., Borger, W., and Korte, F. (1966a). Gaschromatographische Analyse der Inhaltsstoffe des Hanfes. *Liebigs Ann. Chem.* **693**, 158–64.

Claussen, U., Fehlhaber, H.-W., and Korte, F. (1966b). Haschish. 11: Massenspektrometrische bestimmung von Haschisch-Inhaltsstoffen–2. *Tretrahedron* 22, 3535–43.

Coffman, C. B., and Gentner, W. A. (1974). Cannabis sativa. Effect of drying time and temperature on cannabinoid profile of stored leaf tissue. *Bull. Narcot.* **26**, 67–70.

Cook, C. E. (1979). Radioimmunoassay of cannabinoid compounds. In Vinson, J. A. (ed.), *Cannabinoid Analysis in Physiological Fluids*. A.C.S. Symposium Ser. No. 98, pp. 137–154.

Cook, C. E., Hawes, M. L., Amerson, E. W., Pitt, C. G., and Williams, D. (1976). Radioimmunoassay of Δ^9-tetrahydrocannabinol. In Willette, R. E. (ed.), *Cannabinoid Assays in Humans*. Res. Monogr. Ser. No. 7. NIDA, Rockville, pp. 15–27.

Cook, C. E., Seltzman, H. H., Schindler, V. H., Tallent, C. R., Chin, K. M., and Pitt, C. G. (1982). Radioimmunoassays for cannabinoids. In Hawks, R. L. (ed.), *The Analysis of Cannabinoids in Biological Fluids*. Res. Monogr. Ser. No. 42, NIDA, Rockville, pp. 19–32.

Coutts, R. T., and Jones, G. R. (1979). A comparative analysis of cannabis material. *J. Forens. Sci.* **24**, 291–302.

Crombie, W. M. L. (1976). The analysis of cannabis. In Graham, J. D. P. (ed.), *Cannabis and Health*. Academic, London, pp. 21–41.

Crombie, L., and Crombie, W. M. L. (1975). Cannabinoid bis-homologues: miniaturised synthesis and GLC study. *Phytochemistry* **14**, 213–20.

Davis, K. H., Jun., Martin, N. N., Pitt, C. G., Wildes, J. W., and Wall, M. E. (1970). The preparation and analysis of enriched and pure cannabinoids from marihuana and hashish. *Lloydia* **33**, 453–60.

De Clercq, H., Massart, D. L., and Vercruysse, A. (1973). Fluorimetric identification reaction of cannabis constituents. *J. Pharm. Belg.* **28**, 437–44.

De Faubert Maunder, M. J. (1969a). Two simple colour tests for cannabis. *Bull. Narcot.* **21(4)**, 37–43.

De Faubert Maunder, M. J. (1969b). Simple and specific test for cannabis. *J. Assn. Publ. Analysts* 7, 24–30.

De Faubert Maunder, M. J. (1969c). Simple chromatography of cannabis constituents. *J. Pharm. Pharmacol.* **21**, 334–5.

De Faubert Maunder, M. J. (1970). A comparative evaluation of the Δ^9-tetrahydrocannabinol content of cannabis plants. *J. Assn Publ. Analysts* **8**, 42–7.

De Faubert Maunder, M. J. (1974a). Preservation of cannabis thin layer chromatograms. *J. Chromatogr.* **100**, 196–9.

De Faubert Maunder, M. J. (1974b). Improved procedure for the field testing of cannabis. *Bull. Narcot.* **26(4)**, 19–26.

De Faubert Maunder, M. J. (1976). The forensic significance of the age and origin of cannabis. *Med. Sci. Law* **16**, 78–90. (*Chem. Abstr.* **90** (1979) 17336v.)

De Ropp, R. S. (1960). Chromatographic separation of the phenolic compounds of Cannabis sativa. *J. Amer. Pharm. Assoc.* **49**, 756–8.

Detrick, R., and Foltz, R. (1976). Quantitation of Δ^9-tetrahydrocannabinol in body fluids by gas chromatography/chemical ionization–mass spectrometry. In Willette, R. E., (ed.), *Cannabinoid Assays in Humans*. Res. Monogr. Ser. No. 7. NIDA, Rockville, pp. 88–95.

De Zeeuw, R. A., Malingre, Th. M., and Merkus, F. W. H. M. (1972). Δ^1-Tetrahydrocannabinolic acid, an important component in the evaluation of cannabis products. *J. Pharm. Pharmacol.* **24**, 1–6.

De Zeeuw, R. A., Wijsbeek, J., and Malingre, Th. M. (1973). Interference of alkanes in the gas chromatographic analysis of cannabis products. *Ibid.*, **25**, 21–6.

Dionyssiou-Asteriou, A., and Miras, C. J. (1974). Fluorescence of cannabinoids. *Ibid.*, **27**, 135–7.

Duquenois, P., and Moustapha, H. N. (1938). Identification and assay of Cannabis indica. *J. Egypt Med. Assn* **21**, 224–7.

El-Feraly, F. S., Elsohly, M. A., and Turner, C. E. (1977). Anisaldehyde as a spray reagent for cannabinoids and their methyl ethers. *Acta. Pharm. Jugosl.* **27**, 43–6.

Elsohly, M. A., El-Feraly, F. S., and Turner, C. E. (1977). Isolation and characterization of (+)-cannabitriol and (–)-10-ethoxy-9-hydroxy-$\Delta^{6a[10a]}$-tetrahydrocannabinol: two new cannabinoids from *Cannabis sativa* L. extract. *Lloydia* **40**, 275–80.

Fairbairn, J. W., and Liebmann, J. A. (1973). The extraction and estimation of the cannabinoids in *Cannabis sativa* L. and its products. *J. Pharm. Pharmacol.* **25**, 150–5.

Fairbairn, J. W., Liebmann, J. A., and Rowan, M. G. (1976). The stability of cannabis and its preparations on storage. *Ibid.* **28**, 1–7.

Fairlie, K., and Fox, B. G. (1976). Rapid quantitative determination of tetrahydrocannabinol in marihuana by gas chromatography. *J. Chromatogr. Sci.* **14**, 334–5.

Fenimore, D. C., Freeman, R. R., and Loy, P. R. (1973). Determination of Δ^9-THC in blood by electron capture GLC. *Analyt. Chem.* **45**, 2331–5.

Fenimore, D. C., Davis, C. M., and Horn, A. H. (1976). Determination of Δ^9-tetrahydrocannabinol in human blood serum by electron capture gas chromatography. In Willette, R. E. (ed.), *Cannabinoid Assays in Humans*. Res. Monogr. Ser. No. 7. NIDA, Rockville, pp. 42–7.

Fetterman, P. S., and Turner, C. E. (1972). Constituents of Cannabis sativa L., 1: propyl homologues of cannabinoids from an Indian variant. *J. Pharm. Sci.* **61**, 1476–7.

Fetterman, P. S., Keith, E. S., Waller, C. W., Guerrero, O., Doorenbos, N. J., and Quimby, M. (1971a). Mississippi grown *Cannabis sativa* L.: preliminary observations on chemical definition of phenotype and variations in tetrahydrocannabinol content versus age, sex and plant part. *Ibid.* **60**, 1246–9.

Fetterman, P. S., Doorenbos, N. J., Keith, E. S., and Quimby, M. W. (1971b). A simple gas liquid chromatography procedure for determination of cannabinoidic acids in Cannabis sativa L. *Experientia* **27**, 988–9.

Fish, F. (1974). Gas chromatography of cannabis constituents. *Chromatographia*, **7**, 311–5.

Fishbein, L., (1982). *Chromatography of Environmental Hazards*, vol. 4, *Drugs of Abuse*. Elsevier, Amsterdam, pp. 395–423.

Fochtman, F. W., and Winek, C. L. (1971). Duquenois–Levine test for marijuana. *Clin. Toxicol.* **4**, 287–9.

Foltz, R. L., and Hidy, B. J. (1982). Quantitative analysis for Δ^9-THC, 11-hydroxy-Δ^9-THC, and 9-carboxy-Δ^9-THC in plasma using GC/CI-MS. In Hawks, R. L. (ed.), *The Analysis of Cannabinoids in Biological Fluids*. Res. Monogr. Ser. No. 42, NIDA, Rockville, 99–118.

Foltz, R. L., Clarke, P. A., Hidy, B. J., Lin, D. C. K., Graffeo, A. P., and Petersen, B. A. (1979). Quantitation of Δ^9-tetrahydrocannabinol and 11-norΔ^9-tetrahydrocannabinol-9-carboxylic acid in body fluids by GC/CI–MS. In Vinson, J. A., (ed.), *Cannabinoid Analysis in Physiological Fluids*. A.C.S. Symp. Ser. No. 98, 59–71.

Foltz, R. L., McGinnis, K. M., and Chin, D. M. (1983). Quantitative measurement of Δ^9-tetrahydrocannabinol and two major metabolites in physiological specimens using capillary column gas chromatography negative chemical ionization mass spectrometry. *Biomed. Mass Spectrom.* **10**, 316–23.

Fonseka, K., Widman, M., and Agurell, S. (1976). Chromatographic separation of cannabinoids and their monooxygenated derivatives. *J. Chromatogr.* **120**, 343–8.

Forrest, I. S., Green, D. E., Rose, S. D., Skinner, G. C., and Torres, D. M. (1971). Fluorescent-labeled cannabinoids. *Res. Commun. Chem. Pathol. Pharmacol.* **2**, 787–92.

Fowler, P. B., Gihooley, R. A., and Baker, P. B. (1979). Thin layer chromatography of cannabinoids. *J. Chromatogr.* **171**, 509–11.

Friedrich-Fiechtl, J., Spiteller, G., Just, W. W., Werner, G., and Wiechmann, M. (1973). Zu Nachweis und Indentifizierung von Tetrahydrocannabinol in Biologischen Flussigkeiten. *Naturwissenschaften* **60**, 207–8.

Fulton, C. C. (1970). Furfural test for cannabis resin. *Bull. Narcot.* **22**(2), 33.

Gaoni, Y., and Mechoulam, R. (1964). Isolation, structure and partial synthesis of an active constituent of hashish. *J. Amer. Chem. Soc.* **86**, 1646–7.

Gaoni, Y., and Mechoulam, R. (1966). Cannabichromene, a new active principle in hashish. *Chem. Commun.* 20–1.

Gaoni, Y., and Mechoulam, R. (1971). The isolation and structure of Δ^1-tetrahydrocannabinol and other neutral cannabinoids from hashish. *J. Amer. Chem. Soc.* **93**, 217–24.

Garrett, E. R., and Hunt, C. A. (1973). Picogram analysis of THC and application to biological fluids. *J. Pharm. Sci.* **62**, 1211–4.

Garrett, E. R., and Hunt, C. A. (1974). Physicochemical properties, solubility and protein binding of Δ^9-tetrahydrocannabinol. *Ibid.* **63**, 1056–64.

Garrett, E. R., and Hunt, C. A. (1976). Separation and sensitive assay of THC in biological fluids by HPLC and GLC. Willette, R. E. (ed.), *Cannabinoid Assays in Humans*. Res. Monogr. Ser. No. 7. NIDA, Rockville, pp. 33–41.

Garrett, E. R. and Hunt, C. A. (1977a). Pharmacokinetics of Δ^9-tetrahydrocannabinol in dogs. *J. Pharm. Sci.* **66**, 395–407.

Garrett, E. R., and Hunt, C. A. (1977b). Separation and analysis of Δ^9-tetrahydrocannabinol in biological fluids by high pressure liquid chromatography and GLC. *Ibid.* **66**, 20–26.

Garrett, E. R., and Tsau, J. (1974). Stability of tetrahydrocannabinols, 1. *Ibid.* **63**, 1563–74.

Garrett, E. R., Gouyette, A. J., and Roseboom, H. (1978). Stability of tetrahydrocannabinols, 2. *Ibid.* **67**, 27–32.

Ghamrawy, M. A. (1937). The detection of cannabis Indica. A new test. *J. Egypt Med. Assoc.* **20**, 193–208.

Gough, T. A., and Baker, P. B. (1982). Identification of major drugs of abuse using chromatography. *J. Chromatogr. Sci.* **20**, 289–314.

Goutam, M. P., and Agnihotri, V. B. (1981). Different Indian essential oils react positively to the Duquenois–Levine test of cannabis. *Seifen, Oele, Fette, Wachse.* **107**, 124–5 (*Chem. Abstr.* **95** (1981) 1293w.)

Grant, J. D., Gross, S. J., Lomax, P., and Wong, R. (1972). Antibody detection of marihuana. *Nature, New Biol.* **236**, 216–7.

Green, D. E. (1976). Quantitation of cannabinoids in biological specimens using probability based matching GC/MS. In Willette, R. E. (ed.), *Cannabinoid Assays in Humans*. Res. Monogr. Ser. No. 7. NIDA, Rockville, 70–87.

Green, D. E., Chao, F.-C., Loeffler, K. O., and Kanter, S. L. (1979). Quantitation of Δ^9-tetrahydrocannabinol and its metabolites in human urine by probability based matching GC/MS. In Vinson, J. A. (ed.), *Cannabinoid Analysis in Physiological Fluids*. A.C.S. Symp. Ser. No. 98, 93–113.

Grlic, L. (1970). A simple thin layer chromatography of cannabinoids by means of silica gel sheets treated with amines. *J. Chromatogr.* **48**, 562–4.

Grlic, L. (1971). Highly-sensitive chromatographic detection of cannabis constituents by means of silica gel sheets treated with silver nitrate. *Eur. J. Toxicol.* **4**, 43–5.

Grlic, L. (1974). Identification of cannabis users by detecting cannabinoids in biological media. *Acta Pharm. Jugosl.* **24**, 63–72.

Gross, S. J., and Soares, J. R. (1976). Separate radioimmune measurements of body fluid Δ^9-THC and 11-nor-9-carboxy-Δ^9-THC. In Willette, R. E. (ed.), *Cannabinoid Assays in Humans*. Res. Monogr. Ser. No. 7. NIDA, Rockville, 10–14.

Gross, S. J., Soares, J. R., Wong, S.-L. R., and Schuster, R. E. (1974). Marijuana metabolites measured by a radioimmune technique. *Nature* **252**, 581–2.

Grote, H., and Spiteller, G. (1978). New cannabinoids, 2. *J. Chromatogr.* **154**, 13–23.

Gudzinowicz, B. J., and Gudzinowicz, M. J. (1980). Natural pyrolytic and metabolic products of tobacco and marijuana. *Analysis of Drugs and Metabolites by Gas Chromatography–Mass Spectrometry*, vol. 7. Dekker, New York.

Gudzinowicz, B. J., Gudzinowicz, M. J., Hologgitas, J., and Driscoll, J. L. (1980). The analysis of marijuana cannabinoids and their metabolites in biological media by GC and/or GC–MS techniques. *Adv. Chromatogr.* **18**, 197–265.

Hackel, R. (1972). Detection of cannabinoids in the saliva following use of hashish. *Arch. Toxicol.* **29**, 341–4.

Harvey, D. J. (1976). Characterization of the butyl homologues of Δ^1-tetrahydrocannabinol,

cannabinol and cannabidiol in samples of cannabis by combined gas chromatography and mass spectrometry. *J. Pharm. Pharmacol.* **28**, 280–5.

Harvey, D. J. (1977). Cyclic alkylboronates as derivatives for the characterization of cannabinolic acids by combined gas chromatography and mass spectrometry. *Biomed. Mass Spectrom.* **4**, 88–93.

Harvey, D. J. (1978). Comparison of fourteen substituted silyl derivatives for the characterization of alcohols, steroids and cannabinoids by combined gas–liquid chromatography and mass spectrometry. *J. Chromatogr.* **147**, 291–8.

Harvey, D. J. (1980). Stereospecific elimination of deuterium as a method for determining the stereochemistry of a number of metabolites of the tetrahydrocannabinols. *Biomed. Mass Spectrom.* **7**, 28–34.

Harvey, D. J. (1981a). Analytical studies on marihuana. *Trends Analyt. Chem.* **1**, 66–71.

Harvey, D. J. (1981b). The mass spectra of the trimethylsilyl derivatives of Δ^1- and Δ^6-tetrahydrocannabinol. *Biomed. Mass Spectrom.* **8**, 575–8.

Harvey, D. J. (1981c). The mass spectra of the trimethylsilyl derivatives of the hydroxy and acid metabolites of Δ^1- and Δ^6-tetrahydrocannabinol. *Ibid.* **8**, 579–88.

Harvey, D. J. (1981d). The mass spectrs of the trimethylsilyl derivatives of *cis*- and *trans*-hexahydrocannabinol and their hydroxy and acid analogues. *Ibid.* **8**, 366–72.

Harvey, D. J., and Paton, W. D. M. (1975). Use of trimethylsilyl and other homologous trialkylsilyl derivatives for the separation and characterization of mono- and di-hydroxy-cannabinoids by combined gas chromatography and mass spectrometry. *J. Chromatogr.* **109**, 73–80.

Harvey, D. J., and Paton, W. D. M. (1980). The use of deuterium labelling in structural and quantitative studies of tetrahydrocannabinol metabolites by mass spectrometry. *Adv. Mass Spectrom.* **8**, 1194–1203.

Harvey, D. J., Martin, B. R., and Paton, W. D. M. (1977). Identification of di- and tri-substituted hydroxy and ketone metabolites of Δ^1-tetrahydrocannabinol in mouse liver. *J. Pharm. Pharmacol.* **29**, 482–6.

Harvey, D. J., Martin, B. R., and Paton, W. D. M. (1979). Identification and measurement of cannabinoids and their in vivo metabolites in liver by gas chromatography–mass spectrometry. In Nahas, G. G., and Paton, W. D. M. (eds), *Marihuana: Biological Effects*. Pergamon, Oxford, pp. 45–62.

Harvey, D. J., Leuschner, J. T. A., and Paton, W. D. M. (1980). Measurement of Δ^1-tetrahydrocannabinol in plasma to the low picogram range by gas chromatography–mass spectrometry using metastable ion detection. *J. Chromatogr.* **202**, 83–92.

Harvey, D. J., Leuschner, J. T. A., and Paton, W. D. M. (1982). Gas chromatographic and mass spectrometric studies on the metabolism and pharmacokinetics of Δ^1-tetrahydrocannabinol in the rabbit. *J. Chromatogr.* **239**, 243–50.

Hauck, G., and Moll, H. R. (1974). Tests for the determination of the cannabis contents of exhaled air. *Beitr. Gerichtl. Med.* **32**, 221–6 (*Chem. Abstr.* **88** (1978) 164979u.)

Hawkins, B. L., and Roberts, J. D. (1973). NMR spectroscopy ^{13}C Fourier transform spectra of Δ^8- and Δ^9-THC. *Proc. Nat. Acad. Sci.* **70**, 1027–29.

Hawks, R. L. (1982). *The Analysis of Cannabinoids in Biological Fluids*. Res. Monogr. Ser. No. 42. NIDA, Rockville.

Heaysman, L. T., Walker, E. A., and Lewis, D. T. (1967). The application of gas chromatography to the examination of the constituents of Cannabis sativa L. *Analyst* **92**, 450–5.

Hendriks, H., Batterman, S., Bos, R., Huizing, H. J., and Malingre, Th.M. (1981. Use of Amberlite XAD-2 columns for the separation of cannabinoids from *Cannabis* extracts. *J. Chromatogr.* **205**, 444–50.

Hively, R. L., Mosher, W. A., and Hoffmann, F. W. (1966). Isolation of trans-Δ^6-tetrahydrocannabinol from marijuana. *J. Amer. Chem. Soc.* **88**, 1832–3.

Hoffman, N. E., and Yang, R. K. 91972). Gas chromatography of Δ^1-tetrahydrocannabinol. *Analyt. Letters.* **5**, 7–11.

Hollister, L. E., Kanter, S. L., Board, R. D., and Green, D. E. (1974). Marihuana metabolites in urine of man. 3: Unchanged delta-9-tetrahydrocannabinol. *Res. Commun. Chem. Pathol. Phamacol.* **8**, 579–84.

Hughes, R. B., and Kessler, R. R. (1979). Increased safety and specificity in the thin-layer chromatographic identification of marihuana. *J. Forensic Sci.* **24**, 842–6.

Hughes, R. B., and Warner, V. J. (1978). A study of false positives in the chemical identification of marihuana. *Ibid.* **23**, 304–10.

Hunt, D. F., and Crow, F. W. (1978). Electron capture negative ion chemical ionization mass spectrometry. *Analyt. Chem.* **50**, 1781–4.

Inayama, S., Sawa, A., and Hosoya, E. (1976). Mass spectrometry of oxidation products of Δ^1- and Δ^6-tetrahydrocannabinols. *Chem. Pharm. Bull.* **24**, 2209–18.

Johnson, E., Abu-Shumays, A., and Abbott, S. R. (1977). Use of fluorescence detection in high-performance liquid chromatography. *J. Chromtogr.* **134**, 107–9.

Jones, G., Widman, M., Agurell, S., and Lindgren, J.-E. (1974). Monohydroxylated metabolites of Δ^1-tetrahydrocannabinol in mouse brain. Comparison with *in vitro* liver metabolites. *Acta. Pharm. Suecica* **11**, 283–94.

Jones, A. B., Elsohly, M. A., Bedford, J. A., and Turner, C. E. (1981). Determination of cannabidiol in plasma by electron-capture gas chromatography. *J. Chromatogr.* **226**, 99–105.

Just, W. W., Werner, G., and Wiechmann, M. (1972). Bestimmung von Δ^1- and $\Delta^{1(6)}$-tetrahydrocannabinol in Blut, Urin und Speichel von Huschisch-rauchern. *Naturwissenschaften* **59**, 222.

Just, W. W., Filipovic, N., and Werner, G. (1974). Detection of Δ^9-tetrahydrocannabinol in saliva of men by means of thin-layer chromatography and mass spectrometry. *J. Chromatogr.* **96**, 189–94.

Kaistha, K. K., and Tadrus, R. (1982). Semi-quantitative thin-layer mass screening detection of 11-nor-Δ^9-tetrahydrocannabinol-9-carboxylic acid in human urine. *Ibid.* **237**, 528–533.

Kanter, S. L., Hollister, L. E., Moore, F., and Green, D. E. (1974a). Marihuana metabolites in urine of man. 4: Extraction procedures using diethyl ether. *Res. Commun. Chem. Pathol. Pharmacol.* **9**, 205–13.

Kanter, S. L., Hollister, L. E., Moore, F., and Green, D. E. (1974b). Marihuana metabolites in urine of man. 2: Undescribed metabolite following oral ingestion of delta-9-tetrahydrocannabinol. *Ibid.* **7**, 79–84.

Kanter, S. L., Hollister, L. E., and Moore, F. (1975). Marihuana metabolites in urine of man. 5: Characterization and separation of polar metabolites of delta-9-tetrahydrocannabinol. *Ibid.* **10**, 215–18.

Kanter, S. L., Hollister, L. E., and Loeffler, K. O. (1978). Marihuana metabolites in the urine of man. 8: Identification and quantitation of Δ^9-tetrahydrocannabinol by thin-layer chromatography and high-pressure liquid chromatography. *J. Chromatogr.* **150**, 233–7.

Kanter, S. L., Musumeci, M. R., and Hollister, L. E. (1979). Quantitative determination of Δ^9-tetrahydrocannabinol and Δ^9-tetrahydrocannabinolic acid in marihuana by high-pressure liquid chromatography. *Ibid.* **171**, 504–8.

Kanter, S. L., Hollister, L. E., and Williams, M. (1982a). Extraction of glucuronide metabolites of Δ^9-tetrahydrocannabinol by diethyl ether. *Ibid.* **234**, 255–60.

Kanter, S. L., Hollister, L. E., and Musumeci, M. (1982b). Marijuana metabolites in urine of man. 10: Identification of marijuana use by detection of Δ^9-tetrahydrocannabinol-11-oic acid using thin-layer chromatography. *J. Chromatogr.* **234**, 201–8.

Karasek, F. W., Karasek, D. E., and Kim, S. H. (1975). Detection of lysergic acid diethylamide, Δ^9-tetrahydrocannabinol and related compounds by plasma chromatography. *Ibid.* **105**, 345–52.

Knaus, E. E., Coutts, R. T., and Kazakoff, C. W. (1976). The separation, identification and quantitation of cannabinoids and their *t*-butyldimethylsilyl, trimethylsilyl and diethylphosphate derivatives using high-pressure liquid chromatography, gas liquid chromatography and mass spectrometry. *J. Chromatogr. Sci.* **14**, 525–30.

Kolsek, J., Maticic, M., and Repic, R. (1962). Paper chromatography of the constituents of Cannabis sativa. *Arch. Pharm.* **295**, 151–7.

Korte, F., and Sieper, H. (1960). Papierchromatographische Charakterisierung von Haschischinhaltsstoffen. *Tetrahedron* **10**, 153–9.

Korte, F., and Sieper, H. (1964). Zur chemischen Klassifizierung von Pflanzen, 24. Untersuchung von Haschish-Inhaltsstoffen durch Dünnschichtchromatographie. *J. Chromatogr.* **13**, 90–8.

Krejci, Z., and Hanus, L. (1976). Identification of cannbinoidic acids by thin-layer chromatography of their methyl esters. *Acta. Univ. Palacki. Olomuc.* **76**, 145–52.

Kreuz, D. S., and Axelrod, J. (1973). Delta-9-tetrahydrocannabinol: localization in body fat. *Science* **179**, 391–3.

Lau-Cam, C. A. (1978). Coffee as an interference in the Duquenois test: a differential test. *Clin. Toxicol.* **12**, 535–41.

Lau-Cam, C. A., and McDonnell, J. (1978). The furfural test for cannabis: an evaluation and modification. *Bull. Narcot.* **30**(2), 63–68.

Lau-Cam, C. A., and Pizzitola, V. (1979). Simple field test for marijuana. *J. Pharm. Sci.* **68**, 976–8.

Law, B., Mason, P. A., Moffat, A. C., and King, L. J. (1982a). Preparation of 2[^{125}-I]-iodohistamine-labelled Δ^8-tetrahydrocannabinol-11-oic acid for use in cannabinoid radioimmunoassay. *J. Lab. Compds Radiopharmaceut.* **19**, 915–28.

Law, B., Pocock, K., and Moffat, A. C. (1982b). An evaluation of a homogeneous enzyme immunoassay (EMIT) for cannabinoid detection in biological fluids. *J. Forens. Sci. Soc.* **22**, 275–81.

Lemberger, L., Silberstein, S. D., Axelrod, J., and Kopin, I. J. (1970). Marihuana: Studies on the disposition and metabolism of delta-9-tetrahydrocannabinol in man. *Science* **170**, 1320–2.

Lerner, P. (1969). The precise determination of tetrahydrocannabinol in marijuana and hashish. *Bull. Narcot.* **21**(3), 39–42.

Liu, J. H., Fitzgerald, M. P., and Smith, G. V. (1979). Mass spectrometric characterization of cannabinoids in raw *Cannabis sativa* L. samples. *Analyt. Chem.* **51**, 1875–7.

Lombrozo, L., Kanter, S. L., and Hollister, L. E. (1976). Marihuana metabolites in urine of man. 6: Separation of cannabinoids by sequential thin layer chromatography. *Res. Commun. Chem. Pathol. Pharmacol.* **15**, 697–703.

McCallum, N. K., (1973). The measurement of cannabinols in the blood by GC. *J. Chromatogr. Sci.* **11**, 509–11.

McCallum, N. K., and Shaw, S. M. (1981). Chromatographic analysis for Δ^1-tetrahydrocannabinol in blood and brain. *J. Analyt. Toxicol.* **5**, 148–9.

McCallum, N. K., Cairns, E. R., Ferry, D. G., and Wong, R. J. (1978). A simple gas chromatographic method for routine Δ^1-tetrahydrocannabinol analysis of blood and brain. *Ibid.* **2**, 89–93.

McCarthy, T. J., and Van Zyl, J. D. (1972). Breath analysis of cannabis smokers. *J. Pharm. Pharmacol.* **24**, 489–90.

Machata, G. (1969). Analytical procedure for the identification and estimation of hashish. *Arch. Toxicol.* **25**, 19–26.

Marks, V., Teale, J. D., and King, L. J. (1976). Radioimmunoassay of cannabis products in blood and urine. In Nahas, G. G. (ed.), ***Marihuana: Biological Effects***. Springer, New York, pp. 71–85.

Martin, L., Smith, D. M., and Farmilo, C. G. (1961). Essential oil from fresh *Cannabis sativa* and its use in identification. *Nature* **191**, 774–6.

Martone, G., and Della Casa, E. (1975). Identification of the active constituents of Indian hemp from forensic samples. *Zacchia* **11**, 197–206. (*Chem. Abstr.* **84** (1976) 69919L.)

Masoud, A. N., and Doorenbos, N. J. (1973). Mississippi grown *Cannabis sativa* L. 3: Cannabinoid and cannabinoid acid content. *J. Pharm. Sci.* **62**, 313–5.

Masoud, A. N., and Wingard, D. W. (1979). High performance liquid chromatography with electrochemical detection. 1: Separation of cannabis constituents and quantitation of Δ^9-tetrahydrocannabinol. *J. High Res. Chromatogr.* **2**, 118–22.

Mechoulam, R. (1970). Marihuana Chemistry. *Science* **168**, 1159–66.

Mechoulam, R., and Gaoni, Y. (1967). Recent advances in the chemistry of hashish. *Fortschr. Chem. Org. Naturst.* **25**, 175–213.

Mechoulam, R., Ben-Zvi, Z., and Gaoni, Y. (1968). Hashish. 13: On the nature of the Beam test. *Tetrahedron* **24**, 5615–24.

Mechoulam, R., Ben-Zvi, Z., Yagnitinsky, B., and Shani, A. (1969). A new tetrahydrocannabinolic acid. *Tetrahedron Letts.* **28**, 2339–41.

Mechoulam, R., McCallum, N. K., and Burstein, S. (1976). Recent advances in the chemistry and biochemistry of cannabis. *Analyt. Chem.* **76**, 75–112.

Melikian, A. P., and Forrest, I. S. (1973). Dansyl derivatives of Δ^9-and Δ^8-tetrahydrocannabinols. *J. Pharm. Sci.* **62**, 1025–6.

Merkus, F. W. H. M. (1971). Thin layer chromatography of cannabis constituents. *Pharm. Weekblad.* **106**, 49–55.

Miller, I. J., McCallum, N. K., Kirk, C. M., and Peake, B. M. (1982). The free radical oxidation of the tetrahydrocannabinols. *Experientia* **38**, 230–1.

Miras, C., Simas, S., and Kiburis, J. (1964). Comparative assay of the constituents from the sublimate of smoked cannabis with that from ordinary cannabis. *Bull Narcot.* **16**, 13–15.

Mobarak, Z., Zaki, N., and Bieniek, D. (1974). Chromatographic aspects of hashish analysis. *Forensic Sci.* **4**, 161–9.

Mobarak, Z., Bieniek, D., and Korte, F. (1978). Some chromatographic aspects of hashish analysis. 2. *Ibid.* **11**, 189–93.

Moffat, A. C., Williams, P. L., and King, L. J. (1982). Combined high performance liquid chromatography and radioimmunoassay method for the analysis of Δ^9-tetrahydrocannabinol and its metabolites in plasma and urine. In Hawks, R. L. (ed.), *The Analysis of Cannabinoids in Biological Fluids, Res. Monogr. Ser.* **42**, NIDA, Rockville, 56–68.

Mole, M. L., Jun., and Turner, C. E. (1974). Phytochemical screening of *Cannabis sativa* L. 1: constituents of an Indian variant. *J. Pharm. Sci.* **63**, 154–6.

Nahas, G. G. (1973). From Bhang to delta-9-THC: four thousand years of history. *Marihuana–Deceptive Weed*. Raven, New York, pp. 1–58.

Nakamura, G. R. (1969). Forensic aspects of cystolith hairs of cannabis and other plants. *J. Assoc. Official Analyt. Chem.* **52**, 5–16.

Nickolls, L. C. (1936). Note on Beam's test for hashish (Indian hemp). *Analyst* **61**, 604.

Nielsen, E. (1970). Thin layer chromatographic analysis of cannabis from Danish and other sources. *Dansk. Tidsskr. Farm.* **44**, 359–64.

Noirfalise, A., and Lambert, J. (1978). Proof of the consumption of cannabis. *Bull. Narcot.* **30**(3), 65–7.

Nojima, A., and Shoyama, M. (1980). Fluorometric analysis of the major constituents of cannabis sativa L. *Bunseki Kagaku,* **29**, 436–40 (*Chem. Abstr.* **93** (1980) 198605n).

Nordqvist, M., Lindgren, J.-E., and Agurell, S. (1976). Identification of a major metabolite of tetrahydrocannabinol in plasma and urine from cannabis smokers. In Frigerio, A., and Ghisalberti, E. L. (eds), *Mass Spectrometry in Drug Metabolism.* Plenum, New York, pp. 441–8.

Nordqvist, M., Lindgren, J.-E., and Agurell, S. (1979a). Acidic metabolites of Δ^1-tetrahydrocannabinol isolated from rabbit urine. *J. Pharm. Pharmacol.* **31**, 231–7.

Nordqvist, M., Agurell, S., Rydberg, M., Falk, L., and Ryman, T. (1979b). More acidic metabolites of Δ^1-tetrahydrocannabinol isolated from rabbit urine. *Ibid.* **31**, 238–43.

Novotny, M., Lee, M. L., Low, C. E., and Raymond, A. (1976). Analysis of marijuana samples from different origins by high-resolution gas–liquid chromatography for forensic applications. *Analyt. Chem.* **48**, 24–9.

Novotny, M., Merli, F., Wiesler, D., Fencl, M., and Saeed, T. (1982). Fractionation and capillary gas chromatographic–mass spectrometric characterization of the neutral components in marijuana and tobacco smoke condensates. *J. Chromatogr.* **238**, 141–50.

O'Connor, J. E., and Rejent, T. A. (1981). EMIT Cannabinoid assay: confirmation by RIA and GC/MS. *J. Analyt. Toxicol.* **5**, 168–173.

Ohlsson, A., Lindgren, J.-E., Leander, K., and Agurell, S. (1976a). Detection and quantification of tetrahydrocannabinol in blood plasma. In Willette, R. E. (ed.), *Cannabinoid Assays in Humans.* Res. Monogr. Ser. No. 7. NIDA, Rockville, pp. 48–63.

Ohlsson, A., Lindgren, J.-E., Leander, K., and Agurell, S. (1976b). Detection and quantification of cannabinoids in human blood plasma. In Frigerio, A., and Ghisalberti, E. L. (eds). *Mass Spectrometry in Drug Metabolism*. Plenum, New York, pp. 429–40.

Ohlsson, A., Agurell, S., Lindgren, J.-E., and Leander, K. (1979). Improvement of the mass fragmentographic technique for quantification of tetrahydrocannabinol in human blood plasma. In Vinson, J. A. (ed.), *Cannabinoid Analysis in Physiological Fluids*. ACS, Symp. Ser. No. 98, pp. 73–9.

Ohlsson, A., Lindgren, J.-E., Wahlen, A., Agurell, S., Hollister, L. E., and Gillespie, H. K. (1982). Single dose kinetics of deuterium labelled Δ^1-tetrahydrocannabinol in heavy and light cannabis users. *Biomed. Mass Spectrom.* **9**, 6–10.

Owens, S. M., McBay, A. J., Reisner, H. M., and Perez-Reyes, M. (1981). ^{125}I-radioimmunoassay of Δ^9-tetrahydrocannabinol in blood and plasma with a solid phase second antibody separation method. *Clin. Chem.* **27**, 619–24.

Owens, S. M., McBay, A. J., and Reisner, H. M. (1982). Radioimmunoanalysis of delta-9-THC in blood by means of an ^{125}I tracer. In Hawks, R. L. (ed.), *The Analysis of Cannabinoids in Biological Fluids*. Res. Monogr. Ser. No. 42, NIDA, Rockville, pp. 33–43.

Paris, M. R., and Paris, R. R. (1973). Importance of chromatography for studying the constituents of Cannabis sativa. *Bull. Soc. Chim. Fr.*, 118–22.

Parker, J. M., and Fiske, H. L. (1972). Thin layer chromatography of marihuana. *J. Assn. Official Analyt. Chem.* **55**, 876–79.

Parker, J. M., and Stembal, B. L. (1974). Review of gas liquid chromatography of marihuana. *Ibid.*, **57**, 888–92.

Parker, K. D., Wright, J. A., Halpern, A. F., and Hine, C. H. (1968). Preliminary report on the separation and quantitative determination of cannabis constituents present in plant material and when added to urine, by thin layer and gas chromatography. *Bull. Narcot.* **20**(4), 9–14.

Parker, J. M., Borke, M. L., Block, L. H., and Cochran, T. G. 1974). Decomposition of cannabidiol in chloroform solution. *J. Pharm. Sci.* **63**, 970–1.

Patterson, D. A., and Stevens, H. M. (1970). Identification of cannabis. *J. Pharm. Pharmacol.* **22**, 391–2.

Peat, M. A., Finkle, B. S., and Deyman, M. E. (1982). Laboratory immunoassay kits for the detection of cannabinoids in biological fluids. In Hawks, R. L. (ed.), *The Analysis of Cannabinoids in Biological Fluids*. Res. Monogr. Ser. No. 42, NIDA, Rockville, pp. 85–98.

Petcoff, D. G., Strain, S. M., Brown, W. R., and Ribi, E. (1971). Marihuana: Identification of cannabinoids by centrifugal chromatography. *Science* **173**, 824–6.

Pirl, J. N., Papa, V. M., and Spikes, J. J. (1979). The detection of delta-9-tetrahydrocannabinol in postmortem blood samples. *J. Analyt. Toxicol.* **3**, 129–32.

Pitt, C. G., Hendron, R. W., and Hsia, R. S. (1972). Specificity of the Duquenois color test for marihuana and hashish. *J. Forens. Sci.* **17**, 693–700.

Pitt, C. G., Seltzman, H. H., Setzer, S. R., and Williams, D. L. (1980). The preparation of 5′-iodo-I-125-delta-8-THC. A radioligand for the radioimmunoassay of cannabinoids. *J. Lab. Compds Radiopharmaceut.* **17**, 681–9.

Pranitis, P. A. F., and Kornfield, J. M. (1982). New approach to the visualization and identification of cannabinoids in plant material by thin-layer chromatography. *J. Chromatogr.* **247**, 197–200.

Rao, N. V. R. (1977). 1-Nitroso-2-naphthol as a spray reagent for the detection of cannabis on thin layer plates. *Curr. Sci.* **46**, 140.

Rasmussen, K. E. (1975a). Analysis of cannabinoids in cannabis by means of gas–liquid chromatography and solid injection. Improvements to the method. *J. Chromatogr.* **109**, 175–6.

Rasmussen, K. E. (1975b). On-column silylation of cannabinoids after injection of solid plant material and cold trapping. *Ibid.* **114**, 250–54.

Rasmussen, K. E., and Aaro, B. (1977). A combination of TLC and GLC using direct transfer of the TLC spot into gas chromatograph. *Medd. Norsk. Farm. Selskop.* **39**, 22–31.

Rasmussen, K. E., Rasmussen, S., and Svendsen, A. B. (1972). Gas–liquid chromatography of cannabinoids in micro quantities of cannabis by solid injection. *J. Chromatogr.* **69**, 381–4.

Razdan, R. K., Puttick, A. J., Zitko, B. A., and Handrick, G. R. (1972). Hashish. 6: Conversion of (−)-$\Delta^{1(6)}$-tetrahydrocannabinol to (−)-$\Delta^{1(7)}$-tetrahydrocannabinol. Stability of (−)-Δ^1- and (−)-$\Delta^{1(6)}$-tetrahydrocannabinols. *Experientia* **28**, 121–2.

Razdan, R. K., Dalzell, H. C., and Handrick, G. R. (1974). Hashish: a simple one-step synthesis of (−)-Δ^1-tetrahydrocannabinol (THC) from *p*-mentha-2,8-dien-1-ol and olivetol. *J. Amer. Chem. Soc.* **96**, 5860–5.

Ribi, E., Smith, R. F., Strain, S. M., Petcoff, D. G., Parker, R., Goode, G., and Sorvall, I. (1973). Purification of Δ^9-THC, an active constituent of marihuana, by accelerated microparticulate gel chromatography. *Prep. Biochem.* **3**, 209–20.

Robinson, J. D., Aherne, G. W., Teale, J. D., Morris, B. A., and Marks, V. (1975). Problems encountered in the use of radioiodination tags in radioimmunoassays for drugs. In

Pasternak, C. A. (ed.), ***Radioimmunoassay in Clinical Biochemistry***. Heyden, London, 113–23.

Rogers, R., Crowl, C. P., Eimstad, W. M., Hu, M. W., Kam, J. K., Ronald, R. C., Rowley, G. L., and Ullman, E. F. (1978). Homogenous enzyme immunoassay for cannabinoids in urine. *Clin. Chem.* **24**, 95–100.

Rosenfeld, J. (1977). The simultaneous determination of Δ^9-tetrahydrocannabinol and 11-hydroxy-Δ^9-tetrahydrocannabinol in plasma. *Analyt. Letters.* **10**, 917–30.

Rosenfeld, J. (1979). A general approach to the analysis of cannabinoids from physiological sources. In Vinson, J. A. (ed.), ***Cannabinoid Analysis in Physiological Fluids***. A.C.S. Symp. Ser. No. 98, 81–91.

Rosenfeld, J. M., and Taguchi, V. Y. (1976). Mass fragmentographic assay for 11-hydroxy-delta-9-tetrahydrocannabinol in plasma. *Analyt. Chem.* **48**, 726–9.

Rosenfeld, J. J., Bowins, B., Roberts, J., Perkins, J., and MacPherson, A. S. (1974). Mass fragmentographic assay for Δ^9-tetrahydrocannabinol in plasma. *Ibid.* **46**, 2232–4.

Rosenthal, D., Harvey, T. M., Bursey, J. T., Brine, D. R., and Wall, M. E. (1978). Comparison of gas chromatography mass spectrometry methods for the determination of Δ^9-tetrahydrocannabinol in plasma. *Biomed. Mass Spectrom.* **5**, 312–6.

Rowley, G. L., Armstrong, T. A., Crowl, C. P., Eimstad, W. M., Hu, W. M., Kam, J. K., Rogers, R., Ronald, R. C., Rubenstein, K. E., Sheldon, B. G., and Ullman, E. F. (1976). Determination of THC and its metabolites by EMIT homogenous enzyme immunoassay: a summary report. In Willette, R. E. (ed.), ***Cannabinoid Assays in Humans***. Res. Monogr. Ser. No. 7. NIDA, Rockville, pp. 28–32.

Rubenstein, K. E. (1979). Determination of cannabinoids in urine by EMIT homogenous enzyme immunoassay. In Nahas, G. G., and Paton, W. D. M. (eds.), ***Marihuana: Biological Effects***. Pergamon, Oxford, pp. 89–99.

Salaschek, M., Matte, A., and Seifert, R. (1973). Uber die Problematik des Nachweises von Haschischgenuss durch Dunnschichtchromatographische Urinuntersuchungen. *J. Chromatogr.* **78**, 393–400.

Scherrmann, J. M., Hoellinger, H., Nguyen-Hoang-Nam, Bourdon, R., and Fournier, E. (1977). Methodology for the detection and quantitation of Δ^9-tetrahydrocannabinol in plasma by dansylation and double labelling. *Clin. Chim. Acta.* **79**, 401–9.

Scherrmann, J. M., Hoellinger, H., Sonnier, M., Hoffelt, J., and Nguyen-Hoang-Nam (1980). Simple, rapid method for extraction of urinary cannabinoids by liquid-solid chromatography. *J. Chromatogr.* **196**, 342–6.

Schou, J., Steentoft, A., Worm, K., Morkholdt Andersen, J., and Nielsen, E. (1971). A highly sensitive method for gas chromatographic measurement of tetrahydrocannabinol (THC) and cannabinol (CBN). *Acta Pharmacol. Toxicol.* **30**, 480–2.

Schultz, O. E., and Mohrmann, H. L. (1962). Beitrag zur Papierchromatographie der Inhaltstoffe des deutchen Faserhanfes–Cannabis sativa L. *Arch. Pharm.* **295**, 66–7.

Segelman, A. B. (1973). ***Cannabis sativa*** L. (Marijuana). 3: The RIM test: a reliable and useful procedure for the detection and identification of marijuana utilizing combined microscopy and thin-layer chromatography. *J. Chromatogr.* **82**, 151–7.

Segelman, A. B., and Segelman, F. P. (1976). ***Cannabis sativa*** L. (Marijuana). 7: The relative specificity of the RIM test. *Ibid.* **123**, 79–100.

Segelman, A. B., Babcock, P. A., Braun, B. L., and Segelman, F. H. (1973). ***Cannabis sativa*** L. (Marijuana). 2: standardized and reliable microscopic method for detection and identification of marijuana. *J. Pharm. Sci.* **62**, 515–6.

Shoyama, Y., Yamauchi, T., and Nishioka, I. (1970). Cannabis 5: Cannabigerolic acid monomethyl ether and cannabinolic acid. *Chem. Pharm. Bull.* **18**, 1327–30.

Shoyama, Y., Oku, R., Yamauchi, T., and Nishioka, I. (1972). Cannabis. 6: Cannabicyclolic acid. *Ibid.* **20**, 1927–30.

Skinner, R. F. (1971). Analysis of marihuana. *Proc. West. Pharmacol. Soc.* **14**, 4–9.

Smith, R. N. (1975). High-pressure liquid chromatography of cannabis. Identification of separated constituents. *J. Chromatogr.* **115**, 101–6.

Smith, R. N., and Vaughan, C. G. (1976). High-pressure liquid chromatography of cannabis. Quantitative analysis of acid and neutral cannabinoids. *J. Chromatogr.* **129**, 347–54.

Smith, R. N., and Vaughan, C. G. (1977). The decomposition of acidic and neutral cannabinoids in organic solvents. *J. Pharm. Pharmacol.* **29**, 286–90.

Soares, J. R., and Gross, S. J. (1976). Separate radioimmune measurements of body fluid Δ^9-THC and 11-nor-9-carboxy-Δ^9-THC. *Life Sci.* **19**, 1711–18.

Soares, J. R., Grant, J. D., and Gross, S. J. (1982). Significant developments in radioimmune methods applied to Δ^9-THC and its 9-substituted metabolites. In Hawks, R. L., *The Analysis of Cannabinoids in Biological Fluids*. Res Monogr. Ser. No. 42. NIDA, Rockville, pp. 44–55.

Stearn, W. T. (1970). The cannabis plant: botanical characteristics. In Joyce, C. R. B., and Curry, S. H. (eds), *The Botany and Chemistry of Cannabis*. Churchill, London, pp. 1–10.

Straight, R., Wayne, A. W., Lewis, E. G., and Beck, E. C. (1973). Marihuana extraction and purification for oral administration of known amounts of Δ^9-tetrahydrocannabinol (THC). *Biochem. Med.* 8, 341–4.

Stromberg, L. E. (1971). Minor components of cannabis resin. 1: Their separation by gas chromatography, thermal stability and protolytic properties. *J. Chromatogr.* **63**, 391–6.

Teale, J. D., Forman, E. J., King, L. J., and Marks, V. (1974a). Radioimmunoassay of cannabinoids in blood and urine. *Lancet* 1974 **(ii)**, 553–5.

Teale, J. D., Forman, E. J., King, L. J., and Marks, V. (1974b). Production of antibodies to tetrahydrocannabinol as the basis for its radioimmunoassay. *Nature* **249**, 154–5.

Teale, J. D., Forman, E. J., King, L. J., Piall, E. M., and Marks, V. (1975). The development of a radioimmunoassay for cannabinoids in blood and urine. *J. Pharm. Pharmacol.* **27**, 465–72.

Teale, J. D., Clough, J. M., King, L. J., Marks, V., Williams, P. L., and Moffat, A. C. (1979). Antisera raised against tetrahydrocannabinol in the radioimmunoassay of cannabinoids. In Vinson, J. A. (ed.), *Cannabinoid Analysis in Physiological Fluids*. A.C.S. Symposium Ser. No. 98, pp. 155–73.

Terlouw, J. K., Heerma, W., Burgers, P. C., Dijkstra, G., Boon, A., Kramer, H. F., and Salemink, C. A. (1974). The use of metastable ion characteristics for the determination of ion structures of some isomeric cannabinoids. *Tetrahedron* **30**, 4243–8.

Tewari, S. N., and Sharma, J. D. (1979). Specific color reactions for the detection and identification of microquantities of cannabis preparations. *Pharmazie* **34**, 196–7.

Tewari, S. N., Harpalani, S. P., and Sharma, S. C. (1974). Separation and identification of the constituents of hashish (Cannabis Indica) by thin-layer chromatography and its application in forensic analysis. *Chromatographia* 7, 205–6.

Tsui, P. T., Kelly, K. A., Ponpipom, M. M., Strahilevitz, M., and Sehon, A. H. (1974). Δ^9-tetrahydrocannabinol–protein conjugates. *Can. J. Biochem.* **52**, 252–8.

Turk, R. F., Dharir, H. I., and Forney, R. B. (1969). Simple chemical method to identify marihuana. *J. Forensic Sci.* **14**, 389–92.

Turk, R. F., Manno, J. E., Jain, N. C., and Forney, R. B. (1971). The identification, isolation and preservation of Δ^9-tetrahydrocannabinol (Δ^9-THC). *J. Pharm. Pharmacol.* **23**, 190–5.

Turner, C. E., and Elsohly, M. A. (1979). Constituents of *Cannabis sativa* L. 16: A possible decomposition pathway of Δ^9-tetrahydrocannabinol to cannabinol. *J. Heterocyclic Chem.* **16**, 1667–8.

Turner, C. E., and Hadley, K. (1973a). Constituents of *Cannabis sativa* L. 2: Absence of cannabidiol in an African variant. *J. Pharm. Sci.* **62**, 251–5.

Turner, C. E., and Hadley, K. W. (1973b). Constituents of *Cannabis sativa* L. 3: Clear and discrete separation of cannabidiol and cannabichromene. *Ibid.* **62**, 1083–6.

Turner, C. E., and Henry, J. T. (1975). Constituents of *Cannabis sativa* L. 9: Stability of synthetic and naturally occurring cannabinoids in chloroform. *Ibid.* **64**, 357–9.

Turner, C. E., Hadley, K. W., and Davis, K. H. (1973a). Constituents of *Cannabis sativa* L. 5: Stability of an analytical sample extracted with chloroform. *Acta. Pharm. Jugoslav.* **23**, 89–94.

Turner, C. E., Hadley, K., and Fetterman, P. S. (1973b). Constituents of *Cannabis sativa* L. 6: Propyl homologues in samples of known geographical origin. *J. Pharm. Sci.* **62**, 1739–41.

Turner, C. E., Hadley, K. W., Henry, J., and Mole, M. L. (1974). Constituents of *Cannabis sativa* L. 7: Use of silyl derivatives in routine analysis. *Ibid.* **63**, 1872–6.

Turner, C. E., Elsohly, M. A., and Boeren, E. G. (1980a). Constituents of *Cannabis sativa* L. 17: A review of the natural constituents. *J. Nat. Prods* **43**, 169–234.

Turner, C. E., Bouwsma, O. J., Billets, S., and Elsohly, M. A. (1980b). Constituents of

Cannabis sativa L. 18: Electron voltage selected ion monitoring study of cannabinoids. *Biomed. Mass Spectrom.* **7**, 247–56.

Turner, J. C., and Mahlberg, P. G. (1982). Simple high-performance liquid chromatographic method for separating acidic and neutral cannabinoids in *Cannabis sativa* L. *J. Chromatogr.* **253**, 295–303.

Twitchett, P. J., Williams, P. L., and Moffat, A. C. (1978). Photochemical detection in high-performance liquid chromatography and its application to cannabinoid analyses. *Ibid.* **149**, 683–91.

Valentine, J. L., and Psaltis, P. (1979). Detection of marijuana use in human saliva using a fluorometric assay based on cannabinol decomposition. *Analyt. Lett.* **12**, 855–66.

Valentine, J. L., Bryant, P. J., Gutshall, P. L., Gan, O. H. M., Lovegreen, P. D., Thompson, E. D., and Niu, H. C. (1977). High pressure liquid chromatographic mass spectrometric determination of Δ^9-tetrahydrocannabinol in human plasma following marijuana smoking. *J. Pharm. Sci.* **66**, 1263–6.

Valentine, J. L., Gan, O. H. M., Niu, H. C., and Thompson, E. D. (1979a). HPLC analysis of Δ^9-tetrahydrocannabinol and 11-nor-Δ^9-tetrahydrocannabinol-9-carboxylic acid in human plasma. In Vinson, J. A. (ed.) *Cannabinoid Analysis in Physiological Fluids*. A.C.S. Symp. Ser. No. 98, pp. 175–205.

Valentine, J. L., Bryant, P. J., Gutshall, P. L., Gan, O. H. M., and Hiu, H. C. (1979b). Detection of Δ^9-tetrahydrocannabinol in human breath following marijuana smoking. *Analyt. Lett.* **12**, 867–80.

Verwey, A. M. A., and Witte, A. H. (1972). Thin layer and gas chromatographic analysis of illicit hashish samples. *Pharm. Weekblad.* **107**, 153–63.

Vinson, J. A. (ed.) (1979). *Cannabinoid Analysis in Physiological Fluids*. A.C.S. Symp. Ser. No. 98.

Vinson, J. A., and Hooyman, J. E. (1975). Studies in laboratory-use reagents. 3: Simple thin-layer chromatographic system for the separation of cannabinoids. *J. Chromatogr.* **106**, 196–9.

Vinson, J. A., Patel, D. D., and Patel, A. H. (1977). Detection of tetrahydrocannabinol in blood and serum using a fluorescent derivative and thin layer chromatography. *Analyt. Chem.* **49**, 163–5.

Vree, T. B. (1977). Mass spectrometry of cannabinoids. *J. Pharm. Sci.* **66**, 1444–50.

Vree, T. B., and Nibbering, N. M. M. (1973). Phenolic proton transfer to the 1, 2-double bond in the molecular ion of *trans*-1,2-tetrahydrocannabinol. *Tetrahedron* **29**, 3849–52.

Vree, T. B., Breimer, D. D. van Ginneken, C. A. M., van Rossum, J. M., de Zeeuw, R. A., and Witte, A. H. (1971). Identification of cannabivarins in hashish by a new method of combined gas chromatography mass spectrometry. *Clin. Chim. Acta* **34**, 365–72.

Vree, T. B., Breimer, D. D., van Ginneken, C. A. M., and van Rossum, J. M. (1972a). Identification in hashish of tetrahydrocannabinol, cannabidiol and cannabinol analogues with a methyl side-chain. *J. Pharm. Pharmacol.* **24**, 7–12.

Vree, T. B., Breimer, D. D., van Ginneken, C. A. M., and van Rossum, J. M. (1972b). Gas chromatography of cannabis constituents and their synthetic derivatives. *J. Chromatogr.* **74**, 209–24.

Vree, T. B., Breimer, D. D., van Ginneken, C. A. M., and van Rossum, J. M. (1973). Gas chromatography of cannabinoids. *Ibid.* **79**, 81–90.

Wall, M. E., and Brine, D. R. (1976). Identification of cannabinoids and metabolites in biological materials by combined gas–liquid chromatography–mass spectrometry. In Nahas, G. G. (ed.), *Marihuana: Chemistry, Biochemistry and Cellular Effects*. Springer, New York, pp. 51–62.

Wall, M. E., and Brine, D. R. (1979). Applications of mass spectrometry in cannabinoid research. In Nahas, G. G., and Paton, W. D. M. (eds), *Marihuana; Biological Effects*. Pergamon, Oxford, pp. 15–43.

Wall, M. E., and Perez-Reyes, M. (1981). The metabolism of Δ^9-tetrahydrocannabinol and related cannabinoids in man. *J. Clin. Pharmacol.* **21**, 178S–89S.

Wall, M. E., Harvey, T. M., Bursey, J. T., Brine, D. R., and Rosenthal, D. (1976). Analytical methods for the determination of cannabinoids in biological media. In Willette, R. E. (ed.), *Cannabinoid Assays in Humans*. Res. Monogr. Ser. No. 98. NIDA, Rockville, 107–17.

Wall, M. E., Brine, D. R., Bursey, J. T., and Rosenthal, D. (1979). Detection and quantitation of tetrahydrocannabinol in physiological fluids. In Vinson, J. A. (ed.), *Cannabinoid Analysis in Physiological Fluids*. A.C.S. Symp. Ser. No. 98, 39–57.

Waller, C., Hadley, K., and Turner, C. (1976). Detection and identification of compounds in cannabis. In Nahas, G. G. (ed.), *Marihuana: Chemistry, Biochemistry and Cellular Effects*. Springer, New York, pp. 15–30.

Wenkert, E., Cochran, D. W., Schell, F. M., Archer, R. A., and Matsumoto, K. (1972). CMR Spectral analysis of tetrahydrocannabinol and its isomers. *Experientia* **28**, 250–1.

Wheals, B. B., and Smith, R. N. (1975). Comparative cannabis analysis. A comparison of high-pressure liquid chromatography with other chromatographic techniques. *J. Chromatogr.* **105**, 396–400.

Willette, R. E. (ed.) (1976). *Cannabinoid Assays in Humans*. Res. Monogr. Ser. No. 7. NIDA, Rockville.

Williams, P. L., and Moffat, A. C. (1980). Identification in human urine of Δ^9-tetrahydrocannabinol-11-oic acid glucuronide: a tetrahydrocannabinol metabolite. *J. Pharm. Pharmacol.* **32**, 445–8.

Williams, P. L., Moffat, A. C., and King, L. J. (1978). Combined high-pressure liquid chromatography and radioimmunoassay method for the quantitation of Δ^9-tetrahydrocannabinol and some of its metabolites in human plasma. *J. Chromatogr.* **155**, 273–83.

Williams, P. L., Moffat, A. C., and King, L. J. (1979). Combined high-performance liquid chromatography and radioimmunoassay for the analysis of Δ^9-tetrahydrocannabinol metabolites in human urine. *Ibid.* **186**, 595–603.

Willinsky, M. D. (1973). Analytical aspects of cannabis chemistry. In Mechoulam, R. (ed.), *Marijuana: Chemistry, Pharmacology, Metabolism and Clinical Effects*. Academic, New York, pp. 137–65.

Willinsky, M., and Di Simone, L. (1973). Rapid simultaneous determination of the cannabinoids. *Il Farmaco, Ed. Prat.* **28**, 441–448.

Wong, A. S., Orbanosky, M. W., Reeve, V. C., and Beede, J. D. (1982). Stability of delta-9-tetrahydrocannabinol in stored blood and serum. In Hawks, R. L. (ed.), *The Analysis of Cannabinoids in Biological Fluids*. Res. Monogr. Ser. No. 42. NIDA, Rockville, 119–124.

Yeager, E. P., Goebelsmann, U., Soares, J. R., Grant, J. D., and Gross, S. J. (1981). Δ^9-tetrahydrocannabinol by GLC–MS validated radioimmunoassay of hemolyzed blood or serum. *J. Analyt. Toxcicol.* **5**, 81–4.

Yotoriyama, M., Ito, I., Takashima, D., Shoyama, Y., and Nishioka, I. (1980). Plant breeding of cannabis. Determination of cannabinoids by high-pressure liquid chromatography. *Yakugaku-Zasshi* **100**, 611–4.

Index